Springer Series on Family Violence

2002   **Serving Mentally Ill Offenders**
Gerald Landsberg, DSW, Marjorie Rock, PhD, Lawrence K.W. Berg, PhD, Esq, and Amy Smiley, PhD

2001   **Sexual Violence on Campus**
Allen J. Orrens, PhD, and Kathy Hotelling, PhD, ABPP, Editors

1998   **The Heart of Inmate Abuse: New Interventions in Child Welfare, Criminal Justice, and Health Settings**
Linda G. Mills, PhD, LCSW, JD

1998   **Preventing Teenage Violence: An Empirical Paradigm for Schools and Families**
John S. Wodarski, PhD, and Lois A. Wodarski, PhD

1998   **Battered Women and Their Families: Intervention Strategies and Treatment Programs, Second Edition**
Albert R. Roberts, PhD, Editor

Serving Mentally Ill Offenders

Challenges and Opportunities for Mental Health Professionals

Gerald Landsberg, DSW
Marjorie Rock, Dr. PH
Lawrence K.W. Berg, PhD, Esq.
Amy Smiley, PhD

Editors

 Springer Publishing Company

Springer Publishing Company, Inc.
536 Broadway
New York, NY 10012-3955

Acquisitions Editor: Sheri W. Sussman
Production Editor: Janice G. Stangel
Cover design by Susan Hauley

00 01 02 03 04 / 5 4 3 2 1

Library of Congress Cataloging-in-Publication Data

Serving mentally ill offenders : challenges and opportunities for mental health professionals / Gerald Landsberg . . . [et al.].
    p.   cm.
    Includes bibliographical references and index.
    ISBN 0-8261-1504-7
    1. Mentally ill offenders—Care—United States. 2. Mentally ill offenders—Service : for—United States. I. Landsberg, Gerald.
    RC451.4.P68 S46 2001
    362.2'086'9270973—dc21   2001034487

Printed in the United States of America by Sheridan Books, Inc.

CONTENTS

Contributors   *xi*

Introduction   1

SECTION I   JAIL/PRISON SERVICES FOR INCARCERATED POPULATIONS

1 Lane County Adult Corrections Mental Health Services,
   Lane County, Oregon   25
   Richard K. Sherman

2 Oswego Mental Health Forensic Mental Health
   Program, Oswego, New York   35
   Joette Deane

SECTION II   COMMUNITY-BASED DIVERSION PROGRAMS

1.   Police/Mental Health Linked Programs

3 Overview: The Law Enforcement Response to Social
   Problems: Mental Health As a Case in Point   47
   George T. Patterson

4 The Development and Implementation of a Police/
   Mental Health Training Program in a Large Urban
   Environment   51
   Marjorie Rock

5 The Memphis CIT Model   59
   Randolph T. Dupont and Charles S. Cochran

6 The Birmingham Police Department Community
   Service Officer Unit   70
   *Vickie B. Burnett, Bennie C. Henderson, Susan D. Nolan,
   Cynthia M. Parham, Leslie Gregg Tucker, and Craig Young*

2. Community Programs

7 Criminal Justice Diversion of Individuals with
Co-Occurring Mental Illness and Substance Use Disorders:
An Overview   83
Nahama Broner, Randy Borum, and Kristen Gawley

8 Jail Diversion in a Managed Care Environment:
The Arizona Experience   107
Michael Franczak and Michael S. Shafer

9 Friends of Island Academy: Providing Youth With
Positive Opportunities After Jail   120
Beth Navon

10 Broward's Mental Health Court: An Innovative
Approach to the Mentally Disabled in the Criminal
Justice System   128
Ginger Lerner-Wren

11 Preventing Incarceration of Adults With Severe
Mental Illness: Project Link   133
J. Steven Lamberti and Robert L. Weisman

12 New York City's System of Criminal Justice Mental
Health Services   144
Stacy S. Lamon, Neal L. Cohen, and Nahama Broner

SECTION III   SERVING EMOTIONALLY DISTURBED WOMEN

13 Overview: Working With Women in Jails: Developing
A Gender-Based Network of Services for Strengthening
Women and Their Families   159
Susan Salasin

14 Maryland's Programs for Incarcerated Women With
Mental Illness and Substance Abuse Disorders   165
Joan Gillece and Betty G. Russell

15 A Gender-Specific Intervention Model for Incarcerated
Women: Women's V.O.I.C.E.S. (Validation Opportunity
Inspiration Communication Empowerment Safety)   172
Kate DeCou with Sally Van Wright

SECTION IV   SERVING THE VICTIMS OF
MENTALLY ILL OFFENDERS

16   Elder Abuse and Forensic Mentally Ill Abusers   193
Pat Brownell, Jacquelin Berman, Aurora Salamone,
and Adele Welty

17   Identifying and Addressing the Needs of Victims of
Mentally Ill Offenders   215
Gerald Landsberg and Marjorie Rock

SECTION V   PERSPECTIVES FROM THE LEGAL SYSTEM:
ISSUES FOR MENTAL HEALTH PROFESSIONALS

18   A Judge's Perspective   225
Martin G. Karopkin

19   Social Workers as Advocates for Mentally Ill Criminal
Defendants/Inmates   229
Heather Barr

20   Observations of a Criminal Defense Attorney   246
Mary Elizabeth Anderson

21   Someone Had to Stop the Spinning: The Prosecutor's Role
in an Unlikely Alliance Called "Mental Health Court"   258
Lee Cohen and Lourdes Roberts

22   A Personal Experience   270
The Honorable Sol Wachtler

23   Implementing Kendra's Law   274
Neal L. Cohen, Stacy S. Lamon, and Norman Katz

SECTION VI   SCREENING INSTRUMENTS

24   A Review of Screening Instruments for Co-occurring Mental
Illness and Substance Use in Criminal Justice Programs   289
Nahama Broner, Randy Borum, Laura Whitmire,
and Kristen Gawley

Conclusion   338
Gerald Landsberg

Index   *343*

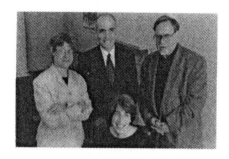

Gerald Landsberg, DSW, is Professor, Chair of Social Policy and Director of the Institute Against Violence at the Ehrenkranz School of Social Work of New York University. He holds a DSW degree (CUNY, 1979), an MPA (NYU, 1979), and an MSW (NYU, 1967). Prior to this academic appointment in 1991, Dr. Landsberg had an extensive administrative and research professional career in mental health. These included serving as an Associate Commissioner for the New York City Department of Mental Health (1987–1991), Director of Ulster County Mental Health Services (1979–1987), and the Director of Research and Evaluation of Maimonides Community Mental Center (1968–1978). In his professional roles at Ulster County Mental Health Services and with the New York Department of Mental Health, Dr. Landsberg oversaw forensic mental health services. Dr. Landsberg is and has conducted significant research in this area—e.g., an evaluation of alternatives to incarceration, victims of mentally ill offenders. He is the author of numerous books and articles and has made presentations of forensic mental health. He is the editor of forensic mental health newsletter.

Lawrence K.W. Berg, MSW, JD, PhD, entered law after more than 20 years of direct experience in the health, mental health, and human service fields. He practices in the areas of Behavioral Health Law and Health Law, as well as in the areas of Disability Law. For more than 18 years, he was the Director of Mental Health, Mental Retardation and Developmental Disabilities, and Alcohol and Substance Abuse Services in Columbia County, NY., where he was responsible for the design and implementation of a wide range of mental health services to criminal offenders in the county jail and in the community. He also served as the county's Public Health Director. In addition to his executive leadership positions, Dr. Berg has conducted research, has published, and has made numerous presentations on legal and ethical matters in health, forensic and other mental health services. His clinical and administrative experience in the behavioral health system makes him knowledgeable about the many legal and operational issues facing clinicians, managers and executives. Dr. Berg is currently in the faculty of the Ehrenkranz School of Social Work of the New York University as a Clinical Associate Professor. His prior legal experience being an associate with a major health law firm in Albany, NY. He now has his own firm in New York and Massachusetts. His practice includes providing legal and management consultation services to healthcare and behavioral healthcare professionals, organizations and networks of providers. Dr. Berg has a BA degree in Psychology from the City College of New York and holds a MSW degree from Yeshiva University, NY. He earned his PhD at the University of Chicago and was awarded his JD cum laude from Western New England College of Law. He is a certified Social worker in New York State, and is also admitted to the Bar in New York and Massachusetts.

Marjorie Rock, DrPH, is an Associate Professor at the Ehrenkranz School of Social Work where she teaches courses in Social Policy, Mental Health and Research at the Masters and Doctoral level. She has more than 25 years of experience in public mental health and, for the last 14 years, she has conducted research and provided training in the area of forensic mental health. Prior to her full time academic affiliation, Dr. Rock served as the Director of Research and Training for the New York City Department of Mental Health, Mental Retardation and Alcoholism Services. In this capacity she developed, implemented, and evaluated a model police-mental health training program. This program received a Certificate of Significant Achievement from the Institute on Hospital and Community Psychiatry in 1989. Dr. Rock has written extensively about forensic mental health issues and is currently the Director of the Forensic Mental Health Certificate Training Program at the Ehrenkranz School of Social Work's Institute Against Violence. This purpose of this program is train staff in the criminal justice, substance abuse and mental health system with respect to both clinical and systems aspects so that they may work together more effectively. Dr. Rock has served as a consultant to several juvenile and criminal justice agencies. Dr. Rock received her MSW from the Adelphi University school of Social Work and her Doctorate in Public Health from Columbia University School of Public Health.

Amy Smiley, PhD. Amy Smiley received her PhD from the Université de Paris VII (1990) in the Science of Texts and Documents. A former professor of Twentieth-Century French Studies at Johns Hopkins University, she published a book and numerous articles in her areas of specialization including the French Resistance and French colonialism in North Africa. Since 1999, she has been a Research Associate at the Institute Against Violence at NYU's Ehrenkranz School of Social Work, where she is also pursuing her MSW. Among other activities at the Institute, Smiley coordinated the Second International Conference on Forensic Mental Health. She also analyzed and reported on survey results regarding mental health services in the jails of New York State. She is Assistant Editor of the *Community Mental Health Report,* and is co-editor of two major publications on forensic mental health.

CONTRIBUTORS

Mary Elizabeth Anderson, BA, JD
Senior Attorney
The Legal Aid Society
New York, New York

Heather Barr, JD, MA
Staff Attorney
Urban Justice Center
Mental Health Project
New York, New York

Jacquelin Berman, PhD
Director of Research
Department for the Aging
Adjunct Professor
Fordham University
New York University
New York, New York

Randy Borum, PsyD
Associate Professor
Department of Mental Health Law
    & Policy
Louis de la Parte Florida Mental
    Health Institute
University of South Florida
Tampa, Florida

Nahama Broner, PhD
Research Director
Forensic Mental Health and Dual
    Disorders Projects
Ehrenkranz School of Social Work
New York University
New York, New York

Patricia Brownell, PhD, CSW
Graduate School of Social Work
Fordham University
New York, New York

Vickie Broadnax Burnett, MSW
Community Service Officer
Birmingham Police Department
North Precinct
Birmingham, Alabama

Major Sam Cochran, MS
Coordinator
Crisis Intervention Team,
Critical Incident Services, and
    Hostage Negotiation Team
Memphis Police Department
Memphis, Tennessee

Lee G. Cohen, Esq.
Assistant State Attorney
Broward County Courthouse
Fort Lauderdale, Florida

Neal L. Cohen, MD
Commissioner
New York City Department of
    Health and Mental Health
Mental Retardation and
    Alcoholism Services
Associate Clinical Professor
Mount Sinai School of Medicine
New York, New York

Joette Dean, MS
Director of Community Services
Oswego County Mental Health
  Department
Oswego, New York

Kate Decou, LICSW
Assistant Deputy Superintendent
Hampden County Correctional
  Center
Springfield, Massachusetts

Randolph Dupont, Ph.D
University of Tennessee College of
  Medicine
Department of Psychiatry
Memphis, Tennessee

Michael Franczak, PhD
Chief for Clinical Services
Arizona Department of Health
Division of Behavioral Health
Phoenix, Arizona

Michele Frank, CSW
Private Practice
Professor
New School University
New York, New York

Kristen Gawley
Doctoral Candidate
School of Applied and
  Professional Psychology
Rutgers University
New Brunswick, New Jersey

Dr. Joan Gillece, MA, PhD
Director for Special Needs
  Populations
Mental Hygiene Administration
Maryland Department of Health
  and Mental Hygiene
Jessup, Maryland

**Bennie Carol McGhee Henderson,
  MEd**
Community Service Officer
Birmingham Police Department
West Precinct
Birmingham, Alabama

Martin Karopkin, JD
Criminal Court of the City of
  New York
New York, New York

Norman Katz, PhD
Consultant on Mental Health
  Issues
Past Director of Public Education
  for Department of Mental
  Health
New York, New York

J. Steven Lamberti, MD
Associate Professor
Associate Chair for Clinical
  Programs
Universtiy of Rochester Medical
  Center
Department of Psychiatry
Rochester, New York

Stacy Lamon, PhD
Forensic Coordinator
NYC Department of Mental Health
New York, New York

Ginger Lerner Wren, BA, JD
Criminal Court Judge
17th Judicial Circuit
Administrative Judge
Broward Mental Health Court
Fort Lauderdale, Florida

Beth Navon, MS, ACSW
Executive Director
Friends of Island Academy
New York, New York

Susan D. Nolan, BSW, MTS
Birmingham Police Department
M/Power Ministries, Inc.
Birmingham, Alabama

Cynthia Parham, BSW, MPPM
Birmingham Police Department
North Precinct
Birmingham, Alabama

George T. Patterson, PhD, MSW
Assistant Professor
New York University
Ehrenkranz School of Social
    Work
New York, New York

Lourdes Fernandez Roberts, Esq.
Assistant State Attorney
Mental Health Division
Broward County State Attorney's
    Office
Fort Lauderdale, Florida

Betty G. Russell, PhD
Former Director, Trauma
    Services
Division of Special Populations
Mental Hygiene Administration
Maryland Department of Health
    and Mental Hygiene
Jessup, Maryland

Aurora Salamone, MPS
Director
Elderly Crime Victims Resource
    Center
New York City Department for the
    Aging
New York, New York

Susan Salasin
Director
Women and Violence Mental
    Health Program
and Mental Health and Criminal
    Justice Program
Center for Mental Health
    Services
Rockville, Maryland

Michael S. Shafer, PhD
Director
Community Rehabilitation
    Division
School of Public Administration
    and Policy
College of Business and Public
    Adminstration
The University of Arizona
Phoenix, Arizona

Richard Sherman, MS
Supervisor
Lane County Sheriff's Office
Eugene, Oregon

**Leslie Gregg Tucker, MSW, ACSW,
    LCSW, PIP**
Senior Community Service
    Officer
Unit of the Birmingham Police
    Department
South Precinct
Birmingham, Alabama

Sol Wachtler, BA, LL.B., LLD
Chief Judge of the State of New
    York
and the New York Court of
    Appeals (retired)
Chairman of the Board
Law and Psychiatry Institute
Professor
Touro Law School
New York, New York

Robert L. Weisman, DO
Assistant Professor of Psychiatry
University of Rochester School of
    Medicine and Dentistry
Co-Director of Project Link,
Strong Ties Community Support
    Program
Rochester, New York

Adele Welty, CSW
Supervisor
Elder Abuse Services
New York City Department for the
    Aging
New York, New York

Laura E. Whitmire, PhD
Private Practice
New York, New York

Sally Van Wright, MSW, LICSW
Hampden County Sheriff's
    Department and Correctional
    Center
Ludlow, Massachusetts

Craig S. Young, BSW
Community Service Officer
Birmingham Police Department
West Precint
Birmingham, Alabama

INTRODUCTION

This collection of essays address the problem of the criminalization of mentally ill offenders in the United States and the ways in which social workers and other mental health professionals can best channel their efforts to work towards a solution to this problem. The purpose of this book is, first, to elucidate the impact of this policy on American society, as the numerous offenders in this population seek reintegration into our communities following discharge from jail or prison. It also identifies the hardships endured by these individuals who, in most cases, face a criminal sentence that leads to inadequate treatment, and often aggravation, of the mental disorder in the environment of incarceration. "It seems to be a nearly universal opinion that no state prison system in this country handles mentally ill prisoners in a way that comports with minimum mental health standards of treatment" (Anderson, Section 5, Chapter 20). Second, and of equal importance, the studies that follow represent some of the best practices across the United States whose common purpose is to change the status quo. Specialists in law enforcement (police), community-based mental health and outreach workers, the legal community (judges, prosecutors, defenders), the corrections environment, and substance abuse providers have set up programs that offer rehabilitating alternatives to mentally ill offenders. As this book will make clear, such alternatives can be realized only through the collaboration of the partners working in these different areas. Indeed, as Henry J. Steadman pointed out in his keynote address at the Second International Forensic Mental Health Conference held at NYU (June, 2000), the fragmentation of, or lack of coordination between, these partners who exert considerable influence on the mental health field has served only to abet the criminalization of the mentally ill. When diversion or alternative-to-incarceration programs are successful, they are highly cost-effective, dramatically reduce the rates of recidivism and rehospitalization, and help reintegrate individuals back into the community. It is, therefore, the hope of the editors that the readers of this book will not only gain insight into the complexities of the trend and consequences of the criminalization of the mentally ill during the last few decades but also learn, on a practical level, what sources to turn to and what strategies to employ to best work with this population, which has grown tragically and disconcertingly. In this introduction, we will look more closely at the roots and repercussions of the criminalization of the mentally ill and then highlight the ways in which the programs described in each chapter specifically offer an alternative solution to this grave social problem.

* The Criminalization of the Mentally Ill: A Background

Forensic mental health professionals identify serious mental illness as that class of disorders described in the *Diagnostic and Statistical Manual of Mental Disorders* as schizophrenia, major depression, or mania/bi-polar disorder (Monahan, 1992; Lamb & Weinberger, 1998). (For further details on prevalence and types of mental disorders, see Broner, Borum & Gawley, Criminal Justice Diversion of Individuals with Co-Occurring Mental Illness and Substance Use Disorders in Chapter 7.) With a national incarcerated population at a record high of 2,026,596 at the end of 1999 (Butterfield, August, 2000), the percentage of seriously mentally ill in jails and prisons has had, and will long continue to have, dire effects on our society. Lamb and Weinberger (1998) conclude that approximately 6 to 15 percent of city and county inmates, and 10 to 15 percent of prison inmates, are seriously mentally ill. Teplin et al. (1996) estimate that, on a given day, 9 percent of the male and 18.5 percent of the female offenders entering local jails have serious mental illness. This gender discrepancy is partly based on the fact that, from 1983 to 1998, the rate of the incarcerated female population in jails rose from 7.1 to 12 percent—a rate faster than that of males. This was due, for the most part, to the war on drugs and "tough-on-crime" legislation which began with the Reagan Administration in the eighties (see DeCou's study, Section 3, Chapter 15). As Allen and Bell (1998a, p. G3) point out, "in 1980, prisons and jails held about a half-million inmates. By 1997 that number had more than tripled to 1.7 million."

More recently, Dean and Steadman et al. (1999) suggest that mental illness is present in 7 percent of the jail population, a figure confirmed by the latest findings of the Bureau of Justice Statistics (2000). Seven percent, or 700,000 persons, describes a large population with active symptoms of severe mental illness (Dean, Steadman, et al., 1999; Morris et al., 1997). It is crucial to note that the majority of these offenders (four out of five inmates, according to Hogan, 2000) are convicted not of felonies but of misdemeanors—i.e., non-violent crimes, usually trespassing or shoplifting.[1] To some extent, the incarceration of this category of offenders reflects the general trend of an exploding prison population. The fact that a thousand beds are added to correctional facilities every week (Skolnick, 1998b) eloquently demonstrates this phenomenon. However, in comparison to the general population, the seriously mentally ill are incarcerated two to three times more often (Teplin et al., 1996; Lamb & Weinberger, 1998). It is for this reason that, in keeping with Abramson's 1972 study (in which the expression was first coined), specialists speak of the criminalization of the mentally ill, especially when the criminal justice system sentences the mentally ill to serve time in a corrections environment for misdemeanor offenses.

Such criminalization has been even easier because of the extreme vulnerability—not only psychological, but legal—of this population. Most mentally ill offenders are poor and homeless; they live either on the streets or in shelters. According to a study conducted by Martell, Rosner and Harmon (1995) on the prevalence of homelessness in the offending mentally ill population in New York City (a problem common to United States cities), the figures are staggering. Among the homeless mentally ill, as compared to the domiciled mentally ill, the rate was 27 times higher for non-violent crimes and 40 times higher for violent crimes (p. 598). As the authors point out, homelessness adds tremendous stress—and therefore, destabilization—to the life of a mentally ill person. Not only is the stressful condition of homelessness a major contributor to the onset of mental illness, but it "exacerbates psychiatric disorders" (Martell, Rosner & Harmon, p. 599). And what happens to these offenders when their cases get processed by the criminal justice system? Whitmer (1983, p. 217) writes that, although judges have become more educated in the problems facing the mentally ill, the courts, more often than not, don't have the resources to provide for appropriate interventions. Because of their poverty, these offenders, when convicted, "are represented by public defenders or other court-appointed counsel" (see Anderson's chapter, here). Although there are noteworthy public defenders who take the mentally ill client's case to heart, there are many who either do not understand the effects of mental illness on behavior or who find it difficult to work with this population (Anderson, here). The poverty-stricken client—mentally ill or not—cannot afford to hire an attorney who would be more attentive to his or her case. It is beyond question that the poor end up doing jail time more often than those who benefit from proper defense. As a case in point, we can look to a report released on December 19, 2000 by the non-partisan group, the Texas Appleseed Foundation, which states that Texas spends only $4.65 per poor person for his or her defense. This state, as we know, has the largest prison system in the country (study cited in Butterfield, December 20, 2000).

• The Impact of the Corrections Environment

The authors of the studies cited in this Introduction are unanimous in their contention that the corrections environment is not a suitable setting for those severely mentally ill who have been convicted of misdemeanors (see also Laberge & Morin, 1995; Goldstrom et al., 1998).

First of all, jails and prisons often do not provide adequate mental health treatment which can result in the exacerbation of symptoms. In

1998, two articles written by Andrew A. Skolnick in the *Journal of the American Medical Association* and a series of reports in a special issue of the *St. Louis Post-Dispatch*—"Health Care Behind Bars"—point to privatized health services as a major contributing factor to this problem. (These reports, as well as others, recognize that government-run facilities are also responsible for inadequate services.) Both the *Journal of the American Medical Association* and the *St. Louis Post-Dispatch* report single out one HMO as having a particularly poor record in the treatment of mentally ill inmates.[2] There have been an increasing number of suits across the country filed against this private, for-profit HMO, the nation's largest correctional health care firm, located at 341 sites in 30 states and serving one out of every six inmates across the country (Allen & Bell, 1998a). As Skolnick points out, this HMO applies special licensing arrangements, enabling it to employ— at a lower cost—convicted physicians who, by law, cannot treat the mentally or physically ill in the public sector (1998a). As a case in point, two wrongful death suits of inmates at the Kilby Correctional Facility in Alabama revealed that the chief psychiatrist and mental health director for Alabama's prisons was someone who had lost his medical license twice for sexual misconduct in other states (Skolnick, 1998a). It is not only this particular HMO, however, that takes advantage of such licensing arrangements. E. Fuller Torrey remarks that this practice is neither rare nor confined to any particular region of the country (Skolnick, 1998a, p. 1388). "The use of special licensing arrangements that allow physicians who cannot be licensed to treat the public to treat sick and mentally ill inmates in prisons or jails is a scandal. It is a scandal that is being tolerated because we don't care what happens to these people" (Skolnick, 1998b, p. 1392). No one disputes the facts that there are competent doctors in corrections, and that all jails and prisons across the country do not share such a bleak reality. However, it is the case that both substandard treatment and deliberate curtailment of treatment—for economic reasons—have contributed to inadequate services in many of them.

Secondly, the pervasive violence to which inmates are subjected (Allen & Bell, 1998a) also contributes to mental and physical deterioration. James Gilligan (1997) offers the conservative estimate of nine million rapes a year among male inmates. Although there are approximately two million incarcerated men in this country, there are about eight million more in short-term incarceration environments awaiting sentencing. Among this total of ten million inmates, 18 are raped every minute, which comes to, roughly, nine million rapes (Gilligan, 175–176). This type of violence is overwhelmingly tolerated and even encouraged by corrections officers. It is not surprising that corrections centers in the United States, compared to those in other countries (such as Sweden and England), increase the likelihood of violence by the mentally ill (Marzuk, 1996). "Punishment is a form of violence in itself. . . . Punishment stimulates violence. . . . The more punitive our society has become, the higher our rate of violence (both criminal and noncriminal)" (Gilligan, 1997, p. 184). In this light, The *Human Rights Watch World Report 2001* cites serious human rights violations in the United States criminal system, such as "abusive conditions of confinement," and highlights a statement released in May, 2000 from the U.N. Committee against Torture which identifies violations of the Convention Against Torture.[3] It is no surprise that violence is most often self-inflicted. Between 75 and 95 percent of those inmates who commit suicide in jail have mental illness (Goldstrom et al., 1998, p. 177).

- Link between Violence and Mental Illness

The strongest and most frequent argument in favor of incarcerating mentally ill offenders is public safety, meaning that it is the duty of law enforcement officers to protect citizens from danger. (See Chapter 18 for Judge Karopkin's discussion of public safety as a factor in judicial decisions). Civil commitment laws, such as Kendra's Law, have been implemented to ensure the institutionalization of mentally ill persons presenting a threat to themselves or to others.[4] (See Cohen, Lamon and Katz's study, here, on the implementation of Kendra's Law in New York State). Fear of the mentally ill has increased since deinstitutionalization. As Lamb and Weinberger point out (1998, p. 488), there is little tolerance for mental illness; the public desires ever greater measures of detention and punishment. Politicians and political candidates—Republicans and Democrats alike—predicate their reputations as guardians of order by supporting incarceration. Rather than treat and educate, our society punishes. It is an authoritarian culture, Gilligan argues, structured to keep the ruling class in place. The overwhelming majority of inmates are poor and non-Caucasian. A recent report by the Department of Justice indicates that in federal prisons, black men, ages 25 to 29, were incarcerated at a rate 10% higher than white men (cited in Butterfield, Aug., 2000). Black women were eight times more likely to end up in jail than white women (*Human Rights Watch World Report 2001*).

It is important, however, not to dismiss the argument of public safety, not only because it is a driving force of law and policy regarding the mentally ill but also because we must determine the extent to which this argument is well-founded. If the claim of an implicit link between mental illness and violence is based more on reality than myth, then the public's desire to be protected from danger must indeed be taken seriously. Correctional facilities do offer this protection to the public although they do not offer it to mentally ill offenders.

This possible link between violence and mental illness has been central to research conducted by forensic mental health specialists for the past decade. John Monahan's seminal 1991 American Psychological Association Award Address represents a turning point in the assessment of the relationship between mental disorder and violent behavior (Monahan, 1992). Having previously believed that there was no such relationship—and he was only one of many social scientists and advocates who held this belief—, he came to a different conclusion after studying the results of some major studies conducted in the United States. (For the most recent findings on this crucial subject, see Monahan, Steadman, et al.'s ground-breaking work, *Rethinking Risk Assessment: The MacArthur Study of Mental Disorder and Violence*, 2001, Oxford University Press.[5]) Among the studies that Monahan and other specialists cite, and which offer convincing evidence that a sub-group of violent mentally ill does exist, include those conducted by: 1) Klassen and O'Conner (1988, 1990) who found that 25 to 30 percent of male subjects with at least one violent incident in their past committed a violent act in the year following their release from incarceration; 2) Swanson, Holzer, Ganju, and Jono (1990) who concluded that, among a sample of 10,000 offenders, the categories of those most prone to committing violent acts were males with a substance abuse disorder and males with a major mental disorder; 3) Link, Cullen, & Andrews (1992) who observed that, for the most part, violence could be accounted for in the mentally ill only when psychotic symptoms were active; and 4) Mulvey's 1994 study which corroborated the finding that "a general measure of symptom severity over the six-month period was positively associated with the likelihood of a violent incident."

All of these studies have their drawbacks because of selection criteria and treatment biases. However, after careful reflection, Monahan concludes that "the currently mentally disordered—those actively expressing serious psychotic symptoms—are involved in violent behavior at rates several times higher than those of nondisordered members of the general population, and that this difference persists even when a wide array of demographic and social factors are taken into consideration" (1992, p. 517). Although Monahan identifies the existence of this sub-group of violently mentally disordered individuals, he states forcefully that *the overwhelming majority of the mentally ill are not violent* (our emphasis). Yet, because this violent sub-group does exist, Monahan advocates better mental health services in the community and in corrections environments in order to relieve those symptoms that may lead to violence. Likewise, Dvoskin and Steadman point out that "people with mental illness, especially those with histories of violent behavior, most often require continuous rather than episodic care" (1994, p. 680). Swanson et al. (1997, p. 18) concur, on the basis of their evidence that "mentally ill individuals with no treatment contact in the past six months had significantly higher odds of violence in the long term."

An additional facet to the problem is addressed by E. Fuller Torrey (1994, p. 653) who is very concerned about the stigma associated with the mentally ill as necessarily violent which, he argues, can be just as debilitating as the illness itself. The media, as many have pointed out, substantially contribute to this stigma. While there are outstanding journalists dedicated to serious reporting on the mentally ill (such as Michael Winerip, Fox Butterfield, and Nina Bernstein at *The New York Times*), it is often the case that sensationalist coverage misrepresents the facts about the mentally ill, due both to ignorance and to the commercial pressures of market-driven journalism.

Torrey agrees that there does exist a small minority of the mentally ill who are violent. According to him, this behavior is due to drug and/or alcohol abuse and to non-compliance in taking medication. Swanson et al.'s findings (1997, p. 16) support this conclusion in stating that "among the clinical correlates of violence, co-morbid substance abuse is by far the strongest—producing nearly a four-fold increase in the odds of violence." In fact, the overwhelming majority—75 percent (Bernard Aron's Congressional testimony, September 21, 2000; Steadman et al., 1999)— of incarcerated mentally ill offenders have co-occurring drug/alcohol abuse disorders. It is therefore critical that we reverse the trend of treating substance abuse separately from mental illness. The dually diagnosed should be treated in the context of their co-occurring disorder (Swanson et al., 1997, p.19).

Mulvey (1994) points out that, although there is evidence of a link between mental illness and violence in the sub-groups mentioned above, the exact causality has yet to be determined. Marzuk talks about evidence for a biological propensity toward violence: "Low serotonin level has been linked with impulsive violence and suicidality" (1996, p. 483). However, he also argues that, when there are genetic or bio-chemical dispositions for violence in the mentally ill, they cannot be dissociated from environmental factors. Swanson et al. (1997, p. 6) concur and challenge researchers to broaden their scientific inquiry into the realm of social circumstance by asking the following inter-related questions: "1) what specific kinds of psychopathology are most related to violent behavior?, 2) at what levels of severity and functional impairment?, and 3) under what social circumstances?"

While all of these specialists agree that a sub-group of violent mentally ill does exist, and that specific treatment policy must be enacted to reverse the conditions that lead to violence, they also are unanimous in their contention that *this sub-group represents a very small percentage of the population and therefore does not justify the high rate of incarceration of the mentally ill.* Indeed, as Marzuk wrote in an editorial in 1996, "violent and criminal acts directly attributable to mental illness account for a very small proportion of all such acts in the United States. . . . Most persons with mental illness are not criminals, and of those who are, most are not violent" (p. 485).

- Historical Precedent to the Incarceration of Mentally Ill Offenders

Monahan (1992) points out that the association of mental illness with violence is transcultural and transhistorical. One can look to references in the Western world as far back as Plato, or, in the East, to villages in present-day Laos where the association is also commonplace. But whether this association is based on scientific observation or on myth, the problem that interests us here is the incarceration of the mentally ill as a method of treatment. In this light, in *Madness and Civilization*, Michel Foucault speaks of a powerful epistemological divide—originating with the Enlightenment —between Reason and Madness. This divide, he argues, is predicated on the oppression of the insane who found themselves on the other side of an ideological barrier, whose tangible reality is evidenced in the erection of hospitals, asylums or prisons. "In the serene world of mental illness, modern man no longer communicates with the madman," writes Foucault (1973, p. *x*). This code of silence not only has obliterated the lives of those who are locked away from society, but also has penetrated prison walls, as Foucault went on to demonstrate 10 years later in *Discipline and Punish* (1979). In the late Eighteenth and early Nineteenth Centuries in the United States, "a rule of absolute, total silence" was put into practice in two prisons in Philadelphia. "The convicts were to be locked in cells that would prevent all external communication with each other," Foucault writes. Solitary confinement in contemporary prisons has ensured this silence and isolation. And, as Jay Neugeboren expresses so movingly in *Imagining Robert* (1997), the use of seclusion and restraint in institutional settings is barely different from the punishing environment of prison. He bitterly recounts the plight of his brother, Robert, a schizophrenic, who, during one of his stays in a psychiatric facility in New York, was left alone in a bare room in which the only piece of furniture was a mattress to which he was bound by his wrists and ankles. In the locked ward in which this room was located, even when he was free to circulate he was often not allowed to use a pay phone to contact the outside world.

The historical precedent for the incarceration of the mentally ill shows the extent to which fear of this population has produced a policy of punishment rather than treatment and eventual reintegration of the mentally ill into the community. However, we need to look at the more recent phenomenon of deinstitutionalization in order to understand today's enormous numbers of mentally ill inmates. According to Lamb & Weinberger (1998), the number of state hospital beds has decreased over the past 40 years from 339 to 29 per 100,000, while, as we have pointed out, the number of beds in correctional facilities skyrockets weekly. We see from these figures that state hospitals have been replaced by jails and prisons.

The policy of deinstitutionalization grew out of the post-World War II climate of acute attention to mental hygiene, from which emerged the creation of the National Institute of Mental Health. In 1963, President John F. Kennedy signed the Community Mental Health Centers Act which inaugurated the era of deinstitutionalization. This act was precipitated by the work of a tireless movement of reform that called for the total reconceptualization of the state mental hospital, which was seen as a "costly kind of jail" (Whitmer, 1983, p. 218). The goal was eventually to replace state hospitals—where conditions were notoriously barbaric—with community-based treatment, thus enabling the reintegration of the mentally ill into society. Deinstitutionalization of juvenile correctional institutions followed in the early seventies through the efforts of Jerome Diller, Commissioner of the Massachusetts Department of Youth Services. Expansion of community-based treatment for juveniles throughout the United States did not begin until the 1980s (Roberts & Brownell, 1999). However, as with the adult population, deinstitutionalization of the juvenile population also failed. Now, obtaining a bed either in a state hospital or in a community facility requires years of waiting, and when patients do profit from treatment, their release often lacks crucial follow-up through case management. It is most often for these reasons that the mentally ill end up in jails or prisons.

These dire consequences were surely unforeseen by the reformers of the deinstitutionalization era. While there is evidence of a desire to treat the mentally ill humanely in our society, we must note that the creation of adequate facilities in the community has not occurred. This is due to the emphasis on curtailing services for both political and economic reasons under Reagan and Bush during the 1980s, the changing nature of clients as the use of illegal substances became more widely available, and the fear of integration of the mentally ill into the community. But even with a change in administration under Clinton and a booming economy, it remained the policy (with some exceptions) to incarcerate the mentally ill instead of treating them. While we are aware of the record of high incarceration and meager legal support given to public defendants under Governor Bush in Texas, we have yet to see how he will approach this problem on a federal level.

Many see the policy of incarceration as dangerously short-sighted, since 12 million offenders are released back into society every year (Allen & Bell, 1998). For the mentally ill offenders, the negative consequences are far too real; many reappear in far worse shape than when they entered prison, and therefore are at high risk of recidivism. It is suggested that if governments were serious about public safety, they would focus on *properly treating the mentally ill offender to prevent criminal behavior and encourage a positive reintegration back into the community*. Indeed, as Judge Sol Wachtler pointed out in his prison memoirs, a "new philosophy based on public

safety rather than punishment" (1994, pp. 266–268) is urgently needed
to guide policy in American society. Wachtler points to a number of critical areas in which public safety policy should be adopted: through the
creation of alternative programs and rehabilitative services for non-violent offenders, the elimination of mandatory drug sentences, and the
funding of federal, state or private systems *only* if they provide treatment
for substance/alcohol abusers. As Franczak and Shafer point out in their
contribution to this book, in relation to the mentally ill offender, this
would entail the provision of integrated treatment for the dually diagnosed. James Gilligan has also forcefully argued for models that are non-
moralistic, and which approach the problem of treating the mentally ill
offender as a necessity of public health, through preventive medicine and
other related forms of community action. It is our sense that the programs
described here in this book embody such models—or promising practices—of public health, to which all of us in the profession can turn for
inspiration and guidance.

• Promising Practices
How to read this book
At the core of the promising practices identified in this book are collaborative systems that partner community services, law enforcement, the
legal community, consumers, victims, corrections, hospitals, and all others who are involved with or affected by the mentally ill offender. As we
have remarked, such collaboration is crucial to the conceptualization and
implementation of these programs. It is for this reason that the task of
presenting the essays in this book with traditional chapter divisions was
daunting. Since all areas of specialization overlap, what divisions, if any,
would make sense? After much debate, we decided that it was important
to identify programs in terms of the systems, institutions or, in some cases,
the populations that predominantly define them, i.e., jail/prison services;
community-based diversion, including police/mental health linked programs; serving emotionally disturbed women; victims of mentally ill offenders; and perspectives from the legal system. One additional chapter, which
speaks to another essential aspect of the problem, was added to further
instruct the readers of this book: screening for co-occurring mental illness and substance abuse. The different chapter divisions will be useful
to readers specializing, or who have an interest, in a particular area.
However, it should be kept in mind that, to a certain extent, these divisions are artificial in light of their fundamental interdependence.

The aims and importance of these programs
We will briefly introduce the programs that follow, chapter by chapter,
in an effort to ground the reader in the material in question and to relate

these programs directly to the consequences of the criminalization of the mentally ill as described in this Introduction. Moreover, we will point out some of the major ways in which the chapters intersect and fit together as a whole, thereby demonstrating the essential importance of collaborative organization. Social workers and other mental health professionals will gain a sense, perhaps more than ever before, of the necessity of branching out beyond one's specialization and adopting a true systems approach to serve mentally ill offenders.

The book purposely begins with Jail/Prison Services for Incarcerated Populations (Section I) and a discussion of the vast and complex problem of forensic mental health within the incarceration environment. As noted in this Introduction, the high numbers of mentally ill inmates present a need for systematic and proper treatment. As Richard Sherman points out in his chapter, Lane County Adult Corrections Mental Health Services, Oregon places great emphasis on initial assessment and screening in order to identify, from the outset, evidence of mental illness and/or substance abuse and suicide risk in order to respond to the special needs of this population and provide enhanced supervision when necessary. Readers should turn their attention to the final chapter on screening for a detailed analysis of these crucial tools. Among the jail mental health services in Lane County are alternatives to incarceration, thanks to a grant from SAMHSA (Substance Abuse and Mental Health Services Administration) in 1997. In his recent congressional testimony (September 21, 2000), the Executive Director of SAMHSA, Bernard Arons, advocates both further implementation of diversion programs in the United States in order to place non-violent offenders in community-based services and evaluation of the effectiveness of these programs in order to assist policy makers in their implementation. For a national perspective on this subject, the reader should refer to Broner, Borum and Gawley's study on diversion in Chapter 7 and, for a local perspective, to Judge Lerner-Wren's description of incarceration prevention in the Broward Mental Health Court. See also Judge Karopkin's discussion in Chapter 18 of his role in the Brooklyn night arraignment court for insight into the complex task of assessing mental illness and the ways in which arraignment can provide alternatives to jail.

To return to the programs in Section I, Joette Deane, Director of Community Services for the Oswego Forensic Mental Health Program in New York, highlights in her description the comprehensive suicide prevention and crisis intervention training implemented in the Oswego Corrections Facility. As a result, corrections officers and jail medical and mental health personnel have become more sensitive to the serious problems arising in the mentally ill inmate population and are better equipped to handle difficult situations. Both Deane's and Sherman's chapters emphasize their linkages to community services for mentally ill offenders which create a transition back into the community and ensure their support during their time in jail or prison and when they depart.

Section II—Community-Based Diversion Programs—addresses this major aspect of services for this population, whose value and importance was at the heart of the original movement of deinstitutionalization. The first part of this section—Police/Mental Health Linked Programs—has a chronological logic in that police are often the first to have contact with the mentally ill offender. Therefore, law enforcement agents, with the proper training and support, are major contributors to the prevention of incarceration by linking the offender to treatment rather than categorically resorting to jail (for non-violent offenses). As the authors point out in Section IV, it is for this very reason that family victims of mentally ill offenders resist contacting the police when their safety is threatened to avoid having their loved ones given jail/prison time when there is a dire need for treatment. The three chapters in Section II on police programs, along with George Patterson's overview, stress the importance of partnerships with mental health systems and human service agencies to assist this population of offenders. Marjorie Rock describes a model police/mental health training program in New York City developed by the Department of Mental Health and the New York City Police Department and implemented at John Jay College. Rock offers keen insight into the complexities of creating such a program and the necessity of cultivating a close, collaborative relationship among the different partners involved. The curriculum itself emphasizes ways in which officers can best approach problems of anti-social behavior, violence, and substance and/or alcohol abuse when dealing with the mentally ill population. Importantly, it also recognizes the high levels of stress for officers who do this kind of work and helps them deal with their own responses. The Memphis CIT (Crisis Intervention Team) model, as described by Dupont and Cochran, ensures both public safety and emergency mental health care for the offender. Moreover, the CIT program partners with consumers and family members, which, from the family member point of view, is essential to treatment since that family member is directly involved and affected by the behavior of the offender (see Landsberg, Rock & Frank's study, Chapter 17). Training for CIT officers is conducted by mental health professionals, giving officers a special expertise in crisis response to mental illness. Finally, as Dupont and Cochran point out, social workers can play a vital role in community-based services through case management which needs to partner with law enforcement in order to be truly efficacious.

In their discussion of the Birmingham Police Department's Community Service Officer (CSO) Unit, Burnett et al. explain how their program grew out of a series of collaborative experiments which sought to team up police

officers with social workers in the master's program at the University of
Alabama; these social workers provide aide of a psycho-social nature for
the crisis situation. Today, crisis management is still handled through this
approach, i.e., pairing Community Service Officers (trained social workers) with uniformed officers who work as a team. The CSOs provide an
essential link between the police department and the community. In these
two chapters, we see the ways in which social workers can play an essential role in aiding the mentally ill offender.

The second part of Section II—Community Programs—focuses on other
local, community-based diversion initiatives. Beth Navon, Executive Director
of Friends of Island Academy (FOIA) in New York City, describes the program's unique services for juveniles leaving Rikers Island who have completed their jail sentence. FOIA provides crucial services in which social
workers play a key role, as in the mentoring project, case managers, and
discussions groups that take up problems facing these youths. FOIA partners with other community services to create employment, housing, and
educational opportunities. The youth are encouraged to transform their
lives and become leaders in their communities, the highest form of community integration possible.

Franczak & Shafer present the jail diversion program in Arizona from
another progressive point of view, one that critically involves managed
care. In this Introduction, we have seen how managed care may have dire
effects in both the jail/prison environment if there is inadequate treatment. And, as Cypress, Landsberg & Spellman (1997) explain, managed
care can also affect community mental health services: the escalating trend
toward brief therapy does not work well for patients with severe mental
illness. However, in the case of jail diversion in Arizona, managed health
care, when delivered appropriately, can be a strong partner in diversion.
in Tucson and Phoenix jails the Regional Behavioral Health Authorities
have implemented a formalized, three-tiered diversion program. Managed
care is instrumental in the first tier: the mentally ill, in the post-booking
phase, are released from jail for further evaluation/treatment which is
administered by managed care. The second tier entails deferred prosecution, while the third tier allows for summary probation. The Arizona
program drives home the importance of systems collaboration in which
community-based health services, police, hospital emergency departments,
the fire department, and prosecutors, along with managed care, work
together to ensure the best possible treatment and services for the mentally ill. Such extraordinary collaborative networking is at the core of the
highly successful Project Link in Rochester, New York. In Chapter 11, project director Steven Lamberti and co-director Robert Weisman describe
the ways in which a university-led consortium (at the University of
Rochester), in conjunction with community health care, social services,

and the criminal justice system, has successfully diverted the mentally ill from the incarceration environment. Key to Project Link is case management, specifically designed to help restabilize and reintegrate the mentally ill in the community. In a study of four programs across the country, Phyllis Solomon (1992) concludes that case management reduces the rates of rehospitalization and the length of hospital stay; it is therefore cost-effective. Dvoskin & Steadman (1994) found that intensive case management was intrinsic to reducing violent acts in the community by the mentally ill. In Rochester's Project Link, case managers play the role of an "advocate team." They have been chosen because they are members of minority groups, with special sensitivity to minority offenders' needs. As we pointed out earlier in this Introduction, there is a highly disproportionate representation of minorities in jail and prison inmate populations in the United States. The choice of Project Link to use case managers from minority groups has contributed to the success of the program. On its end, the Broward Mental Health Court is designed to divert mentally ill defendants with misdemeanant charges through a court that is uniquely sensitive to the needs of this population. In its application of Therapeutic Jurisprudence, the court acts as a therapeutic agent in the recovery process. Its goal is to reduce, and eventually eliminate, recidivism. Lamon, Cohen, and Broner's section on New York City's system of criminal justice mental health services (Chapter 12) draws our attention to the fact that forensic mental health in this major city is a particularly important problem in view of the 15,000 mentally ill people who return to the city from New York City jails each year, one-third of whom are homeless. The authors discuss the NYC LINK program which provides discharge planning, court diversion, and community case management for those leaving jail, with a special program for adolescents. They also point out that while LINK is designed to serve misdemeanant offenders, another program in New York City (the Nathaniel Project) provides diversion services to felony offenders. This project is particularly commendable in view of the rare efforts in the United States on behalf of this population. Importantly, this essay discusses the stigma on the mentally ill population in New York City and stresses the vital role of public education to help transform community attitudes. Moreover, as Gilligan points out (1997), there is also a dire need for education for inmates: "The single most effective factor which reduces the rate of recidivism in the prison population is education, and yet education in the prisons is the first item to be cut when an administration 'gets tough on crime.'" The features of these local programs are explored nationally and in depth in Broner et al.'s section (Chapter 7) on diversion which stresses coordination among multiple systems and describes in detail diversion's different forms, i.e., pre-booking, post-booking, and specialized courts.

Section III is a unique feature of this book in its focus on the much-ignored population of mentally ill women offenders. Indeed, as Decou and Van Wright point out, nearly all corrections programming targets male offenders. Similar to the need to match minority populations with case managers whose ethnic backgrounds give them particular insight into the special needs of offenders from African-American or Hispanic backgrounds, as in the Rochester Link Program, so too do gender-specific models need to be utilized in corrections and community settings. This section discusses such a model, *V.O.I.C.E.S.*, which has been implemented in the Hampden County Correctional Center and explains how women benefit from therapeutic treatment and other community support that address their problems as mothers and victims of domestic violence as well as their traumatic histories of sexual abuse. On their end, Gillece and Russell discuss the implementation of two diversion programs specifically designed for women in Maryland. The Phoenix Project serves women on the Eastern Shore of Maryland who committed non-violent crimes and who have a serious mental illness and a co-occurring substance abuse disorder. These women benefit from case management and clinical interventions in their homes, and remain with their children. Further, these women, as well as their children, are linked to community services. This program thus recognizes the value of treating women as individuals and in relation to their children. The TAMAR Project—implemented in three Maryland counties—is also unique to women in that it pays special attention to the histories of violence in the lives of mentally ill, substance-abusing women inmates. This program serves women who are involved in the criminal justice system by offering them treatment while incarcerated and linkages to trauma specialists in the community after their release. In her overview to this section, Susan Salasin points out that only gender-based programs can help women cope with the corrections environment, and, upon the release of women into the community, are necessary to help them as single mothers and as patients recovering from traumatic events.

Like Section III, Section IV also treats a population which suffers from lack of programs and which has been neglected by research: the Victims of Mentally Ill Offenders. Both chapters in this section make clear that it is difficult to gauge the number of family victims in this population since feelings of guilt and the desire to protect the abuser from criminal punishment inhibit their asking for help, despite the disastrous consequences that may ensue. In their section on Elder Abuse and Forensic Mentally Ill Abusers, Brownell et al. point to the particular vulnerability of this elderly population who are subject to financial neglect and/or physical or psychological abuse. Traditional aging services are too limited to aid these elder victims whose service needs require help from mental health, substance, and criminal justice systems. The role of social workers in this area has become extremely important and represents a major new direction in the field. As the authors suggest, social service intervention strategies can bring much required aid to victims through protective, community-based, and victim services. The second chapter of this section, written by Landsberg, Rock, and Frank, provides a broader analysis of victims' issues in that it includes an analysis of the special needs of victims who are not family members. Non-family members, who are more likely to press charges, find themselves caught up in the maze of the criminal justice system and feel unsupported. These victims indicate that they feel "doubly victimized" since their need to be involved in the criminal justice process may be denied if the offender is judged to have a condition warranting mental health treatment. In the cases where the perpetrator is a family member or close friend of the family, there are frequently feelings of guilt and shame, along with the stigma of mental illness, which can impede the family members from seeking relief through the legal system. This contribution is noteworthy in particular for the specific recommendations it makes about educating all those who deal or work with victims and offenders and the resources to which it refers the reader. Both chapters of this section highlight the importance of sensitizing the courts to the special needs of both mentally ill offenders and family members.

Section V—Perspectives from the Legal System—offers a rare view into the workings of the criminal justice system in relation to mental illness from the perspectives of all its key players, i.e., the judge, the prosecutor, the advocate, and the defense attorney, and also provides unique insight from a man whose keen understanding of the system is derived from his experience as a judge, on the one hand, and a mentally ill offender, on the other. A final chapter on the implementation of Kendra's Law in New York City closes the section with a discussion of its implications of this law which originated due to a crime committed in this city. All of these contributions make clear that there is much hope for a greater sensitivity to the plight of mentally ill offenders within criminal justice which has a major determining influence on the future of these offenders. The authors also stress the importance of the role of partnering with specialists in mental health and social work communities to find the most humane and appropriate solutions. This section offers brilliant analysis and concrete suggestions for social workers and other service providers navigating the criminal justice system. Judge Karopkin elucidates the complex problems of public safety and screening in the realm of arraignment court. Heather Barr, staff attorney at the Urban Justice Center/Mental Health Project, guides social workers advocating for a client through the obstacles and intricacies of the criminal justice system. Mary Elizabeth Anderson, public defense attorney at The Legal Aid Society, describes the special challenges of advocating for the mentally ill due to the nature of the illness, problems of homelessness, and the severity of the crime. Anderson also sheds light on the tenuous but often beneficial relationship between social workers and public defenders. Lee Cohen, from the Public Defender's Office in Broward County, discusses how his role of prosecutor has also become that of social worker, case manager, and probation officer with the creation of Broward's Mental Health Court. Cohen argues that this specialized court has greatly enhanced public safety because the mentally ill are taken out of the jail setting and given proper treatment. While recidivism has not been completely eliminated, its rate has considerably lessened. This is due, to a great extent, to the commitment made on the part of defendants to engage in treatment and therefore take responsibility for their mental health and well-being. Judge Wachtler analyzes the plight of the mentally ill in prison and argues for a reappraisal of the insanity defense in order to procure necessary treatment for this population. Cohen, Lamon and Katz, in their discussion of the implementation of Kendra's Law in New York City, highlight the complex issues related to this law that allows for services to be ordered by civil courts for the non-compliant mentally ill. The authors make the important point that Kendra's Law will have a real impact on the judicial system in New York where criminal and civil courts overlap considerably, with judges from one court assigned to duties in the other. Because of growing judicial understanding of the problem of criminalization of the mentally ill, there is hope that the recommendations for treatment will outweigh those for punishment.

Section VI—A Review of Screening Instruments for Co-occurring Mental Illness and Substance Abuse in Criminal Justice Programs—provides in-depth research into the challenges of diversion of dually diagnosed offenders (who, as already noted, represent the majority of this population). Readers will gain an important understanding of the kinds of instruments employed to screen for mental illness, alcohol and drug abuse, and personality disorders as well as those instruments used to assess psychiatric symptoms and determine diagnoses. As pointed out by all of the authors in this book, integrated treatment is essential for treating the complex problems of this population. In this particular contribution, the authors—Broner et al.—describe in detail the effects of integrated treatment on the reduction of hospital stay and stabilization of the client. They make the point that screening needs to be culturally specific (depending on the ethnic population) and offer a detailed analysis of screening instruments. Social workers and other mental health professionals will find this chapter of considerable use in their work with mentally ill offenders who are often in dire need of proper treatment, which should be the result of an accurate diagnosis of disorders and symptoms.

As the profession of social workers and others in mental health has evolved to accommodate the growing numbers of the incarcerated mentally ill, it has become an essential responsibility for all of us in these fields to gain an understanding of the different legal, community-based, and clinical systems with which offenders and victims become involved. And, as all of the authors in this book can attest, it is only through the cooperation of specialists in these systems that these populations will benefit from better services and treatment. The health of society depends on it.

The Editors

Notes

1. According to the *Human Rights Watch World Report 2001*, "approximately 70 percent of all new admissions to state prison in 1998. . . . were people convicted of nonviolent property, drug or public order offenses."

2. See the articles in *JAMA* and the *St. Louis Post-Dispatch*—cited in the bibliography—for details on legal findings against this HMO and a description of wrongful death and class action suits.

3. The "ill-treatment by . . . prison officials . . . sexual assaults upon female detainees and prisoners and degrading conditions of confinement of female prisoners; the use of electro-shock devices and restraint chairs; the excessively harsh regime of super-maximum security prisons; and the holding of youths in adult prisons," (*Human Rights Watch World Report 2001*).

4. It should be pointed out that in the case of Andrew Goldstein, from which Kendra's Law emerged, Goldstein's request, on a *voluntary* basis, to be institutionalized had been repeatedly rejected. Further, during his hospitalization in the weeks prior to pushing Kendra Webdale onto the subway tracks, he was released while still exhibiting active symptoms (Winerip, 2000).

5. This study was in press during the writing of this Introduction.

REFERENCES

Abramson, M.F. (1972). The criminalization of mentally disordered behavior: Possible side-effects of a new mental health law. *Hospital and Community Psychiatry, 23,* 101–105.

Allen, W. & Bell, K. (1998a). Death, neglect and the bottom line. *St. Louis Post-Dispatch* special report, *Health Care Behind Bars.* September 27: G1–3.

Allen, W. & Bell, K. (1998b). Business is booming for CMS due to states' efforts to cut costs and lots of inmates. *St. Louis Post-Dispatch* special report, *Health Care Behind Bars.* September 27: G4.

Allen, W. (1998). Alabama teen died in isolation seven weeks after sentence began. *St. Louis Post-Dispatch* special report, *Health Care Behind Bars.* September 27: G6–7.

Arons, B. (September 21, 2000). Mental health and criminal justice. A testimony before the Subcommittee on Crime of the Committee on the Judiciary United States House of Representatives.

Butterfield, F. (2000). Number in prison grows despite crime reduction. *The New York Times*, August 10: A10.

Butterfield, F. (2000). Texas spends little on public defenders for poor criminal defendants, report says. *The New York Times*, December 20.

Cypress, A., Landsberg, G. & Spellmann, M. (1997). The impact of managed care on community mental health outpatient services in New York State. *Administration and Policy in Mental Health, 24*(6), 509–521.

Deane, M.W., Steadman, H.J., Borum, R., Veysey, B.M. & Morrissey, J.P. (1999). Emerging partnerships between mental health and law enforcement. *Psychiatric Services, 50*(1), 99–101.

Dvoskin, J.A. & Steadman, H.J. (1994). Using intensive case management to reduce violence by mentally ill persons in the community. *Hospital and Community Psychiatry, 45*(7), 679–684.

Foucault, M. (1973). *Madness and Civilization.* New York: Vintage.

Foucault, M. (1979). *Discipline and Punish.* New York: Pantheon.

Goldstrom, I. D., Henderson, M., Male, A. & Manderscheid, R. (1998). Jail mental health services: A National survey. In R. Manderscheid & M. Henderson (Eds.), Mental Health, United States, 1998 (pp. 176–187). DHHS Pub. No. (SMA) 99-285. Washington, DC: U.S. Government Printing Office.

Gilligan, J. (1997). *Violence. Reflections on a National Epidemic.* New York: Vintage.

Hogan, M.F. (September 21, 2000). The "mental illness problem" is severe in criminal justice, and in society. A testimony before the Subcommittee on Crime of the Committee on the Judiciary United States House of Representatives.

Human Rights Watch World Report 2001: United States: Human Rights Developments. http://www.hrw.org/wr2k1/usa/index.html#conditions.

Klassen, D. and O'Connor, W. (1988). Crime, inpatient admissions, and violence among male mental patients. *International Journal of Law and Psychiatry, 11*, 305–312.

Klassen, D. and O'Connor, W. (1990). Assessing the risk of violence in released mental patients: A cross-validation study. *Psychological Assessment: A Journal of Consulting and Clinical Psychology, 1*, 75–81.

Laberge, D. and Morin, D. (1995). The overuse of criminal justice dispositions: Failure of diversionary policies in the management of mental health problems. *International Journal of Law and Psychiatry, 18*(4), 389–414.

Lamb, H.R. and Weinberger, L.E. (1998). Persons with severe mental illness in jails and prisons: A review. *Psychiatric Services, 49*(4), 483–492.

Link, B.G., Andrews, H. & Cullen, F.T. (1992). The violent and illegal behavior of mental patients reconsidered. *American Sociological Review, 57,* 275–92.

Martell, D.S., Rosner, R. & Harmon, R.B. (1995). Base-rate estimates of criminal behavior by homeless mentally ill persons in New York City. *Psychiatric Services, 46*(6), 596–600.

Marzuk, P.M. (1996). Violence, crime, and mental illness. *Archives General Psychiatry, 53,* 481–486.

Monahan, J. (1992). Mental disorder and violent behavior. *American Psychologist, 47*(4), 511–521.

Morris, S.M., Steadman, H.J. & Veysey, B.M. (1997). Mental health services in United States jails: a survey of innovative practices. *Criminal Justice and Behavior, 24,* 3–19.

Mulvey, E.P. (1994). Assessing the evidence of a link between mental illness and violence. *Hospital and Community Psychiatry, 45*(7), 663–668.

Neugeboren, J. (1997). *Imagining Robert.* New York: Henry Holt.

Roberts, A.R. & Brownell, P. (1999). A century of forensic social work: Bridging the past to the present. *Social Work, 44*(4), 359–366.

Skolnick, A.A. (1998a). Prison deaths spotlight how boards handle impaired, disciplined physicians. *Journal of the American Medical Association, 280*(16), 1387–1390.

Skolnick, A.A. (1998b). Critics denounce staffing jails and prisons with physicians convicted misconduct. *Journal of the American Medical Association, 280*(16), 1391–1392.

Skolnick, A.A. (1998c). Physicians with troubled pasts have found work behind bars. *St. Louis Post-Dispatch* special report, *Health Care Behind Bars.* September 27, p. G9.

Skolnick, A.A. (1998d). Two key posts in Alabama were filled by doctors with checkered histories. *St. Louis Post-Dispatch* special report, *Health Care Behind Bars.* September 27, p. G9.

Solomon, P. (1992). The efficacy of case management services for severely mentally disabled clients. *Community Mental Health Journal* 28(3):163–180.

Solomon, P. & Draine, J. (1995). Issues in serving the forensic client. *Social Work, 40*(1), 25–33.

Steadman, H.J. (2000). National Perspectives on Forensic Mental Health. Keynote address at the Second Annual International Forensic Mental Health Conference, New York University.

Steadman, H.J., Deane, M.W., Morrissey, J.P., Westcott, M.L., Salasin, S. & Shapiro, S. (1999). A SAMHSA research initiative assessing the effectiveness of jail diversion programs for mentally ill persons. *Psychiatric Services, 50*(12), 1620–1623.

Swanson, J., Estroff, S., Swartz, M., Borum, R., Lachicotte, W., Zimmer, Ca. & Wagner R. (1997). Violence and severe mental disorder in clinical and community populations: The effects of psychotic symptoms, comorbidity, and lack of treatment. *Psychiatry, 60,* 1–22.

Teplin, L.A., Abram, K.M. & McClelland, G.M. (1996). Prevalence of psychiatric disorders among incarcerated women. *Archives General Psychiatry, 53,* 505–512.

Torrey, E.F. (1994). Violent behavior by individuals with serious mental illness. *Hospital and Community Psychiatry, 45*(7), 653–662.

Trattner, W.I. (1989). *From Poor Law to Welfare State.* New York: The Free Press.

Winerip, M. (2000). The role of the media. Keynote address at the Second Annual International Forensic Mental Health Conference, New York University.

Whitmer, G.E. (1983). The development of forensic social work. *Social Work,* May–June, 217–223.

SECTION I
Jail/Prison Services for Incarcerated Populations

1

Lane County Adult Corrections Mental Health Services, Lane County, Oregon

Richard K. Sherman

PURPOSE OF PROGRAM

The Mental Health Services Section of Lane County Adult Corrections attempts to identify people with a mental disorder and/or a substance abuse problem among those who are booked into the jail. After identifying them, we make every effort to stabilize their condition and mental status, divert them to appropriate services or facilities when appropriate, and assist the criminal justice system in finding appropriate dispositions to resolve their criminal cases. As individuals leave the jail facility, we help them connect to appropriate community-based services so as to maintain their stability and reduce the possibility of recidivism.

COMMUNITY CONTEXT

Lane County, Oregon has a population of 308,500 in a geographic area of 4,575 square miles, roughly the size of Connecticut, and stretches from the summit of the Cascade Mountains to the Pacific Ocean. Approximately 180,000 of Lane County residents reside in the county's two largest cities, Eugene and Springfield, which are located on opposite sides of the Interstate 5 highway dividing eastern and western Lane County. Most of the other Lane County residents live in the other 11 incorporated cities within the county. About 95,000 residents reside in unincorporated areas along river valleys.

Until the early 1980s, the entire county was heavily dependent on a timber-based economy. Over the past 15 years, the problem of sufficient timber, combined with increasing public concerns for the health of the ecosystem, have resulted in a forced transition to a more diversified, service-based workforce. The principal industries in Lane County remain agriculture, lumber, recreation, and tourism. In 1995, the per capita income was $19,917. The unemployment rate in that same year was 5.7%. Among registered voters about 83,000 are Democrats, 61,000 are Republicans, and 41,000 are unaffiliated with any party.

In 1994, Lane County ranked third in the country in the production and distribution of methamphetamine, according to Drug Enforcement Agency data. More recently, Lane County has seen a dramatic shift, with heroin rapidly becoming the substance of choice among drug abusers. In 1999, heroin deaths in Lane County had increased eleven-fold since 1986. This trend is consistent with a state-wide trend. According to the state medical examiner's office, a record 246 people died from drug-related causes in Oregon in 1999. Seventy-nine percent of those deaths were due to heroin.

The interstate highway that divides Lane County and the train tracks that parallel the highway stretch from Mexico to the Canadian border. The highway and freight trains serve as a thoroughfare for drug trafficking as well as for homeless men and women. There is a large incidence of mental illness among this transient population. Oregon, like the rest of the country, has seen a significant downsizing of its state mental hospitals. The resulting impact of the trend of "deinstitutionalization" is well-documented elsewhere (see Abramson, 1972; Butterfield, 1999; Lamb, 1998; Penrose, 1939; Torrey, 1992; Torrey, 1995). The same number of mentally ill persons book into the Lane County jail as on a nationwide basis. Of the 15,619 screenings that were conducted at booking in 1999, 32% of them were identified with a mental health or substance abuse-related problem.

THE JAIL PHYSICAL PLANT

The Lane County Jail was constructed and occupied in 1979. In addition to the jail itself, an 18-bed, acute care psychiatric hospital was also constructed as a wing to the jail. In fact, the jail and the hospital facility share the same front door. The psychiatric hospital is owned by the county and is operated today as a 12 bed, acute-care facility under contract by the local hospital, Sacred Heart Medical Center. Sacred Heart Medical Center also has a psychiatric unit in its own facility which is a less secure facility than the Lane County Psychiatric Hospital. The Lane County Psychiatric Hospital is a fully locked and secure facility with the jail operating the entrance and exit doors. The jail correctional staff also provide support for patients needing to be restrained.

An additional 88 beds were added to the jail in 1988. In 1999, a 152-bed addition was constructed as well. Today the capacity of the jail is 485 beds. The jail continues to operate under a Federal court order that limits the jail population on any given day to 421. In 1999, there were 4,475 persons who were released from the jail under the terms of that court order as a result of overcrowding. There are an additional 32 beds in the jail that are part of a residential alcohol and drug treatment program for fully sentenced jail inmates. Other "alternative programs" for fully sentenced inmates include a forest work camp which is currently funded to operate with 30 beds (but which has a much larger capacity), a road crew, and a community corrections center. The community corrections center has a capacity of 116 beds. The combination of beds in the jail and these alternative programs brings the total number of beds available for jail inmates to 631.

SERVICES PROVIDED

Lane County Adult Corrections' mental health staff train corrections officers in the identification and recognition of persons suffering from mental illness, substance intoxication, and suicide risk warning signs. As offenders enter the jail facility, arresting officers are queried as to their knowledge of the presence of a mental health or substance intoxication issue with each inmate. In addition, these trained corrections deputies question the newly booked inmates and make their own observations of the individuals' behavior and indicators of mental illness, intoxication, or suicide risk. These observations, along with the responses of the inmates and arresting officer inquiries, are recorded on an Initial Assessment Screening Form. Based on the outcome of this screening, a review of an inmate's previous institutional records, the nature of the charges, and the individual's behavior, the corrections staff make an initial decision about where in the facility an inmate is to be housed and under what degree of restrictions. The jail operates a "Special Management Unit" for inmates identified as having special needs or requiring an increased level of supervision. This unit is a single-cell housing unit that operates with "direct supervision," meaning that a corrections officer is assigned and posted inside the housing unit itself so that he/she can closely monitor inmates. Generally, persons who are on suicide precautionary status and those demonstrating overt signs and symptoms of mental illness are initially housed in this special management unit. A copy of the Initial Assessment Screening Form accompanies the inmate which allows for additional observations to be made and recorded by corrections staff over the course of the first 24 to 48 hours that the inmate remains in custody.

Another copy of the form is routed to mental health staff. A third copy is routed to medical staff. Jail mental health and medical staff review copies of this initial screening form for all persons who are booked into the jail. Based on the recorded comments and observations, these professional staff members make a decision regarding further screening or assessment. In the case of mental health-related screening, mental health staff look for indicators of previous mental health treatment or current mental health-related concerns, such as aberrant or unusual behavior, peculiar statements or the use of psychotropic medications. The jail mental health staff have access to the county's Community Mental Health Clinic's client database. If there is an indicator that an inmate has a mental health related problem, mental health staff access that database to determine if the person is currently in treatment at the local mental health clinic. Contact will be made with mental health providers and prescribers of any medications in order to obtain a brief history and confirm medication orders. Mental health providers, doctors, and family members also frequently contact the mental health staff to provide information and to express their concerns about the newly booked inmate. After reviewing all of the information, mental health staff may contact the individual and conduct a more in-depth assessment.

Mental health staff have several goals and interests when conducting their own assessment of an identified mentally ill inmate. There is a primary interest in the person's mental status and the degree to which he/she can be safely managed in the facility. Persons who are deemed to be very psychotic are assessed to determine if their psychosis is organic in nature and possibly substance-induced. If it can be determined that they are under the influence of a substance, mental health staff coordinate with medical and security staff to initiate appropriate detoxification protocols, monitor the inmates condition, and manage the detoxification in a safe manner. In 1999, 1,888 persons (12% of the population booking into the jail) were identified as detoxifying from some substance and requiring close supervision and monitoring.

In addition to safely detoxifying intoxicated persons, mental health staff are always vigilant about the possibilities of suicidal ideation and risk. All staff in the jail are trained to identify suicide risk warning signs and to take preventive action. Persons who are identified as being "at risk" for suicide are placed on a "suicide watch." They are moved to a specialized housing unit where they can be monitored more closely. Mental health staff conduct a further assessment of the degree of risk and offer recommendations and directions on how the security staff can best manage the inmate. Items generally issued to the inmates, such as clothing, sheets, blankets, and toiletries, might be restricted from suicidal inmates to prevent them from harming themselves if there is an indication that they are thinking of using those items to do so. Medications might be ordered after consultation with the psychiatrist, or the person might need counseling. Providing the person with information about the legal process is usually helpful as well. In general, the passage of time, with close monitoring, helps to alleviate the suicide risk as persons regain their judgement (if under the influence of substances) and sense of hope for the future. If persons are actively attempting to harm themselves, they might be placed in restraints until they regain control of their behavior or until another plan is devised to keep them safe.

A third area of interest in conducting a mental health assessment is whether persons can be safely managed in the jail facility if they are psychotic. Persons who are not compliant with recommended treatment for their mental illness and who demonstrate uncontrollable or extreme behaviors will be considered for transfer to a psychiatric hospital facility. If a person is mentally ill and represents a danger to himself or herself or to others, jail mental health staff are authorized under Oregon law to place an inmate on "mental health holds." The inmate is then transferred to one of the two psychiatric units described above. Under these circumstances, the person is admitted to the hospital by an admitting physician. Arrangements are made to have the court release the person from custody so that hospital admission can occur. In the case of the secure facility next door to the jail, a court-ordered release is not required and persons can simply be transferred there to be returned to the jail upon their discharge from the hospital. In many cases, mentally ill persons are arrested for non-violent nuisance types of offenses in which case the charges are frequently dismissed before their transfer to the hospital. Such hospital transfers do occur quickly however, within 24 hours in most cases. In 1999, 27 persons were psychiatrically hospitalized on this basis.

In cases where the criminal charges are more significant and the defendant in custody appears to be psychotic or otherwise mentally ill, jail mental health staff will conduct an assessment to determine if the individual is competent and "fit to proceed" with the criminal trial. If it is determined that the person lacks the ability to understand the nature of the proceedings or is unable to aid and assist counsel or participate in his/her own defense, mental health staff will appear before the court and advise the court of the concerns. This generally happens at the first appearance before the court. Mental health staff will ask the court to appoint an attorney in order to protect the inmate's rights. Once an attorney is appointed, a hearing is convened to determine the fitness issue. Generally, mental health staff provide their findings based on the assessment and a review of the person's mental health and psychiatric history. It is rare that such findings by the mental health staff are contested by either the prosecutors or the court. Once the court finds that the inmate is "unfit to proceed," the court orders the defendant transferred to the Oregon State Hospital forensic ward for care and treatment. The person will return to the jail upon regaining his/her capacity to aid and assist in his/her defense. We hospitalize about 14 persons a year through this criminal commitment process.

Other persons book into the jail with a mental disorder or with a mental disorder co-occurring with a substance abuse problem, but psychiatric hospitalization is not indicated. If they are in custody for a low-level offense, generally non-violent in nature, they may be eligible for our Co-occurring Disorders Diversion Program. In this program, if defendants are interested and the prosecuting attorney is also in agreement, they can be placed in an outpatient treatment program designed to treat both their mental illness and their substance abuse problems. Legally, it functions much like the drug court programs that have been touted as so successful around the country. In fact, we created our program based on the drug court model. Essentially, the defendant, in a petition to the court asking to participate in the diversion, admits that the state could prove the charges against him and gives up his right to a trial. The defendant also agrees to participate in the treatment program, stay in contact with the jail mental health staff, and make required court appearances. The judge generally requires at least monthly appearances but may require them to be more frequent if the defendant is not doing well in treatment. Prior to each appearance, the judge receives a written report from the treatment provider which describes how the defendant is progressing. The report indicates if the person is making his group and individual counseling appointments, taking required medications, and if his urinalysis screens are coming back "clean." The judge attempts to encourage continued compliance and participation in treatment or he may sanction non-compliance and lack of participation. Sanctions include verbal reprimands, more frequent court appearances, or even jail time.

Ultimately, the judge can terminate the offender's participation in the diversion program for lack of compliance. Should this occur, the person has already waived the right to trial and stipulated to the facts of the case. The person is found guilty of the crime for which he is charged and the usual sentencing process occurs. In cases where the person successfully completes the treatment program one year after entering the diversion program, the charge is dismissed. An important element of the success of this program is that the jail mental health staff actually case manage each of the defendants in the program. They develop a rapport with the subjects and encourage their continued participation and success. They stay in regular contact with the defendants, encouraging them to keep their appointments, show up for court, take their medication, and not use illegal substances. Another important element in the outcome is the knowledge, skills, and attitude of the judge. As in drug court, the judge should have an understanding of the nature of mental illness and addiction. The judge cannot expect too much progress too soon and must give the participant an opportunity to experience success, and not just failure. In 1999, sixty one persons entered the diversion program. Many of them are still in the program and final outcomes are still being evaluated.

In addition to the jail diversion program, the Mental Health Section of Lane County Jail is also operating a 32-bed residential substance abuse treatment program for men and women. These programs, collectively referred to as the Intensive Treatment Program, are for fully sentenced inmates. Each requires that participants serve a minimum of 180 days in treatment. The program is based on a modified therapeutic community model. It is designed as a positive, supportive environment where people with similar problems, such as alcohol and drug abuse, live and work together to improve their lives. The program follows a "chain of command" in which all residents strive to earn better jobs, privileges and status in the community. The participants are engaged in substance abuse treatment and education groups. They learn about cognitive restructuring and criminal thinking errors. There are also groups devoted to anger management and domestic violence. "Residents" are also required to participate in meditation, art therapy, and self-help groups as well as individual counseling. During the last phase of treatment, they move out of the jail to the Community Corrections Center which is a work release program. Here they work with a transition therapist who helps them establish connections with community-based services that will assist them to make their transition back into the community and to continue a drug- and crime-free lifestyle. They also participate in educational and vocational support activities to assist them in searching for and finding employment. Family members are invited to participate in this last phase of treatment for family counseling related to their substance abuse.

In addition to these programs, the mental health staff in the Lane County Jail work closely with security staff to help manage inmates whose behavior, for whatever reason, is disruptive. Mental health staff also assist the court release officers in making determinations of the appropriateness of releasing individuals who appear to have mental health problems. They are asked to conduct assessments related to the potential dangerousness of defendants being considered for release. They confer frequently with the courts and attorneys regarding referrals to treatment programs and disposition issues related to defendants who have mental health and substance abuse problems. They provide counseling and psycho-educational materials to inmates asking for assistance with such problems as anger management, impulse control, anxiety, and sleep disturbance. They also provide for the coordination of services and access to inmates for community-based mental health providers.

FUNDING SOURCES

In 1973, the Lane County sheriff's office applied for and received a Law Enforcement Administration Act (L.E.A.A.) Grant for alternative programs in the jail. This grant funded two positions which have evolved into the current Mental Health Section of the jail. In 1977, the Oregon legislature passed the Community Corrections Act which moved resources and authority for a range of corrections-related programs from the state to the county. Lane County used these funds to balance sanctions, supervision, and treatment. In 1979, the Lane County Mental Health Division began providing a range of services to offenders including sex offender treatment and alcohol and drug assessments. These services have since expanded to include mental health assessment and treatment for offenders under the supervision of the parole and probation office as well as assessment, referral, and treatment of offenders for such issues as domestic violence and anger management.

In the late 1970s, the new jail facility and adjacent psychiatric hospital were built with funds obtained by the passing of a voter-approved bond measure. The psychiatric hospital was opened and closed twice due to lack of funds. In the mid-1980s, a class action lawsuit was filed by inmates resulting in a court order to demolish the old jail which was still in use and to limit the jail population to prevent overcrowding. Under increasing pressure to allay the lack of sufficient jail beds, the Lane County citizens passed a law enforcement-related serial levy to fund a variety of corrections-related services in 1985. As a result, some of the alternative programs described above were initiated including the Community Corrections Center and the Forest Work Camp. This serial levy also funded a detoxification center operated by a private non-profit agency as the jail was no longer accepting persons for non-criminal detoxification. This levy also helped fund the opening of the Lane County Psychiatric Hospital adjacent to the jail. The levy also provided for funding a respite care facility designed to serve persons with severe mental and emotional illnesses. In 1989, the State Mental Health Division provided additional funds for the operation of the psychiatric hospital.

In 1994, the Lane County Circuit Court obtained a Byrne Grant which was added to money confiscated by the Inter-agency Narcotics Enforcement Team to begin operating a drug court. Today, the drug court operates a diversion program for non-violent drug offenders. We have obtained additional funding (described below) to develop a specialized program for diverting persons with co-occurring mental illness and substance abuse disorders into treatment. The drug court handles these cases as well.

In 1995, the Oregon legislature passed a bill which moved responsibility for all felony offenders whose terms of incarceration were less than one year from the state to the county. Anticipating the resulting increased number of inmates in the local jails, the legislature also provided money for construction of additional jail beds. The Lane County sheriff's office applied for those construction dollars. Together with money obtained under a contract with the United States Marshals to house federal prisoners, the jail built a 152-bed addition which included a space designed for an alcohol and drug treatment unit. However, we did not have funds to operate this unit. In 1997, as construction of the new treatment unit was underway, we applied for a Residential Substance Abuse Treatment Grant to fund the operation of this unit. This grant stems from the Violent Crime Control and Law Enforcement Act of 1994. This law provided funds to the states to develop or enhance substance abuse treatment programs for offenders. The law authorized the Attorney General to award formula grants for substance abuse treatment programs in state and local correctional facilities. We were granted enough funding to hire five therapists and an office assistant in addition to obtaining the various supplies needed to operate an alcohol and drug treatment program. The funding is only offered on a year-to-year basis through a competitive process. The second year funding was reduced from the original grant award, causing us to reduce our staffing and the number of inmates in the treatment program. We are therefore currently looking for a source of continued funding for the operation of this program. The bill passed and funded by the Oregon legislature did provide us with one additional mental health worker.

Also in 1997, we applied for, and received, a three-year grant from the Substance Abuse and Mental Health Services Administration (SAMHSA) to enhance and evaluate the effectiveness of our jail diversion program for persons with co-occurring severe mental illness and substance abuse problems. These funds provided for the addition of two more mental health staff and office support staff to enhance the operation of this diversion program.

To summarize, we are operating today with a mental health supervisor, three therapists, and an office assistant in the alcohol and drug treatment program; two mental health specialists and an office assistant in the co-occurring disorders diversion program; a mental health specialist assigned to suicide prevention and inmate crises-related services.

Ultimately, jail-based mental health services must be viewed and developed within the context of the community and as a part of the continuum of services that are available in the community. The jail must be seen as a part of the community which it serves and the persons in it must be recognized as predominately the community's citizens. Most will eventually be returning to the community. Any services provided while in the jail must be optimized by a smooth transition back to the community.

REFERENCES

Abramson, M.F. (1972). The criminalization of mentally disordered behavior: Possible side-effects of a new mental health law. *Hospital and Community Psychiatry 23,* 101–105.

Butterfield, F. (1999). Mentally ill languishing in nation's prisons. *The New York Times,* July 12.

Lamb, H.R. & Weinberger, L.E. (1998). Persons with severe mental illness in jails and prisons: a review. *Psychiatric services, 49*(4).

Torrey, E.F. et. al. (1992). Criminalizing the seriously mentally ill: the abuse of jails as mental hospitals. A joint report of the National Alliance of the Mentally Ill and Public Citizen's Health Research Group.

Torrey, E.F. (1995). Editorial: jails and prisons—America's new mental hospitals. *American Journal of Public Health 85*(12), 1612.

2

Oswego Mental Health Forensic Mental Health Program, Oswego, New York

Joette Deane

As a response to increasing numbers of suicides in jail and local police lockup facilities statewide, the Suicide Prevention/Crisis Intervention Program was implemented in 1985. Although there had been no suicides in the immediate past prior to the implementation of the program in Oswego County, there was a considerable increase in suicide attempts. Therefore, as New York State took action through its Office of Mental Health and Commission of Corrections, Oswego County was poised and ready to accept the challenge to develop and implement a suicide prevention and crisis intervention program in the jail and police lockups. Oswego County was one of five counties enlisted to partner with the state to operationalize the program. Through this endeavor, and along with its experience as a contractor for the state-wide implementation of the program and consequent refresher course given five years later, Oswego County Mental Health made significant strides in crucial systems change. The Oswego County programs continue to exist well past the implementation phases due to the careful organization, planning, and commitment of all agencies involved. The atmosphere generated by this program enabled Oswego County to take advantage of other beneficial initiatives, such as the police/mental health program and the jail physical plant construction.

PURPOSE OF THE PROGRAM

The purpose of the Mental Health program at the county jail has evolved over time, but its basic tenets are the same:

- Maintain a no suicide rate.
- Reduce suicide attempts.
- Increase timely identification and referral for services for high-risk inmates.
- Increase safe housing within the facility for at-risk inmates.
- Increase ongoing individual and group counseling for inmates.
- Facilitate discharge planning services for inmates.
- Reduce forensic hospitalizations.
- Reduce county liability and consequent litigation.
- Increase communication and coordination at all levels of staff between mental health, corrections, medical, and outside service providers.

As early as 1975, Oswego County mental health provided services to the correctional facility via 24-hour, seven-day-a-week walk-in and telephone crisis services. Corrections officers would transport inmates to the mental health facility. However, timely identification and referral for services for high-risk inmates was still the first step in accessing mental health services. Given the sheer number of inmates, the 24-hour admission process, and most admissions in the high-risk period for suicide (within 3 to 24 hours after intake), improvement in early identification and care of suicidal and seriously mentally ill offenders was needed. Two suicides occurred in the Oswego County Jail in 1978. No others have occurred since. Suicide attempts were at an all-time high when the New York State Office of Mental Health Bureau of Forensics offered grant funding for a pilot program to address suicide prevention and crisis intervention. Oswego was chosen to be one of five counties to pilot the program. Grant funding for the pilot project was $25,000.

GEOGRAPHIC AREA

Oswego County is a mid-sized New York State county (121,000 persons) bordered by Lake Ontario to the north and the city of Syracuse, New York to the south. It is somewhat isolated in nature by its geographical features (40 miles from Syracuse) and inclement weather (240 inches per year average snowfall). It is comprised of two small (under 25,000 persons) cities located on the Oswego River with the remainder of the area being rural.

TARGET POPULATION

Inmates targeted for services are age 16 and older, male and female, who have serious mental illness and are at risk of suicide. Total inmates incarcerated per year are 1,500 with 200 typically served by mental health jail services annually.

NATURE OF SERVICES

Mental health staffing and services to the jail population and the correctional staff have increased over the years.

Before the grant, the mental health staffing for the county jail came from the existing clinic staff and was very crisis-oriented. The pilot program provided justification to hire staff (.5 FTE social worker). Supervision and administration still came from existing county staff. The facility at the time was a turn-of-the-century, three-story brick jail. There were no interview or group rooms. The cafeteria was not used; inmates ate in the small space outside their cells unless they were in lock-down. Medical services were provided part-time by county public health nurses and hourly coverage by a physician.

A four-part strategy was employed to achieve the above stated programs goals:

1. Develop integrated policies and procedures for mental health and the county jail.
2. Train corrections officers and any other staff persons in the jail in suicide prevention and crisis intervention.
3. Screen inmates for high risk of suicide and or serious mental illness at intake 24 hours a day using correction officers.
4. Implement the program and revise as needed.

The first step was to develop policies and procedures. These were developed according to corrections and mental hygiene law between corrections and mental health which also included jail health services. Procedures included: protocols for the use of screening guidelines; emergency and non-emergency mental health referrals; ongoing services and monitoring; dispute resolution; and revision of the coordination efforts. It was necessary to first complete policies and procedures. Such completion informs officers about ways to identify at-risk inmates and levels of supervision for them, and indicates the respective agencies' support for the program. Subsequent review and revision of procedures is built into the policies and procedures. It includes data and system issues analysis. This is accomplished by meetings with the corrections, jail health, and mental health administrations which include line staff, as well as forensic planning council quarterly meetings. All procedures follow standardization from the state agencies and are responsive to unique county needs.

A local forensic planning council was initiated to develop the policies and procedures and oversee the implementation of the project. The county attorney addressed issues such as legal liability during incarceration and post-discharge, confidentiality, and implications of Miranda warnings. The lead agency for the project was, and continues to be, Oswego County Mental Health.

   Trainings were provided for all levels of staff involved in the program.
A one-hour orientation for administrators from corrections, police, mental health, and jail services (jail chaplin, etc.) as well as a specialized
overview for emergency rooms was conducted. Correction officers (40),
jail medical (4), and mental health personnel (15) were trained by a corrections and mental health training team certified by the Office of Mental
Health and Commission of Corrections in the use of the suicide prevention crisis intervention curriculum developed by both state agencies. Police
(18) were also trained at this time in the same curriculum for their lockups. The training modules included suicide myths and misconceptions:
suicide why, when and how; substance abuse and suicide; mental illness
and suicide; screening guidelines; suicide during incarceration; communication skills; and local policies and procedures. The trainers have an
opportunity during the eight-hour training to interact with the corrections officers and supervisors to engage them in open discussion. This
enables them to identify what interventions will be needed to produce
attitude changes about mental illness, suicide, and mental health service.
Initial training with officers are met most often with resistance. Administrative support is one crucial condition for attitude change as to officers' understanding of the reduction in liability the program can offer
them individually. Comments and body language during the training can
help the trainer assess the needed interventions for attitude change. Some
discussion or further clarification with individuals or groups may occur at
break times during the training sessions. The discussions themselves may
be all the intervention needed for certain individuals, while more long-
term interventions requiring structures for communication (bi-monthly
meetings at the jail with administration and line staff) may be required
for other officers. It is critical to engage line supervisors who are highly
influential with staff. Because resistance may be viewed as the manly
response, it is important to show the officers and supervisors how this program will make their work lives easier. Mental health workers may resist
the program by wanting to retain their mental health mystique. However,
clear communication, which helps earn credibility with corrections officers, will ensure the success of the program. After the initial training program, OMH certified curriculum refresher training is provided for
corrections officers. Once the program is fully implemented and accepted,
subsequent training becomes an expected and accepted part of the normal functioning of the jail. Information on the local program operation
is also incorporated into the training. Critical incident stress debriefing
for all staff involved following an inmate suicide, as well as on an ongoing basis, is also recognized as an important component of the training.
   Operationalizing the program was the next implementation step.
Screening of inmates is done upon booking, initially conducted via paper

copies which have now been replaced by computer. Screenings are prioritized and are accessed electronically by the mental health staff who also consult the hard copy correctional case record and referral source and any other pertinent sources of information. It is imperative that all persons involved with the inmate's care communicate so that a complete, real-time total picture of the inmate's situation is available to staff working with him or her. A partial view of the inmate's condition emerging from separate, non-communicating parties can easily lead to a suicide attempt that could have been prevented. The mental health record is only available by hard record in the correctional facility and at the mental health services. The mental health professional works closely with the correctional officers for initial and ongoing referrals. The jail health staff is also a secondary source of referrals. Families may also be referral sources.

Linkages to community resources was given priority in the implementation. The link between case management and community services is crucial. Release planning is very difficult in a jail setting because the inmate may be released at the court hearing with no advance warning. Therefore, early identification of case managed persons or early referrals to case management reduce recidivism in the jail. Within the jail, the mental health professional is engaged in a variety of activities working with the inmate and persons involved with his or her case. The mental health professional evaluates inmates initially and on an ongoing basis for suicide risk and mental health problems. Based on that evaluation, an inmate may be referred for further evaluation by a psychiatrist from the mental health clinic (ex. medications), case management (which will link to other services outside the facility), education services, and groups which are provided within the jail facility (AA, etc). Further, because of the pre-sentence low average length of stay, group work is reviewed on a regular basis to determine need.

Over time, mental health staffing for services was modified due to changes in the physical structure of the jail and the cooperative approach of the mental health and law enforcement systems. The mental health professional staffing was originally a .5 FTE social worker supervised by the Director of Community Services. The position within two years was changed to a full-time social work position because of the increase in referrals from corrections officers and medical staff to mental health services.

Three years later, the need for mental health professional time in the jail diminished due to two significant factors. First, the police mental health project had been in operation for several years. Incarceration of severely mentally ill persons was reduced by diversion of detainees by police for mental health evaluation versus previous practice of admission to the jail. Mental health evaluations were done primarily during typical crisis hours (i.e., evenings and weekends) at the emergency room. A police/mental health agreement was developed to guide the working relationships of police and mental health with policies and procedures. Secondly, the physical plant of the jail was changed. The planning process included input of all persons who worked in the jail. The resultant physical plant now has a mental health /health suite of rooms, multi-purpose group rooms, recreation area, and pod housing with officers in the pods. With the new facility also came new programs in recreation and education. The new method of supervision of inmates changed corrections officers roles and increased communications between officers and inmates. The new reward system for good behavior was more effective in changing most inmates' behavior. Further, the change in name from Oswego County Jail to Oswego County Correctional Facility indicated a greater degree of professionalism. The total facility also houses the courts, the DA's office, and the probation and sheriff's department. Mental health staffing was reduced to a .5 FTE psychologist based on review of the program and staff recruitment efforts. The current psychologist's duties entail implementation of suicide prevention, crisis intervention program, ongoing mental health individual and group services, informal evaluations for the courts, policy and procedure review, training of corrections officers and mental health professionals, service and system reporting, and release planning. Increased staffing for release planning for those individuals who have no mental health case manager is an emerging need.

RESULTS

Inmates are screened (at booking) and referred for service in a timely manner. Forensic admissions went from multiple admissions with high cost (one inmate $19,000 in 1984) to no admissions in 1999. Suicide attempts have decreased with no attempts in 1999. Liability to the county has consequently been reduced. The corrections, medical, and mental health staff are better trained to identify and intervene with inmates. Communication between all services and staff was listed as the greatest improvement. Collection and analysis of the mental health program data has aided in revision of the program. Other events have shaped the mental health services in the correctional facility: the police mental health program diverts inmates from the facility and the redesign of the physical plant provided a more professional, humane facility atmosphere.

CONCLUSION

After the initial three years, the Oswego County Suicide Prevention/Crisis intervention program has become enculturated into the correctional facility program. The program is fully operational. New corrections officers enter employment at the Oswego County Correctional Facility with the understanding that the program is part of their duties. The means and structures necessary for staff to address evolving needs (individual meetings, forensic service council, etc.) are in place.

Improvements to the program are handled as routine business, not as crises. Further, the working relationships developed through the grant funding processes laid the groundwork for taking full advantage of the planning and implementation of the facility physical plant and the police mental health initiative, which both made a great impact on the delivery of service to inmates. Finally, the leadership and standardized products produced by the Office of Mental Health and Commission of Corrections provided leverage to convince Oswego County that this project was timely, cost-effective, and could be flexible to fit Oswego County's needs.

SECTION II
Community-Based Diversion Programs

1. Police/Mental Health Linked Programs

3

Overview:
The Law Enforcement Response
to Social Problems:
Mental Health As a Case in Point

George T. Patterson

Extensive literature shows that as much as 80% of functions performed by law enforcement agencies consist of handling social problems (Trojanowicz and Dixon, 1974; Scott, 1981, Morris and Heal, 1981, Mastrofski, 1983) such as alcohol and substance use and abuse; medical emergencies; mental illness; runaways; family disputes; landlord-tenant disputes and neighbor conflicts; teenage pregnancy; missing persons; and juvenile delinquency. Although this list is not exhaustive, it is characteristic of the range of social problems that police officers are required to handle. Despite improved training for new recruits in many police academies throughout the country and improved in-service training for experienced police officers, many police officers report feeling poorly equipped to address these social problems. This occurs for a variety of reasons. First, police officers may be unfamiliar with the underlying dynamics of social problems and the treatment and resources required to address them. Second, police officers may experience conflict performing their role as law enforcer and resolving social problems using human service agencies for assistance. Third, handling social problems may not be the priority of the law enforcement agency, or these functions may not be significant for the police officer who may feel that, in order to advance within the department, crime-fighting skills, arrest, and citizen complaint history are more important than resolving social problems. Finally, police officers may not have sufficient time to handle social problems since other emergency police calls and needs may arise.

In an effort to manage these social problems and overcome some of these difficulties, models for collaboration and partnership have formed between law enforcement agencies and human service agencies. Numerous examples are found in the literature focusing on social problems such as domestic violence (Holmes, 1982), child abuse (Marans & Berkman, 1997), and youth services (Briar, Hagens, Payne & Hagoski, 1983; Michaels & Treger, 1973; Walinets, 1985). A variety of models exist throughout the country with regards to the staffing of these collaborations and partnerships. Some models employ specially trained, sworn police officers who respond to social problems. Other models use a team approach employing police officers and civilian social workers or mental health professionals who jointly respond to police calls and resolve social problems. Another type of model employs only civilian social workers or mental health professionals who respond to the scene of police calls and provide technical assistance to the police and help citizens in need.

More than 25 years ago, Treger (1975) recognized the value of law enforcement social work collaboration and identified several assumptions regarding these collaborations. First, social workers can assist police officers by diverting individuals away from the criminal justice system to appropriate mental health and other systems. Second, individuals can be immediately linked with service providers at the time of the crisis when the chances are better that they will accept such services. Third, providing social services at the time of contact with the police and having social workers with specialized training in social problems providing these services allows for quicker assessment, early intervention, and treatment for individuals. Although numerous benefits for individuals and law enforcement agencies arising from collaborations have been identified, numerous barriers to effective collaboration also occur which may strain the effectiveness of these collaborations. Thomas (1994) observed that police officers and social workers are often hostile toward each other's role. Police officers may stereotype social workers as naive, accusing them of covering up crimes and labeling them as liberal "do-gooders." Indeed these collaborations can present challenges (Stephens, 1988).

Two of the chapters in this section (5 & 6) illustrate the law enforcement response to the social problem of mental illness. The authors consider the benefits and barriers of collaborations presented above and provide models for collaboration that effectively serve the law enforcement agency and individuals experiencing mental illness and their families. Dupont and Cochran describe a model of law enforcement response to mental illness that employs specially trained police officers who assist the mentally ill through referrals and other services. The Crisis Intervention Team Model (CIT) has been replicated by numerous law enforcement agencies, others are presently developing it, and many more agencies have requested technical assistance regarding this model. The strengths of this model include the provision of an immediate response during the crisis situation, the use of patrol officers with special training, and linkage with a medical center that reduces the emergency room wait time for law enforcement referrals. The authors also emphasize the importance of selecting appropriate police officers to staff these models.

Whether the staff is comprised of police officers, civilians or a combination, the law enforcement response to mental illness requires that staff have knowledge of state mental hygiene laws, community resources, skills in crisis intervention, knowledge about mental illness, and the procedures of the law enforcement agency regarding mental illness. Vickie Burnett, Bennie Henderson, Susan Nolan, Cynthia Parham, Leslie Gregg Tucker, and Craig Young present the Community Service Officers (CSO) model for law enforcement response to mental illness. This model employs social workers responding to police calls and providing technical assistance to police officers and assistance to individuals experiencing mental illness. When civilians are employed within a law enforcement agency, many issues arise that cause concern for both law enforcement officials and civilian workers, such as the personal safety of unarmed civilian staff assisting on police calls. These authors address these issues as they present the guidelines for responding to police calls, the hours of operation for the unit, and social work functions and tasks.

REFERENCES

Briar, K.H., Hagens, N., Payne, T. & Hagoski, N. (1983). Child welfare services in a law enforcement agency. *Children Today*. Nov-Dec: 17–20.

Holmes, S.A. (1982). A Detroit model for police-social work co-operation. *Social Casework*. April, 220–226.

Marons, S. & Berkman, M. (1997). *Child-development-community policing: Partnership in a climate of violence*. Washington, DC: Office of Juvenile Justice and Delinquency Prevention, Office of Justice Programs, U. S. Department of Justice.

Mastrofski, S. (1983). The police and noncrime services. In *Evaluating performance of criminal justice agencies*. By (eds.) Gordon P. Whitaker and Charles David Phillips. Beverly Hills, CA: Sage Publications.

Michaels, R.A. & Treger, H. (1973). Social work in police departments. *Social Work*. 69:67–75.

Morris, P. & Heal, P. (1981). *Crime control and the police*. Home Office Research Study, no. 67.

Scott, E.J. (1981). *Calls for service: Citizen demand and initial police response*. Washington, DC: National Institute of Justice.

Stephens, M. (1988). Problems of police-social work interaction: Some American lessons. *The Howard Journal. 27:* 81–91.

Treger, H. (1975). The police-social work team. Springfield, Ill: Charles C. Thomas.

Trojanowicz, R. C. & Dixon, S.L. (1974). Criminal justice and the community. Englewood Cliffs, NJ: Prentice-Hall.

Walinets, S. (1985). You're on duty. *Social Work Today.* Sept: 14–15.

4

The Development and Implementation of a Police/Mental Health Training Program in a Large Urban Environment

Marjorie Rock

In 1984, an elderly, seriously mentally disturbed women was shot and killed by a New York City police officer in the midst of an eviction proceeding. This critical incident was the impetus for the development of several new initiatives by the New York City Department of Mental Health, Mental Retardation and Alcoholism Services, the New York City Police Department, and the Human Resources Administration. Senior staff of all three agencies responded to the crisis and began the process of reviewing procedures to develop a more coordinated response to incidents involving mentally disturbed individuals in the community. At the time of the incident, the author was the special assistant to the Senior Deputy Commissioner for Program Services of the New York City Department of Mental Health and was asked to work with the New York City Police Department to develop a police/mental health training program as one part of a response to the need. This chapter will describe the program that was developed in response to that critical incident and discuss its relevance for large jurisdictions.

BACKGROUND

Persons with severe mental illness have come into contact with the criminal justice system, including the police, with increasing frequency during the past 25 years. Contributing factors include deinstitutionalization, higher standards for involuntary admission to psychiatric treatment, increasing availability of substance use, a strong policy emphasis on punishment rather than rehabilitation, and other reasons (Rock, 2001; Lamb & Weinberger, 1998; Torrey, 1997; Steadman, Monahan & Dufee, 1984). Although police routinely manage the vast majority of calls for assistance with the mentally ill, there have been widely publicized incidents in which an officer has used deadly force with this population. When this occurs, the media, the public, and mental health professionals call attention to police failure in the management of persons with serious mental illness (Rock, 1990). Despite the criticism of the police by these groups, Hayes has noted that there has been a failure to provide the police with consistent guidelines for working with this population (Hayes, in Murphy, 1986). True to form, the media duly called attention to this critical incident in 1984. As a result of the seriousness of the incident and the desire to remedy the situation, the New York City Department of Mental Health, Mental Retardation and Alcoholism Services was asked by the mayor to work with the Emergency Services Unit of the New York City Police Department to develop a training program for the Emergency Service Unit officers.

PROGRAM DEVELOPMENT

Initial steps in the development of the program involved multiple meetings between the commissioner and the author and senior police department officials. At first it was believed that a "one shot" brief training at the Police Academy would be sufficient to teach officers how to respond to the mentally ill. However, police officials became convinced of the necessity of developing a more thoughtful program that would not only teach officers additional skills but also would promote a better understanding of the complexities of working with persons with serious mental illness and an understanding of the multi-layered mental health system in New York City. A significant part of this early process was a literature review by the author with respect to any training that might be conducted by other Departments of Mental Health with police officers. Concurrent with this author's investigation into the availability of model police-mental health training programs, there was a review of the use of deadly force by police with respect to this population in New York State (Condon, 1985). Among the conclusions in the Condon report were recommendations about the importance of mental health training for the police. In addition to the literature review, calls were made to major urban areas to inquire whether there were police/mental health training models that could be considered applicable to New York City. Concurrently, a member of the NYPD's Emergency Service Unit (ESU) was following up with large urban police departments in order to determine whether there were any models of police/mental health training and collaboration.

During this time period, the Police Executive Research Forum was conducting a national study of police response to the mentally ill because of the increasing involvement of the police with mentally disturbed persons in the community (Murphy, 1986). There were two major models uncovered during this search that did appear to be interesting. However, both models of police/mental health collaboration (the Birmingham CSO Model and a model in rural Texas) were deemed to be inappropriate to New York City due to both the size of the police department and the complexities of the New York City mental health system. While it is beyond the scope of this chapter to fully describe the mental health system in New York City, there are five state-operated inpatient psychiatric facilities for intermediate and longer term care; 11 municipal hospitals for acute care and emergency psychiatric evaluations, several voluntary hospitals providing acute psychiatric beds with emergency evaluation capacity, several hundred outpatient mental health programs ranging from mental health clinics through psycho-social programs, continuing day treatment programs, and so on. In addition, there are case management programs and mobile crisis teams as well as residential programs. All programs are licensed by the State Office of Mental Health, although most of the voluntary providers are also under contract to the New York City Department of Mental Health. Thus, funding and oversight responsibilities are often shared between the city and the state.

As it became clear that New York City needed to develop a program specifically geared to this urban area and to the systems that operated within this context, it also became clear that there could potentially be formidable barriers to the development of such a program. First, the question was: Who should be trained? The answer was clear. It was determined by the police department that, at least initially, the training should be targeted to members of the Emergency Services Unit. This unit is an elite rescue unit serving multiple purposes. However, it is also the unit which is called on by the police to respond to emotionally disturbed persons (EDPs in police language) in the community. It was the Emergency Service Unit that had been involved in the fatal shooting. At the time of this incident, the unit was comprised of 350 officers who met stringent requirements in order to join. These requirements included serving on the NYPD for at least five years, meeting a variety of mechanical and technical skills, undergoing psychological testing, and passing difficult requirements in rescue work including scuba and other such skills.

It was also decided that the Hostage Negotiation Team's (HNT) commanding officer should become involved in the development of the training as well. This unit is comprised of detectives who have volunteered for additional training and who are called in cases of hostage–taking. The Hostage Negotiation Team frequently works with the Emergency Services

Unit, so it was felt that input from the unit's commanding officer would be important.

The next question was: How can we best make this training relevant to the experiences of the members of the ESU? Several issues had become apparent during the initial exploratory period. These issues included the recognition that officers might be somewhat resistant to training in this area. Resistance by police officers to working with the mentally ill and being trained by mental health professionals is not unique to New York City. It is but a clear example of resistance by one group of professionals to the perception that they are being told "how to do their job" by another group of professionals. Literature about police activities with respect to the mentally ill consistently indicates that the police feel "it was not a proper task" to work with this population (Bittner, 1967) but that they had to because "no one else would do it" (Rock, 1990). In fact, as noted by Teplin, the police are the "street corner psychiatrists" and must respond: they cannot refuse a call for assistance (Teplin, 1984).

Initially, members of the Department of Mental Health were invited to view the methods and equipment used by the ESU in its rescue work. This was important because it began to promote an understanding of the roles and dangers faced by the officers as they engaged in their daily activities. It was also realized early that the training itself would have more meaning to officers and more credibility if it was conducted by trainers with a background in both mental health and law enforcement. It was also felt that the training would have more credibility if it was provided by a recognized academic institution. Therefore, it was agreed that the curriculum would be developed and taught by faculty of John Jay College of Criminal Justice with involvement and oversight by both the NYPD and the Department of Mental Health. John Jay is a senior college in the City University of New York system and offers bachelor's, master's, and doctoral degrees in Criminal Justice and related fields. Many of the faculty have law enforcement backgrounds. The Department of Mental Health contracted with the college for these activities and a tri-partite alliance began to take shape.

THE CURRICULUM

After an extensive needs assessment that involved faculty of John Jay and this author riding with the ESU, as well as a survey given to all members of the unit, John Jay faculty developed an initial curriculum. The curriculum is divided into five major units which include: communications skills; assessment of antisocial behavior and violence, including legal rights of the mentally ill; identifying thinking disorders and mood disorders, including the identification of suicidal potential; issues related to alcohol and substance abuse; and management of people under stress. This last section on working with people in stressful situations included a segment on identifying and managing officer stress. This was considered a critical component of the curriculum as it shifted the focus to the officers' issues and allowed the officers to express their feelings about the stress of the job.

The course of training is one full week (38 hours) in the classroom. Classroom activities include lecture and discussion, readings, and exercises. In addition, a unique component of the curriculum included the development of unscripted scenarios based on actual experiences that officers face in working with the mentally ill. In the initial years of the training, professional actor-trainers worked with the officers on the scenarios in the classroom. Police were thus able to role play themselves, while the actor-trainer portrayed the "client." The scenarios were developed in conjunction with the lesson being taught for the day. The actor-trainers worked closely with the teaching faculty to ensure that points stressed in the didactic part of the lesson were covered in the scenario.

Prior to beginning the course, the curriculum was reviewed by staff of the Department of Mental Health and by the police department. The curriculum was taught to small groups of ESU officers (no more than 20 officers in a class) after an initial pilot to 57 new members of the unit. In order to provide the officers with support and recognition, John Jay College agreed that some college credit could be given to officers completing the course. Additionally, a certificate and a pin, designed by an ESU officer and designating officers completing the training as Emergency Psychological Technicians, were awarded to all who completed the curriculum. It can be noted that the initial exploratory and discussion phases with the police department and the curriculum development phase lasted for several months. This should not be considered unusual given the very large systems and the multiple parties that were involved in this process.

Because it was felt that small classes would be appropriate, it took more than one city fiscal year to complete the training of 350 officers. During the second city fiscal year, the funds from the Department of Mental Health were supplemented by funding from the New York City Police Department.

BARRIERS TO TRAINING

As noted previously, police often express resistance to being trained by mental health professionals to do the job they do. While most officers indicate that they want to be police officers in "order to serve," they often feel that fighting crime is what they should be doing. In reality, most police work involves social service–type activities. However, in working with the mentally ill, officers face daunting challenges and their perception is that the mental health system can only make their job more difficult. For example, officers would report that, in order to talk a "jumper" off a bridge, the officer might spend several hours persuading the individual to allow the officer to bring him safely off the bridge. However, when the officer would bring this individual to the psychiatric emergency room for evaluation, the psychiatric staff would release the individual because he did not meet standards for involuntary hospitalization. Additionally, officers are made to wait with the EDP for several hours prior to the evaluation. This takes the officer off the street, which is where he wants to be, and keeps him "cooling his heels" in the psychiatric and/or medical emergency room.

In order to lessen the resistance of the officers to the training, which was apparent in the early weeks of the program, it was decided that a liaison officer from the ESU and a member of the Department of Mental Health (usually the author) would be present for every new class section. Our roles were to ensure that the program had fidelity to the needs of the officers, that it was respectful of the officers, and that it provided information about the mental health system in New York City. This had unexpected and unintended consequences. One of the primary unexpected consequences was that the author gained a significant appreciation for the work of the unit which was important for future cooperation between the two agencies. On the other hand, officers were able to begin to view mental health professionals with more understanding. In addition, officers were allowed to vent their feelings about the problems faced in trying to work within the system. Thus, many of their beliefs were validated even as they were encouraged to use the system on behalf of the citizens of New York City who required their intervention. This exchange of ideas is an important part of any inter-disciplinary training and cannot be overstated. The development of understanding between two disciplines working together is the cornerstone upon which cooperation rests. Without these mutual activities, little can be accomplished.

FOLLOW-UP ACTIVITIES

At the end of the initial training, the police department decide to implement this curriculum for all new ESU officers and new members of the Hostage Negotiation Team. At the time (1986) there were three full police departments in New York City. In addition to the NYPD, the New York City Transit Police Department had primary responsibility for the public transportation system, and the New York City Housing Police Department had primary responsibility within the public housing units. (At this time, there is only the New York City Police Department which has incorporated the

The Development and Implementation of a Police/Mental Health Program   **57**

other two departments). Upon completion of the ESU program, the chief of the Transit Police approached the Department of Mental Health and asked that his officers in the equivalent Emergency Rescue Unit be given the opportunity to receive the training program. This was in recognition that these officers also encountered individuals with mental illness and worked closely with the NYPD. Therefore, it was felt that they should also receive the training. This was accomplished and the following year the chief of the New York City Housing Police Department requested that his officers receive the training program. These trainings were also conducted at John Jay College using the outline of the original curriculum but tailoring it to the needs of each of these departments. In addition, the New York State Office of Mental Health, which had initially provided the funding for the program and was developing a police training program for recruits statewide, incorporated much of the framework as well as some of the unique methods of the training program for police recruits at the state level. This was accomplished through a state-wide advisory committee which included representatives from police and mental health agencies across the state, including the author and several colleagues from the New York City Police Department's Emergency Service Unit.

DISCUSSION

Lessons learned from the development and implementation of this program are clear: personnel must feel involved in their own training—they cannot be subject to outsiders coming in to tell them "how to do their job." Even though there was involvement by all relevant "players" at the top levels, line officers also had to feel that their needs were being addressed. Systemic problems with mental health services were raised, such as long waiting times in emergency rooms for officers who were required to transport persons with mental illness for evaluation. These issues were "heard" by the Department of Mental Health, although no easy solutions were promised. One beneficial result of the training was that all involved in the initial development and subsequent institutionalization of the program learned how important it is to communicate with each other, to be open to understanding the differences in mission and goals of the systems, and to have respect for each other's functions. Clearly, the issue of police/mental health relationships is a continuing story. As long as there are persons with severe mental illness who, for all the reasons known, continue to need assistance in the community and continue to encounter the police as part of the breakdown of the treatment system, there will be a need to continuously work to improve relations between the police and the mental health provider system. The New York City police/mental health training program is certainly not the only model of working with police. The model developed in Memphis, Tennessee, known as the Crisis Intervention Team (CIT) represents another model of police/mental health training that has received much (and well-deserved) attention, as has the Birmingham CSO model discussed in this book. However, the New York City program works well for a large and very complex urban area with multiple layers of mental health services and with an extremely large police department. Each jurisdiction needs to carefully consider what works best in its own city, village and town. But police and mental health personnel will continue to interact, often in emergency and crisis situations. Therefore, it is vitally important for all to consider how best to achieve a productive working relationship.

REFERENCES

Condon, R. (1985). *Police Use of Deadly Force in New York State: Report to Governor Mario M. Cuomo.* New York: New York State Division of Criminal Justice Services.

Lamb, H.R. & Weinberger, L.E. (1998). Persons with severe mental illness in jails and prisons: A review. *Psychiatric Services, 49*(4)483–492.

Murphy, G.R. (1986). *Special Care: Improving the Police Response to the Mentally Disabled.* Washington, D.C.: Police Executive Research Forum.

Rock, M.(2001) Emerging issues with mentally ill offenders: Causes and social consequences. *Administration and Policy in Mental Health,* 28(3), 165–180.

Rock, M. (1990). *An Evaluation of Police Officers' Opinions and Knowledge About Mental Illness.* Unpublished Doctoral Dissertation. New York: Columbia University.

Steadman, H.J., Monahan, J. & Duffee, J. (1984). The impact of state mental hospital deinstitutionalization on United States prison populations, 1968–1978. *Journal of Criminal Law and Criminology, 75,* 474–490.

Teplin, L.A. (1984). *Mental Health and Criminal Justice.* Beverly Hills, CA: Sage Publications.

Torrey, E.F.(1997). *Out of the Shadows: Confronting America's Mental Illness Crisis.* New York: Wiley.

5

The Memphis CIT Model

Randolph T. Dupont and Charles S. Cochran

THE MEMPHIS CIT MODEL

The Crisis Intervention Team model of law enforcement response to mental health emergencies has been described as "policing for the 21st century" by a community policing expert (Police Chief Charles Moose, 1996) and recommended for duplication in "every city in America" by a leading mental health advocate (Torrey, 1996). It has been featured as a best practice model by the White House Conference on Mental Health (1999), the U.S. Department of Justice Bureau of Justice Assistance (Practitioner Perspectives, 2000), and the U.S. Department of Health and Human Services Substance Abuse and Mental Health Services Administration (SAMHSA News, 2000). It has been given special recognition by groups as diverse as the NAMI—National Alliance for the Mentally Ill (1996, 1997), National Association of People of Color Against Suicide (1999), American Association of Suicidology (1997), and Amnesty International USA (1999). This level of recognition has led sociologist Henry Steadman, PhD, a leading researcher in mental illness and co-occurring disorders to characterize the Memphis CIT model as the "most visible pre-booking jail diversion program in the U.S." (Steadman, Deane, Borum & Morrissey, 2000).

This model links law enforcement and mental health systems in a manner that is widespread and diverse. Its purpose is to maintain the safety of both the officer and the consumer while providing a path to emergency mental health care. It is targeted at the severely and persistently mentally ill individual who is in crisis, but intervenes with a variety of behavioral events including suicide, addiction, and developmentally-related behavioral events. It focuses on jail diversion when the charges are minor in nature and do not involve the victimization of others. The nature of the CIT design provides for an operational change in policing methods that leads to police accountability during a mental illness-related crisis. This same change brings about efficiency in the system resulting in similar accountability for the mental health system. This partnership has significant implications for social workers and other mental health professionals in challenging the manner in which they partner with law enforcement around issues of care and treatment of those with mental illness.

This CIT program also partners with consumers and family members to form a third and critical element to the model. This partnership includes all phases of the model including planning, curriculum development, training, maintenance, and systematic feedback. This three-way partnership and the interdependency it has created are perhaps the critical factors in its success and increasing acceptance on the national level. At present, the Memphis CIT program has been replicated in seven cities nationwide (Portland, OR; Albuquerque, NM; Seattle, WA; San Jose, CA; Houston, TX; Logan, UT, Waterloo, IA), is about to be implemented in six more cities (Roanoke, VA; Lee's Summit, MO; Akron, OH; Orlando, FL; Kansas City, MO; Montgomery County, MD), and is in development in four other cities (Toledo, OH; Fort Wayne, IN; Salt Lake City, UT; Minneapolis, MN). The interest in the program is intense, with over 150 municipalities requesting technical assistance in the past year. As more areas of the country attempt to implement a CIT program, it is important to understand the model from both a program content and system development perspective.

BACKGROUND

While the CIT program became operational in May, 1988, its roots are more accurately traced back to advocacy efforts from NAMI (National Alliance for the Mentally Ill) of Memphis. After experiencing difficulties with police response during crisis events, this group began a program aimed at changing the way police interacted with individuals with mental illness. Their initial efforts were met with politeness but minimal response from community leadership. This all changed when a crisis event in 1987 ended in a citizen's death. The citizen had a history of mental illness and substance abuse and was fatally shot while holding a knife. This crisis event was highlighted by considerations involving cultural diversity as the police officers involved were Caucasian and the citizen was an African-American male. The community response was one of outrage, thrusting the city into a political crisis. The mayor turned to NAMI and formed a task force that began the partnership of advocates, police officials, and mental health professionals. The task force was charged with investigating police mental health training as well as law enforcement and mental health crisis intervention programs.

The task force learned that the Memphis Police Department had an academy-based training program with course hours exceeding the national average for that time. Existing crisis intervention programs involved mental health professionals providing the crisis response, whether based in law enforcement (Community Service Officers) or in the mental health system (Mobile Crisis Teams). However, none of the existing models provided for an immediacy of response during the crisis event. As a result, the community task force began to develop a new concept of law enforcement-based crisis intervention which emerged as specialized expertise within the patrol division, allowing for a crisis intervention response in real time.

OPERATIONAL COMPONENTS

Law Enforcement

The officers in the program were designated Crisis Intervention Team officers (i.e., CITS). While they are part of a broader team of experts operating within the geographic boundaries of the police department, they act individually to provide leadership within the patrol division. The CIT officer answers traditional police calls but is designated the leader if a 911 dispatch protocol or a fellow officer identifies elements of the call suggesting a behavioral crisis. Hence, immediacy, expertise, and responsibility come together in one system. The use of patrol officers makes the program cost-effective by eliminating down time between crisis events. It also has the additional benefit of maintaining the officers' identity as "real" police officers within the patrol division. Despite the impressive accomplishments of the social work profession, police resist any label that implies they are social workers or mental health specialists. A second additional benefit is that the model eliminates the potential for isolation from the community that goes with membership in specialized police units such as organized crime and anti-gang units (Dupont & Cochran, 2000a). Such specialized units have come under increasing criticism due to high-profile events in major metropolitan police forces such as New York and Los Angeles.

Mental Health

This system would not succeed without the partnership of a willing mental health receiving facility. Barriers to care, such as excessive wait times, would likely result in criminal arrest charges instead of a health care referral. Officers are given a minimal turnaround time of 15 to 20 minutes at the Regional Medical Center (The MED). The multi-disciplinary staff at the University of Tennessee Psychiatric Emergency Service accept all referrals, regardless of clinical presentation. While there is a high concordance rate between the professional judgement and the officer referrals, the presentation often results in a variety of diagnostic entities, including those requiring traditional medical care, substance abuse and addiction treatment, developmental disabilities interventions, nursing home referrals, social services assistance, legal considerations, and the like. It is simply unfair to expect police services to sort out these complexities on the street. The CIT system requires the health care system to accept responsibility for the patient and to provide a facility capable of triaging this heterogeneous population. Given the complexity of the professional decision-making and the need to avoid patient "dumping," a single source of entry is optimal for the CIT system.

While other CIT programs like Albuquerque's use a university hospital emergency service similar to the Memphis program, Portland, Seattle, and Akron have used a social service-based crisis center in combination with support from hospital-based emergency care and substance abuse treatment services. The Lee's Summit and Kansas City teams will make use of a state psychiatric hospital emergency intake unit working with a nearby general medical hospital. The CIT system requires the ability to handle a diagnostically heterogeneous population. It also requires a willingness to make decisions around risk for violence and involuntary commitment procedures. The challenge is to provide this type of clinical care in an environment that recognizes the need for treatment continuity and makes the greatest degree of choice available to consumers by using community-based care, case management, and supportive social services. The CIT model does not allow the mental health profession the luxury of programmatic distinctions between medical, psychological, addiction, and social services-based systems. It requires a high level of service integration and professional cooperation in order to accommodate the needs of the police, consumer, and family members.

SELECTION AND TRAINING

The CIT program places an emphasis on experienced officers volunteering for this team. As a result, a great deal of self-selection occurs. Reasons for volunteering can include personal experience with those affected by mental illness, recognition of the limits of traditional policing methods, and a desire for recognition of already existing crisis skills. Psychological testing is minimized since extensive psychological assessment is required of all recruits prior to basic training. Instead, the use of an extensive interviewing process, supervisory evaluations, and the officer's history of citizens' complaints or positive feedback play a key role in the selection process. This is the reason the CIT model is not for all officers and not focused on basic academy training. Officers differ in their interaction skills and ability to de-escalate a situation.

Curriculum

The CIT training program emphasizes experiential-based learning. This is based on a 40-hour course with three phases. These phases are structured learning, consumer and family interactions, and intensive scenario workshops. The lectures and workshops emphasize visual and learning materials and cover a wide range of diagnostic issues, psychopharmacology, mental health legal issues, substance abuse, developmental disabilities, co-occurring disorders, community resources, and diversity issues. The interaction phase is a main feature of the training and involves both formal and informal courses with consumers and family members. Much of this is structured in a small group or one to one format. This part comes early in the training and provides much of the motivation for attitude change resulting in new learning on the part of the officers. Although it was not designed as such, these interactions result in an impressive degree of empathy on the part of the officers. Officers come to recognize not only the struggle faced by those with mental illness but also the humanity of these same individuals. It quickly changes from an "us and them" attitude to what one CIT officer described as a realization that "they are just like us."

The next phase of the training involves high intensity role-playing based on scenarios developed from the officers' experiences during previous crisis events. An attempt is made to simulate the intensity of dealing with a mental illness related crisis by having officers interacting in front of the entire class while being critiqued by senior CIT officers and mental health crisis intervention experts. Police training tends to focus on the outcome of an event (i.e., the use of force justified by a citizen's most recent behavior). CIT training broadens that focus, emphasizing the process leading up to that last behavior. This allows the officers to learn that they can impact on the final outcome of a crisis interaction through their own de-escalation skills. These scenarios are designed to illustrate the phases of crisis escalation and to emphasize productive verbal and non-verbal interventions. These skills are then integrated with police training in scene control and officer safety.

PARTNERSHIP

The partnerships inherent in the CIT model occur not only in the development and instructional phase of the program but also throughout the operation phase. The formal agreements that follow the initial task force gave way to joint curriculum planning and development. Operations-level staff established a communication network and a feedback loop that involved all partners. In Memphis this was accomplished on both a formal and informal level. Leaders of all partnership groups met on a regular basis for feedback sessions. This networking extended to monthly meetings between officers, family members, and consumers. These meetings were often organized around continuing education topics. These meetings also provided an opportunity for an essential component of partnership, that of appreciation. Family members and consumers gave testimonials to successful crisis experiences and recognized a CIT officer of the month at each meeting. NAMI-Memphis gave scholarships to their workshops to CIT officers. This not only encouraged formal knowledge but also reinforced the interactions between consumers, family members, and officers that were originally established during CIT training. Mental health professionals establish regular ride-along sessions with CIT officers. The interweaving between formal and informal structures provides CIT with meaningful partnerships and a sense of ownership for all involved.

EVALUATION

There are three major evaluation efforts focusing on the Memphis CIT program. The first is evaluation work through the University of Tennessee. The second involves research from Policy Research Associates funded through a National Institute of Justice grant. The third is a part of a national jail diversion project funded by the Substance Abuse and Mental Health Services Administration (SAMHSA). The first two projects have yielded results that are very encouraging (see Dupont & Cochran, 2000a). The third is ongoing and focuses on both the CIT model and law enforcement and jail-based intervention programs (see Steadman et al., 1999).

A series of articles and presentations (Deane, Steadman, Borum & Morrisey, 1997; Borum, Deane, Steadman & Morrisey, 1998; Steadman et al., 2000) indicate that the CIT program appears to have a positive impact on officers' perceptions related to crisis interventions with the mentally ill and that it well may increase officer confidence in their crisis-related skills. This same study indicated that the program met its goal of expediency with a response time of just over five minutes, much better than that found for other police-based models. CIT officers make a minimal use of arrest as a disposition (2%) when compared with other crisis programs as well as when compared with estimates of the national average (20%) for this type of officer-citizen interaction. The University of Tennessee research group (Dupont & Cochran, 1998; Dupont, Cochran & Bush,1999; Dupont & Cochran, 2000b) has found that the Memphis Police Department is more involved with mental illness crisis events than it was prior to the CIT program. It was also noted that the department is making greater use of health care referrals as a diversion option. Officer injuries have decreased since the start of the program and are now no longer significantly different from general patrol division calls. Finally, the need for TACT (Tactics Apprehension and Containment Team) and hostage negotiations has also decreased since the start of the team. The Memphis TACT program is similar to the SWAT program in other cities (Special Weapons and Tactics). This result has also been reported from other CIT cities as well.

These results are impressive, especially when one considers that this is one of the lowest cost intervention programs available. While the results from the SAMHSA project cost analysis study is in progress, previous estimates of costs per call are less than $10. The marginal costs of the Memphis program run approximately $70,000 and includes over 180 trained officers. It is true that the program could not have been accomplished with the volunteer time from the mental health and advocacy partners in this coalition. Estimates have put those in-kind donated services at between $70,000 and $90,000 per year. While the City of Memphis funded the initial program from its own budget, funding through the Department of Justice Bureau of Justice Assistance and the Health and Human Services SAMHSA has become increasingly available in recent years.

BARRIERS: CIT IMPLEMENTATION

Mental Health

While the CIT program relies on consensus building and a sense of ownership, mental health programs tend to be extremely heterogeneous and can lack systematic planning. Communities that develop the CIT program most quickly (Portland, Seattle, Akron, Toledo) have centralized planning authorities for mental health and substance abuse. However, strong leadership and cooperative efforts appear to be able to overcome these problems (Memphis, Lee's Summit, Kansas City, Albuquerque, Waterloo).

Since the CIT system is efficient at identifying those in crisis, it results in an immediate increase in mental health emergency referrals. In an era of minimal community mental health funding, administrators often resist providing the single source of entry needed. This resistance is increased when faced with the "privatization" of community mental health care. Privatization reinforces the need for cost savings within an agency and provides a disincentive for the costly care needed for severely mentally ill individuals. It also emphasizes services to those with better third party payment plans, a group with high levels of functioning. Programs often resist the inclusion of individuals with the concomitant problems of poor dress, hygiene, and appearance for fear of alienating the better paying and more middle class clientele. This economic prejudice is part of the barrier to care for the severely mentally ill individual.

Clinicians are often reluctant to participate in the high-risk decision making process necessary to properly treat these individuals. Professionals can be fearful of liability when faced with issues around assessing risk for violence, duty to warn third parties, and involuntary commitment. Unfortunately, such front line clinical positions often come with the least financial compensation. When taken together these trends can make for a mental health system that puts up barriers to care and fails to take full responsibility for the individual in crisis.

Police

Police systems tend to function through tradition handed down by generations of police work. Unfortunately, CIT can present challenges wedded to those traditions (Dupont & Cochran, 2000a). Police systems tend to rely on training to solve most problems instead of pairing training with operational changes in police work. Some training methods promote fear of the mentally ill individual as a by-product of the intent to raise awareness of officer safety procedures. Yet, this method can lead officers to rely on more lethal methods of intervention (Fyfe, 2000). Finally, departments resist specialization and hold to the notion that all officers can be equally skilled at all aspects of police work. This ignores legitimate individual differences in such areas as age, experience, and cultural diversity. In contrast, CIT attempts to link training with operational changes in the law enforcement and mental health systems. It focuses on reducing injury through de-escalation skills and relies on specialized expertise within the patrol division to deliver services to those in crisis.

IMPLICATIONS FOR MENTAL HEALTH PROFESSIONALS

The barriers to the implementation of the CIT program suggest the need for mental health professionals to re-conceptualize themselves as partners with law enforcement, consumers, and family members. This will require a paradigm shift on the part of mental health professionals. Mental health professionals tend to view themselves as a guardian of patient rights and welfare, often viewing the police as a "threat" to consumer safety and as an unwelcome "stepchild" in community care. This tension between police and mental health professionals may have been necessary thirty years ago, but it ignores the major changes community policing programs have brought to law enforcement. In the last 30 years the system has turned upside down and now police have become the one who are seeking alternatives to jails (Teplin, 1986). Yet they often find mental health professionals playing the role of "gatekeepers" and denying access to care. Mental health systems need a framework for making community policing a part of the solutions for individuals in crisis. Social work models that emphasize case management services have the potential for bridging some of this gap, given their active involvement in the community. However, they would need to partner with law enforcement in a way in which consumers would view this partnership as increasing their choices rather than furthering the fear that case management approaches are authoritarian or intrusive in nature.

Police are willing to partner and learn from mental health professionals if such professionals take the time to understand and learn from the police culture. Community ride-along programs with law enforcement could become a required part of mental health graduate school training. An understanding of the job faced by police on the street is part of the "police friendly" attitude law enforcement officers look for from their partners. Practicum participation in police training could also be part of the curriculum. Police tend to learn from visual presentation methods (videotape) rather than the lecture format more common to graduate school. The lecture method tends to lend itself to a view that police need to be "educated" about mental health rather than leaving them feeling empowered to use their existing skills. Graduate and professional schools could emphasize continued work in delineating the crisis process. Many clinicians are excellent at using crisis de-escalation skills but lack the ability to teach them to others

Greater involvement of law enforcement in the treatment planning process might well present some challenges, but it should also improve communication between the police and treatment providers. It is very confusing for police officers to hear from mental health professionals that they should arrest the consumer in order for that person to "face the consequences of their action," whereas other professionals encourage the officers toward jail diversion. It is the opinion of the authors that the belief that jail can make a positive change on behavior patterns likely suggests the mental health professional is overworked. These issues can often be solved more effectively by adequate mental health resources and enlightened crisis care.

Mental health professionals have a significant role available as change agents in developing crisis intervention programs. These programs cross many professional boundaries and require leadership from individuals with a broad systems perspective on change (Cochran & Dupont, 2000). Yet many times it is not the mental health professionals but the advocates and law enforcement officers who are providing leadership. Social workers and other mental health professionals have the conceptual framework and clinical skills necessary to become leaders in this field. They have a history of addressing the issues required for crisis intervention models. These issues include the need for community consensus, appreciation for the diversity of those involved, identification of barriers to change, and the development of coherent service delivery systems. If mental health professionals are willing to address these issues, the mental health profession as a whole may be able to make the necessary paradigm shift required to become a true partner in linking with the police.

REFERENCES

Amnesty International (1999). *United States of America: Race, Rights and Police Brutality. Amnesty International Reports AMR51/147/99*, New York.

Borum, R., Deane, M., Steadman, H. & Morrisey, J. (1998). Police perspectives on responding to mentally ill people in crisis: perceptions of program effectiveness. *Behavioral Sciences and the Law 16*, 393–405.

Cochran, S. & Dupont, R. (2000). *Implementing a Crisis Intervention Team Program.* Paper presented at the meeting of Oklahoma State Legislature, Special Session of the Mental Health and Judiciary Committees, Oklahoma City, Oklahoma.

Deane, M., Steadman, H., Borum, R. & Morrisey, J. (1997). *Effective mental health partnerships within community policing initiatives.* Paper presented at the 126th Annual Meeting of the American Public Health Association, Washington, D.C.

Dupont, R. & Cochran, S. (1998). *Results of the Crisis Intervention Team model of jail diversion.* Paper presented at the New York University Annual Forensics Conference, New York.

Dupont, R. & Cochran, S. (2000a). Police Response to Mental Health Emergencies–Barriers to Change. *Journal of the American Academy of Psychiatry and the Law, 28*, 338–344.

Dupont, R. & Cochran, S. (2000b). *A programmatic approach to use of force issues in mental illness events.* Paper presented at the U.S. Department of Justice Conference on Law Enforcement Use of Force, Washington D.C.

Dupont, R., Cochran S. & Bush, A. (1999). *Reducing criminalization among individuals with mental illness.* Paper presented at the U.S. Department of Justice and U.S. Health and Human Services SAMHSA Conference on Forensics and Mental Illness, Washington D.C.

Fyfe, J.J. (2000). Policing the emotionally disturbed. *Journal of the American Academy of Psychiatry and the Law, 28*, 345–347.

Moose, C.A. (1996). Presented at the Portland Police Services Crisis Intervention Training, Portland, OR.

Practitioner Focus (2000). *Memphis, TN, Police Department's Crisis Intervention Team.* U.S. Department of Justice: Bureau of Justice Assistance.

SAMHSA News (2000). *Jail Diversion Programs Enhance Care.* U.S. Department of Health and Human Services: Substance Abuse and Mental Health Services Administration.

Steadman, H., Deane, M., Morrisey, J., Westcott, M., Salasin, S. & Shapiro, S. (1999). A SAMHSA research initiative assessing the effectiveness of jail diversion programs for mentally ill persons. *Psychiatric Services, 50,* 1620–1623.

Steadman, H., Deane, M., Borum, R. & Morrissey, J. (2000). Comparing outcomes of major models of police responses to mental health emergencies. *Psychiatric Services, 51,* 645–649.

Teplin, L. (1986). *Keeping the peace: The Parameters of Police Discretion in Relation to the Mentally Disordered.* National Institute of Justice Report. Washington, D.C.: U.S. Department of Justice.

Torrey, E.F. (1996). Presented at the meeting of the National Alliance for the Mentally Ill, Nashville, TN.

White House Conference on Mental Health (1999). *Working for a Healthier America.* Washington, D.C.

6

The Birmingham Police Department Community Service Officer Unit

Vickie B. Burnett, Bennie C. Henderson,

Susan D. Nolan, Cynthia M. Parham,

Leslie Gregg Tucker, and Craig Young

MISSION STATEMENT

Community Service Officers (CSOs) are the social service component of the Birmingham Police Department, thereby linking the department and the community. As support personnel, CSOs extend beyond the law enforcement realm by providing crisis intervention services to individuals and families who experience psychiatric disorders, substance abuse, domestic violence, and other social disruptions.

Our objective is to stabilize a crisis, attempt to prevent future crises, and enhance our client's well-being. The CSOs network and maintain professional relationships with community resources and strive to provide exemplary crisis intervention services.

HISTORY OF THE PROGRAM

Today's program grew out of a series of collaborative experiments at a time when the Birmingham Police Department was receiving a substantial number of calls involving persons with mental illness. Thus, a pilot program for master's level social work students at the University of Alabama began in 1976. These initial graduate students were assigned to the Birmingham Police Department's East Precinct for one semester. They accompanied police officers and assisted them with calls of a psycho-social nature. The next year, students were assigned to three additional precincts.

The need for the assistance of social workers was related to a number of legal and policy oriented decisions which affected the mentally ill and the community as we can see from the following history.

In 1975, a large population of mentally ill patients in Alabama State Institutions was released in the aftermath of Lynch vs Baxley 1974. The exodus of mentally ill individuals back into the community created a greater demand on the Birmingham Police Department. The department needed to scrutinize and modify the services provided to these individuals. This case also addressed the issue of incarceration of the mentally ill in Alabama and the fact that jails were not the appropriate facility for detaining individuals involved in an involuntary commitment process. Beginning in 1979, the Birmingham City Jail began to utilize in-house social workers in order to respond to the problem of mentally ill inmates. Presently, the Birmingham City Jail has a full-time, in-house social worker and a part-time psychiatrist.

In 1977, eight CSO positions were federally funded by the Comprehensive Employment Training Act (CETA) Title II program. These eight CSOs were placed under the umbrella of the Family Services division of the Birmingham Police Department. Two CSOs were assigned to each precinct and worked Monday through Friday from 1:00 p.m. to 11:00 p.m. The CSOs attended roll calls with uniformed officers to provide information about cases, social programs, and community resources. The CSOs consulted weekly with a psychiatrist from a local mental health center concerning mentally ill clients.

In 1979, the CSO program was changed to a Crisis Management Team. At that time, only six civilian CSOs were available, and two CSOs became sworn officers.

The crisis management concept paired CSOs and uniformed officers to work as a team. The structure allowed for four civilian CSOs to work day shifts at each precinct and continue to respond to calls with police officers.

Four team models were designed. In one model, a sworn officer and a civilian CSO worked as a team. In the second model, two sworn officers worked together. In a third model, a sworn CSO and a civilian CSO worked together. In a fourth model, a sworn CSO and a sworn officer worked together. By comparing the three models, the most effective way of delivering services could be determined. This was important as federal funds were diminishing and it was becoming crucial to evaluate the effectiveness of the service. It was determined that the model utilizing a sworn CSO/civilian CSO was the most effective.

After the CMT program ended, the CSO unit went back to the original CSO model of civilian CSOs providing assistance with calls of a psychosocial nature. Between 1979 and 1986 the number of CSOs working varied from two to three. Beginning in the early 1980s six permanent positions were funded by the City of Birmingham, at a time when the city was experiencing a hiring freeze. Finally, in 1985, the hiring of new CSOs began. By the end of 1986, the CSO unit had a full staff capacity of six. The CSOs continue to provide crisis intervention social services as secondary civilian units, in keeping with the objective of the original model of 1976.

PROFESSIONAL KNOWLEDGE

The CSOs are social workers with theoretical and practical training in crisis and non-crisis situations. They are versed in laws that apply to individuals who are mentally ill and areas that may bear on this population, such as domestic violence. Further, the CSOs have a clear understanding of the specific rules and regulations of the Birmingham Police Department and their application in situations of a psycho-social nature. They are also aware of the various community resource agencies and their specific functions. Within the police department, CSOs are considered experts in crisis management and intervention in the delivery of social services to diverse client populations. They are required to conduct their professional duties with a knowledge of all aspects of social work practice and a considerable degree of independent judgement.

The minimum education and experience required for a Community Service Officer is a bachelors degree in Social Work and one year experience in social work or any combination of education and experience that demonstrates the required knowledge, skills, and abilities (Jefferson County Personnel Board 1997). The minimum education and experience for the Senior CSO is the same, with the added requirement of three years experience as a CSO (Jefferson County Personnel Board 1997). The title of CSO is a secondary title within the police department. The official job titles through the Jefferson County Personnel Board are Senior Police Community Service Worker and Police Community Service Worker.

EDUCATION AND COMMUNITY SERVICE

Two CSOs are board certified instructors and instruct new recruits at the Birmingham Police Academy on effective communication skills; working with the mentally ill; basic psychology; domestic disturbances; conflict management and pertinent laws.

On request, CSOs speak to community groups about social service topics, they are involved with numerous committees, task forces, and community organizations that strive for improvement within the community. The CSO unit also serves as a field placement for masters level social work students.

OPERATIONS

Currently, there are six CSOs within the unit which is attached to the patrol division. The senior CSO serves as the unit's administrator. All members report to the administrative captain in the Deputy Chief of Patrol's office. CSOs are assigned to four major precincts and answer calls in other precinct areas when needed. The regular work schedule includes two shifts of 8:00 a.m. to 4:30 p.m. and 1:30 p.m. to 10:00 p.m. (Monday through Friday). During weekends and holidays a CSO is on call for case consultation and direct service. The on-call periods begin at 10:00 P.M. the night prior to the weekend or holiday and continue until the beginning of the next regular workday. CSOs can be contacted during off-duty hours for emergency disposition of a case. If a CSO is not on duty a referral can be forwarded to a CSO by police officers. The police officer would complete a police incident report and send the report to the CSO.

The narrative section of the report contains a description of the problem and initial outcome of the call which enables the CSO to determine safety issues and the need for a patrol unit's assistance when making a follow-up visit.

Each CSO is assigned a city vehicle, a pager, and a police radio. The majority of the calls answered by CSOs are responding to assist a patrol unit at an incident location. CSOs are civilian employees and primarily depend on police officers for their safety. The police officers remain at the scene until the CSO is comfortable handling the situation. On many occasions the CSO can continue working on a call that requires social service intervention only, allowing the police officer to resume patrol duties. CSOs also receive referrals from other units within the Department, private citizens, other agencies that provide social services, and area businesses. On request, CSOs do debriefing with an officer who has been involved in a critical incident.

CASEWORK FUNCTIONS OF THE CSO

- Respond to calls from law enforcement officers and others to assist or intervene in situations that can include mentally ill persons, domestic violence, child and adult abuse/neglect, runaways, missing persons, victims of sexual assault, substance abuse, and assisting with basic needs.
- Interview clients to obtain psycho-social history information.
- Conduct assessment and referral to appropriate services.
- Crisis intervention counseling.
- Transport client by automobile to referral agencies and accompany

clients during initial agency visit to serve as a facilitator in the referral process.

- Conduct follow-up contact with clients and referral sources by field visit or telephone call to ensure adequate assistance has been provided.
- Counsel with law enforcement officers, clients, and family members, and provide referral to the appropriate agency for psychosocial problems.
- Maintain records of each client indicating the nature of the problem, actions taken, and disposition of the case.
- File petitions of commitment regarding mentally ill individuals. Attend court hearings and testify if needed.
- Provide feedback to police officers concerning case referral and outcome.

GUIDELINES FOR ANSWERING CALLS

- CSOs are not sworn officers and are not required to handle any situation that calls for law enforcement actions to be taken.
- CSOs are called to the scene to assist patrol units. They are not primary response units unless the call is initiated by them and does not require any law enforcement action.
- CSOs are not to interview any individual without an officer present if weapons are known to be present.
- CSOs are not to transport any individual under the influence of alcohol or drugs.
- When a client is transported to a hospital by a CSO or police officer for psychiatric evaluation, the CSO or police officer remains with the client unless hospital staff determine their presence is not needed.
- If the client was taken into custody under the state law (Act 353) and poses a threat to himself/herself or others and/or has been arrested, a police officer must remain with the client and a CSO will assist.
- CSOs are not to transport any individual who has the potential for violence. This decision is at the CSO's discretion.
- CSOs are not to transport children when they are placed in protective custody.
- CSOs only transport children if the call is initiated to assist a parent or person who is legal guardian.
- Additionally, before leaving a person with a CSO, police officers must identify the person by conducting a complete computer check (e.g., wanted/missing person). They should also check for any weapons and remove them, and discuss the case with the CSO on the scene. The CSO will make a decision as to whether or not the presence of a police officer is needed.

CASE STUDY

Community Service Officers answer a wide variety of calls in which they assist all divisions within the Birmingham Police Department. On occasion, the unit will respond to calls when requested by the Birmingham Fire and Rescue Unit and other agencies, according to the situation and the needs of the victim/client, in an effort to help stabilize the crisis by utilizing the best intervention practices. An average day for a Community Service Officer includes networking, being a broker for services, and advocating for the victim/client. The following case study is based on an example of a common call.

A Community Service Officer was requested in the north precinct area to assist an officer with a reported domestic violence situation. After a brief interview with the victim and her mother, the CSO found a number of factors which converged to generate a crisis. The father, who is unemployed, has a history of alcohol abuse and is unable to support the family on $140 per month and food stamps.

The victim, who is 14 years of age, claims that her father slapped her, after he over-heard a conversation during which the victim told her mother that she might be pregnant. The victim's mother was diagnosed with schizophrenia after the death of her younger sister, and takes haldol, risperdal, and cogentin to treat this illness. The mother depends on her small social security check to pay for the medications she needs. The victim's mother does not have enough money left to assist with managing household expenses, which exacerbates some of the family's problems.

Most of the time the mother is either asleep because of the medication or away from the home to avoid verbal and physical abuse from her husband. According to reports, the father also beats and mistreats the four children, ages 14, 12, 8 and 5. Birmingham Fire and Rescue treated the victim for her injuries, which were visible but not severe.

Two patrol units and a patrol supervisor initially responded to the call. Upon assessment of the situation, a CSO was requested to the scene. The father was arrested per Alabama warrantless arrest domestic laws. The officers' total time at the scene was one and one half hours.

The CSO response time to the call was 15 minutes. The CSO initially obtained information from the officers and assessed risk factors. The family members were interviewed by the CSO after the father left with officers going to jail. The CSO time at the scene was two hours. This included interviewing the family and making referrals to community agencies. Thirty minutes were spent transporting the family to a shelter and one hour was spent writing the final report, and taking that report to child welfare.

The following services and referrals were provided by the CSO:
- A mental health agency was notified for case management services with the mother.
- A family member and local shelter assisted the mother and children with shelter.
- A report was filed with the local child welfare agency in reference to the abuse of the children and assessment of the mother's ability to provide continued care.
- A referral was made to the Department's domestic violence program for protection orders and further social services.
- Follow-up on case outcome.

The CSO conducted a follow-up phone call to the mother at the shelter and spoke to a case manager at the shelter. The mother and children were receiving the appropriate service to meet their needs. The older child was being cared for by family members and has been in contact with his mother and siblings on a daily basis. At this time no other CSO services are presently needed by this family since all issues were addressed during the call and referral process.

CONCLUSION

The Community Service Officer unit has undergone some transitions since 1976. However, the unit has become an integral part of the Birmingham Police Department. Although the unit staffing and scheduling has fluctuated at times, the concept of an in-house social service/crisis management delivery system has remained stable. The CSOs continue to provide a comprehensive crisis intervention social service delivery system for the department. Therefore, police officers have been able to utilize CSOs to approach crisis problems from both a criminological and a psycho-social perspective. Many individuals who have to contact police officers are provided access to social services that might not be obtained without the vital link of a CSO. Due to the fact that CSOs are police department employees and have daily contact with police officers, there is a trusting working relationship that enhances teamwork efforts.

When police departments began to explore options to more effectively intervene in cases involving psychiatric crisis, three types of models emerged. These include the Birmingham Police Department CSO Program, The Memphis Police Department Crisis Intervention Teams, and the Knoxville Mobile Crisis Unit. These programs were analyzed and reported on by Steadman, Morrisey, Deane, & Borum (1998).

Additionally, the State of Alabama-Legislative Act 94–690 (1994) set forth provisions that allow for the establishment of Community Mental

Health Officers within the specific counties of Alabama. The education, experience, and duties of Community Mental Health Officers were developed from the CSO program model.

However, Community Mental Health Officers intervene specifically in psychiatric crisis situations whereas CSOs provide comprehensive crisis intervention services. CSOs are not considered Community Mental Health Officers. The development of a psychiatric response unit within a police department will depend on many factors. The CSO model can be explored for developing a comprehensive crisis intervention social service delivery system. The diverse functions of the CSO unit with its vast problem-solving capabilities continues to contribute to the success and feasibility of the program.

REFERENCES

Act 353, H. 944 Volume II *Alabama Laws of the Legislature of Alabama* (1975).
Act 99–690 H.241 Volume II *Alabama Laws of the Legislature of Alabama* (1994).
Borum, R., Deane, M., Morrisey, J. & Steadman, H. (1998). *Police Response to Emotionally Disturbed Persons: Analyzing New Models of Police Interactions with the Mental Health System* Washington D.C: National Institute of Justice
Lynch v. Baxley, 744 f. 2d 1452 (11th Cir. 1984).
The Personnel Board of Jefferson County: Job Description For Police Community Service Worker (1997).

APPENDIX

Statistics

Each CSO completes monthly reports that represent the total number of calls in a specific category. The Senior CSO is responsible for submitting quarterly, biannual, and annual reports from the unit to the Administrative Captain. CSOs are requested in a variety of situations to provide social services. Therefore, the statistics can include many different categories. The following CSO unit's 1999 statistics reflect this variation in calls.

1999 CSO Statistics

• Homicide/Death	5
• Sexual/Rape	11
• Assault	25
• Arson/Fire	3
• Burglary	1
• Larceny/Theft/Unlawful breaking & entering a vehicle	3
• Forgery	1
• Narcotics Complaint/Dangerous Drugs	2
• Sex Offense (not rape)/Indecent Exposure	6
• Domestic Disturbances	192
• Public Intoxication	1
• Wanted Person/Escape	5
• Weapons Offense/Person with a gun	1
• Disorderly Person or Fight	10
• Invasion of Privacy/Trespassing	3
• Conservation/Animal Complaint	2
• Suspicious Person or Vehicle	1
• Traffic Accident	2
• Assist a Citizen	388
• Person Down	1
• Mentally Disturbed Person	604
• Runaway/Missing Person	4
• Desk/Special Assignment	211
• Neighborhood Meetings	3
• Miscellaneous Complaints	530
Total Number of Calls	**2015**

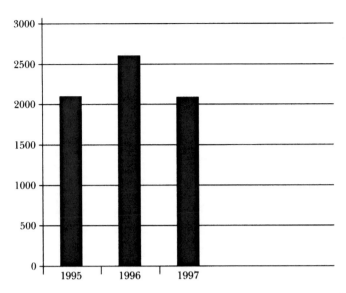

FIGURE 6.1 Birmingham Police CSO Unit Total Calls for Service[1] (1995–1999).

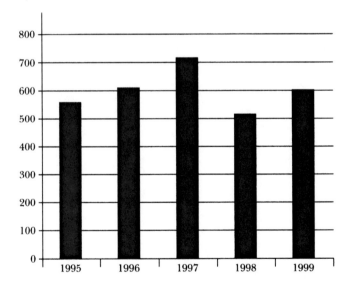

FIGURE 6.2 Birmingham Police CSO Unit Total Calls on Mentally Disturbed Persons[2] (1995–1999),

1. Total Calls 1995–1999: 11,044.
2. Total Calls 1995–1999: 3,052.

2. Community Programs

7

Criminal Justice Diversion of Individuals with Co-Occurring Mental Illness and Substance Use Disorders: An Overview

Nahama Broner, Randy Borum, and Kristen Gawley

This chapter provides an overview of the rates and types of mental illness and co-occurring mental illness and substance abuse in the criminal justice system. We then describe the use of criminal justice diversion programs as a mechanism to reduce the unnecessary incarceration of people with mental illness, highlighting several New York City programs and the type of treatments to which they are diverted. We conclude with a review of core diversion program elements.

CO-OCCURRING MENTAL ILLNESS AND SUBSTANCE USE DISORDERS IN THE CRIMINAL JUSTICE SYSTEM

The steady increase of individuals involved in the criminal justice system presenting with mental illness is well-documented and has various explanations in the literature from public safety initiatives that target nuisance

Preparation of this chapter was supported in part by Grant No. 1-UD8-TI 11213-03, from the U.S. Department of Health and Human Services, Substance Abuse and Mental Health Services Administration, Center for Substance Abuse Treatment and Grant No. MH16242-20, from the National Institute of Mental Health. The opinions expressed in this manuscript are strictly those of the authors and no endorsement by the funding agencies is to be inferred. The authors wish to thank Roger Peters, Ph.D. and Hunter L. McQuisten, M.D. for their review of earlier drafts of this chapter.

crimes (Barnes, 1998; Hiller, Knight, Broome & Simpson, 1996) to dein-
stitutionalization (Hiller et al., 1996) or transinstitutionalization (Shenson,
Dubler & Micheals, 1990; Spence, 1997; cf., Banks, Stone, Pandiani, Cox
& Morschauser, 2000; Rosenheck, Banks, Pandiani & Hoff, 2000). Currently,
approximately 700,000 people with severe mental illness are admitted to
U.S. jails each year. As of 1997, 68% of the 10,000,000 people booked into
U.S. jails during one year were from racial or ethnic minorities (Bureau
of Justice Statistics, 1998; U.S. Department of Justice Statistics, 1997).
National surveys show that between 6% and 15% of all jail inmates and
10% to 15% of prison inmates have a severe mental illness (Lamb &
Weinberger, 1998). Since mentally ill individuals are admitted to jails at
approximately eight times the rate at which they are admitted to public
psychiatric hospitals, there are currently more people with severe mental
illness in U.S. jails than in state hospitals (Torrey et al., 1993). Nearly three
out of four of these people also have a co-occurring alcohol and/or drug
abuse problem (Abram & Teplin, 1991).

Although people with mental illness are at greater risk of arrest than
the general population (Teplin, 1994; Rock & Landsberg, 1998), those
with co-occurring substance use disorders (particularly those who are also
not taking their psychiatric medications) are among the highest risk group,
not only for arrest but also for homelessness, HIV, violent behavior, and
a host of other negative, costly outcomes (Borum, Swanson, Swartz &
Hiday, 1997; Drake, Bartels, Teague, Noordsy, & Clark, 1993; Monahan,
1995; RachBeisel, Scott & Dixon, 1999; Steadman et al., 1998; Swartz,
Swanson, Hiday, Borum & Wagner, 1998). Further, those who use alcohol
or drugs and do not take their prescribed medication are three times more
likely to be arrested than others with mental disorders (Borum et al.,
1997), and their risk for violent behavior significantly increases (Swartz
et al., 1999).

Moreover, the existence of alcohol and drug problems among mental
health clients and the existence of mental health problems among substance abuse clients are both remarkably common. Among people in the
community with a recent substance use disorder, approximately 21% to
39%, will meet criteria for another psychiatric disorder (Kofoed, Kania,
Walsh & Atkinson, 1986), while in a sample of inmates with substance use
disorders, Cote and Hodgins (1990) found that 26% met lifetime diagnostic criteria for affective disorders and 9% had a history of schizophrenia.
Additionally, based on a random sample of individuals receiving services
in New York State, the Center for the Study of Issues in Public Mental
Health (1998) estimated that more than half (57%) of individuals with a
severe mental illness also had a substance abuse problem within the previous five years. The rate for dual diagnosis among individuals in inpatient settings was considerably greater. For current substance abuse, national

studies estimate that among psychiatric inpatients almost half have substantial substance abuse or dependence (Miller & Ries, 1991).

Within the criminal justice system in New York City, as an example of an urban center, the problem is even more complex. Approximately 15,000 to 20,000 people with mental health problems cycle through the city's correctional system each year to the community, with another 1500 mentally ill prisoners returning to New York City annually from state and federal prisons (Lamon, Cohen & Broner, Chap. 12), with a portion of this number likely a duplicative count. Among the approximately 2,000 inmates with mental health problems confined in New York City jails at any one time, almost half are estimated to have been homeless in recent years (Michaels, Zoloth, Alchabes, Braslow & Safyer, 1992). Many, if not most, are repeat offenders. Moreover, 80% to 90% have co-occurring substance abuse problems. The Urban Justice Center, a New York City advocacy group, notes that the city's mentally ill jail inmates spend significantly more time incarcerated—typically 215 days—than do non-mentally ill inmates who average 42 days (Winerip, 1999). A statewide study of New York's mentally ill incarcerated population had similar findings, and noted that alternatives to incarceration programs are less available to those that are mentally (Rock & Landsberg, 1998).

BREADTH OF DISORDERS

With regard to mental health problems, most of the professional literature on the existence of co-occurring disorders in the criminal justice system has focused on the most severe mental disorders—schizophrenia, bipolar disorder, and major depression. However, other "less severe" disorders, such as anxiety disorders, are common among criminal justice samples, "frequently co-exist with substance use disorders," and also affect treatment outcomes (Peters & Hills, 1997, p. 1).

For example, a 1996 survey (Substance Abuse Mental Health Services Administration [SAMHSA], 1997) found that 14% of adults with generalized anxiety disorder also used illicit drugs and 23% used alcohol heavily. Similar relationships existed for other anxiety disorders such as agoraphobia, where 16% used drugs and 14% were heavy alcohol users, and panic disorder, where at least one in five had a substance abuse problem. In a study of a male substance abusing prison therapeutic community population, Wexler and Graham (1993) reported incidences of antisocial personality disorder (52%), attention deficit hyperactivity disorder (42%), phobic disorders (18%), and post-traumatic stress syndrome (16%), in addition to noting the occurrence of depressive disorders (27%). The relationship between anxiety and affective disorders and trauma is well-established and viewed as particularly relevant to urban minority clients who demonstrate a higher rate of witnessing and experiencing violence, and whose condition is often exasperated by poverty and difficulty accessing legal and medical services (Braun, Flanagan & McLeod, 1983; Gelles & Harrop, 1989; Jacobson & Herald, 1990). Ditton (1999) noted the experience of violence as a significant factor in the lives of male mentally ill state prisoners who are more than twice as likely as other males to report a history of physical abuse and almost four times as likely to report prior sexual abuse.

Anxiety disorders, particularly post-traumatic stress disorder (PTSD), are especially a concern among female inmates along with other risk factors (Haywood, Kravitz, Goldman & Freeman, 2000; Henderson, 1997). Research suggests that almost half of the women involved in the criminal justice system have experienced physical and/or sexual violence within and outside families and relationships (Holden, Rann & Van Drasek, 1993; Richie & Johnsen, 1996), and a number of women exposed to such experiences develop PTSD and other anxiety disorders (Jacobson & Herald, 1990). In fact, 22% of women admitted to a large midwestern jail were diagnosed with PTSD, 7% with dysthymia, 2% with generalized anxiety, and 1% with panic disorder. Rates for other psychiatric disorders were also provided (Teplin, Abram & McClelland, 1996). Women who have experienced violence are also more likely to become alcohol and drug abusers (El-Bassel, Gilbert, Schilling, Ivanoff & Borne, 1996; Fullilove et al., 1993; Young & Boyd, 2000), and rates of substance abuse in incarcerated women are particularly high (Jordan, Schlenger, Fairbank & Caddell, 1996; Teplin et al., 1996).

Finally, in discussing prevalence rates for disorders as a basis for guiding the breath of disorders to be considered when defining a co-occurring population in need of particular attention, resource allocation, and treatment, the relationship of diagnosis and race is noteworthy. Researchers have noted that, among African–Americans, anxiety and affective disorders are under-diagnosed while psychotic disorders are over-diagnosed (Fabrega, Mezzich & Ullrich, 1988; Rayburn & Stonecypher, 1996); this problem was also found with substance abusers and the incarcerated mentally ill (Drake, Alterman & Rosenberg, 1993; Fiander & Bartlett, 1997; Paradis, Horn, Yang & O'Rourke, 1999). This discrepancy exists despite evidence from the Epidemiological Catchment Area (ECA) studies that have demonstrated that there are no significant differences in the prevalence rates of major psychiatric illness among different ethnic groups (Myers et al., 1984).

DIVERSION

Policy makers have long recognized the need to reduce the prevalence of severe mental illness and co-occurring substance use disorders in jail by diverting minor offenders away from the criminal justice system into the behavioral health system. This was a major recommendation of the National Coalition for Jail Reform as early as the 1970s. Over the past 30 years, however, the concept of jail diversion has evolved significantly. Initially, jail diversion initiatives focused only on removing mentally ill offenders from the application of criminal law at any stage of the process (McBride, 1978). A more contemporary view, however, focuses not only on "diversion from" a system but also "diversion to" services in other systems. Whether the primary objective is to divert the offender at initial criminal justice contact (Steadman, Morris & Dennis, 1995) or during jail incarceration (Draine & Solomon, 1999), emphasis is now given to linking offenders into community service systems. Viewing diversion as a multi-systems collaboration between criminal justice and community-based agencies allows programs to begin to address potential contributing factors to recidivism such as: a lack of continuity of public assistance; housing; medical benefits and streamlined mechanisms for social service referrals (Barr, 1999; National GAINS Center, 1999a); lack of linkage to programs that provide ongoing psychiatric integrated care in the community (Barr, 1999; Torrey et al., 1993); use of parallel or sequential models of treatment rather than integrated treatment (RachBeisel et al., 1999); and an absence of non-proprietary computerized management information systems to allow efficient, timely, and continuous care (Barr, 1999; National GAINS Center, 1999b; Sherman & Taxman, 1998). Yet, within this framework, diversion initiatives have the potential to: reduce recidivism for high-level misdemeanants and low-level felons (Hoff, Baranosky, Buchanan, Zonana & Rosenheck, 1999); increase the efficiency of criminal justice systems; reduce court backlogs; reduce the costs of criminal justice processing; reduce the impact of and vulnerability to other incarcerated inmates; and help avoid the stigma which may lead to difficulty in obtaining legitimate employment (Inciardi, McBride & Rivers, 1996).

Pre-booking diversion

As jail diversion programs have been extended to serve mentally ill offenders, two major types have emerged; each is categorized according to the point of criminal justice contact at which the diversion occurs as either pre-booking (before arrest) or post-booking (after arrest). Pre-booking diversion occurs before a subject is arrested or formal charges have been filed. The police officer is the primary decision-maker at this point in the process. The American Bar Association's *Criminal Justice Mental Health Standards* posit that "When police custody of a mentally ill or mentally retarded person is based exclusively on either noncriminal behavior or minor criminal behavior, the police should either transport the person to an appropriate facility for evaluation or negotiate a voluntary disposition" (American Bar Association, 1986, p. 40). The success or failure of such a policy depends largely on the degree of cooperation between the law enforcement and mental health systems. The police are unlikely to use a mental health disposition if it is difficult or time-consuming.

A national survey (Deane, Steadman, Borum, Veysey & Morrissey, 1998) of all major police departments investigated the nature and type of law enforcement-mental health partnerships that exist for pre-booking diversion. Although 88% provide some training for officers related to mental illness, only 45% reported having some type of specialized response to mentally ill people in crisis. Results suggest that most police departments with a specialized response conform generally to one of three models:

Police-based specialized police response: These models involve sworn officers who have special mental health training who serve as the first line police response to mental health crises in the community and who act as liaisons to the formal mental health system; 3.4% of police departments had this type of program.

Police-based specialized mental health response: In this model, mental health professionals (not sworn officers) are employed by the police department to provide on-site and telephone consultations to officers in the field; 11.5% of police departments had this type of program.

Mental health-based specialized mental health response: In this more traditional model, partnerships or cooperative agreements are developed between police and mobile mental health crisis teams that exist as part of the local community mental health services system and operate independently of the police department; 30% of police departments had this type of program.

Post-booking diversion

Post-booking diversion occurs after arrest and formal charges have been filed; however, the precise point and locus of diversion varies. Steadman, Barbera & Dennis (1994) identified three core elements of post-booking diversion: 1) screening, 2) mental health evaluation, and 3) negotiation between diversion and legal staffs for a mental health disposition in lieu of prosecution as an alternative to incarceration or in the reduction of charges. Using this working definition, they surveyed 760 U.S. jails. Although 34% reported having some type of jail diversion initiative for inmates with mental illness, only 18% actually had a program that met any of these basic criteria. Many who thought they had a jail diversion program did not have any community-based (non-jail) dispositions. The authors estimated that at the time of their study there were only about 50 formal jail-based diversion programs existing in the U.S.

A number of post-booking programs (along with pre-booking programs) throughout the U.S. have been described (e.g., Borum, 1999; The National GAINS Center, 1999c) and are being evaluated (Steadman et al., 1999). Many of these programs have continued to expand and report new initiatives in their local communities. In New York City, for instance, the number of programs targeting the mentally ill involved with the criminal justice system have increased from one to over 12 in the last few years (Lamon, Cohen & Broner, Chapter 12). One example of a post-booking jail diversion program, the Nathaniel Project (C.A.S.E.S., 2000), begun in 1999, targets a specific population through an adapted alternative to incarceration model. The program targets jail-bound mentally ill felony offenders facing a minimum two-year sentence, the majority of whom have histories of homelessness, alcohol and/or drug use; many have violent offenses and histories. Accepted clients screened in detention are released to the program conditioned upon two-year, court-monitored program participation. As is the focus of many diversion programs in New York City (Lamon et al., Chapter 12), the Nathaniel Project links clients to a comprehensive range of community services; unique for an alternative to incarceration program, intensive case management and supportive counseling are blended by diversion program social work staff. Supportive counseling/case management is provided in benefit offices, shelters, and while clients wait for treatment program interviews. Once clients are successfully placed, contact is gradually reduced. An evaluation is planned but has not yet commenced. Several other New York City programs, which are court-based and have adapted models from the substance abuse diversion field to the co-occurring population, are described below.

Post-booking diversion and specialized courts

While only a small percentage of courts have procedures for formal diversion of the mentally ill and dually diagnosed from a jail setting to community treatment (Bahn & Davis, 1997; Brown, 1997; Center on Crime, Communities & Culture, 1996), there are well-established court diversion models for other populations. For instance, historically, diversion initiatives have been targeted to specific types of offenders in an attempt to identify specific disorders, such as drug abuse or dependence. In 1972, the White House established Treatment Alternatives to Street Crime (TASC) to address the need for court-based screening and case management of substance abusers. According to the National Institute of Justice, TASC

became a "best practice" model in 1986, and at present, there are 195
TASC programs in 26 states and two territories (Anglin, Longshore &
Turner, 1999). Currently, one trend is to adapt substance abuse-focused,
court-based case management models for a co-occurring population, such
as the TASC and Drug Treatment Alternatives to Prison Program(DTAP)
(Sung, Tabachnick & Feng, 1999) models, by honing identification, assessment, and treatment matching procedures to specifically detect mental
illness.

In New York City, the Education and Assistance Corporation (EAC)
adopted the national TASC model. This model consists of pre- and post-
indictment screening through specialty courts and general case finding,
12-month community follow-up for misdemeanants and 24-month follow-
up for felons, monthly case manager meetings with the client in their
placement, weekly calls to the community provider, and intervention in
emergencies. NYC TASC treatment retention for its substance abusers is
70% at the two-year follow-up for placed felony cases (Timler & Linn,
1999). In 1999, NYC TASC added a Mental Health division, starting three
discreet programs which are being evaluated by New York University's
Institute Against Violence. Contracting with New York's Department of
Mental Health, Mental Retardation and Alcoholism Services, they operate the transitional services for NYC–Brooklyn LINK for both court-based
diversion and post-sentenced discharge planning for juvenile and adult
populations as well as an arraignment mental health service that diverts
low-level misdemeanants from the court and "flags" other defendants with
more serious charges for diversion later in the criminal justice process
(Lamon et al., Chapter 12). The third program serving multiple jurisdictions began in January 2000 as a special pilot in the Bronx, with a focus
on Hispanic populations (Broner, Franczak, Dye & McCallister, 2001).
This program integrates best practices of specialized court processing,
TASC community monitoring, and an interdisciplinary, culturally competent screening/assessment treatment planning case management team.
In this program, clients with co-occurring severe mental illness and substance use disorders are adjudicated and monitored in a special mental
health supreme court part for multiple felony offenders with drug indict-
ments. There is also case-by-case review for acceptance of other violent
and non-violent felony and persistent misdemeanor defendants.

With the exception of discharge planning cases, NYC TASC client dispositions are court mandated and include graduated sanctions adapted
for this population (i.e., varying the level of treatment structure and treatment and monitoring intensity, medication petition, jail time, etc.). Across
programs, accepted clients are severely and persistently mentally ill, the
majority with substance use disorders, and have charges ranging from
non-violent misdemeanors to violent felonies. All clients are screened by
supervised case managers and independently assessed by a psychiatrist.

Treatment plans result from a team approach. Innovative are the medication continuity from confinement to community placement, court-based client seeking from arraignment through post-indictment in general and specialty courts, partnerships with community housing and treatment agencies, and the lack of exclusion for difficult to place clients with sex offense or arson charges and clients who have developmental disabilities and mental retardation.

In another initiative, New York City's TASC's Mental Health division has worked in partnership with the Brooklyn District Attorney's Office to develop an innovative, post-booking diversion program called Treatment Alternatives for the Dually Diagnosed (TADD) (Tabachnick, 1999). The TADD program has completed its pilot year and focuses its work on both those with mild mental health problems and those with severe mental illness; a majority of their clients have co-occurring alcohol and/or drug abuse or dependence. Prosecutors first screen the client's legal record, then, if eligible, the client is seen for further screening and assessment by staff in a special court part. This program model blends the best practices of specialty court-based (i.e., drug court) diversion with extensive client outreach and intensive case management (i.e., TASC model) with an enforcement component based upon the DTAP model (Sung et al., 1999). A special warrant enforcement team apprehends program absconders if they have prior felony convictions and are non-compliant with treatment. The TADD program blends these three models and adds enhanced screening, assessment, supervision, and treatment matching to address the special needs of the offenders with co-occurring disorders. Research on the efficacy of both the adaptation of the TASC model to a co-occurring population and this new hybrid model, TADD, is needed.

A second major trend in post-booking diversion approaches has been the emergence of specialized courts to adjudicate certain types of cases. This concept began with the creation of "drug courts" in New York City in the early 1970s (Belenko & Dumanovsky, 1993), with the promise of reduced recidivism due to mandated treatment, faster adjudication, and lowered court costs (Belenko, 1998; Brown, 1997; National Institute of Justice, 1992). Indeed, a study of Florida drug courts indicates significant reductions in recidivism over 30 months when comparing drug court graduates to non-graduates and probationers (Peters & Murrin, 2000). Over time, the courts developed better strategies to address substance abuse, first integrating relapse prevention and treatment retention (Inciardi et al., 1996), and then adding heath and treatment services to the court (Brown, 1997). This latter development, the Boston Model, has been replicated around the country; in New York City, the Center for Court Innovation (CCI) has used this model as a framework for creating treatment (drug), community, domestic violence, and youth courts. In contrast to the TASC and DTAP models, program operations and primary services with non-traditional, community-based partners are court-based (Berman & Andersen, 1999; Gordon, 1994).

An example of a CCI court is Brooklyn Treatment Court (BTC), started in 1996. It diverts men and women charged with drug offenses who present with alcohol and/or drug abuse or dependence to onsite court-based health, treatment, and social services. Through partnerships with the New York City Department of Health, Brooklyn Hospital Center, and New York University Division of Nursing, primary health care and education and testing for HIV, TB, STDs, and pregnancy are provided along with educational and vocational counseling through a job readiness program track. In 1998, to address the mental health problems of these defendants, BTC added a psychiatric nurse practitioner to perform psychiatric assessments and has since adapted a protocol to screen for severe mental illness (i.e., schizophrenias and affective disorders), anxiety, and trauma in addition to its traditional screening for alcohol, drug, and medical disorders along with treatment readiness (Broner, Borum, Whitemire & Gawley, Chap. 24). CCI has ongoing internal program evaluation to examine the effect of expanded program acceptance criteria—clients with co-occurring disorders—on treatment matching, treatment retention, and criminal justice recidivism.

Another development in specialty courts is to focus on mental illness rather than the type of offense. The "Mental Health Court" model, pioneered in Broward County, Florida with mentally ill misdemeanants, operates much like treatment-oriented drug courts (Freidburg, 1997). This court is being evaluated by the Department of Mental Health Law and Policy at the Louis de la Parte Florida Mental Health Institute. Mental health courts have now been implemented in other jurisdictions, and four of these courts (Anchorage, Alaska; San Bernardino, California; Broward County, Florida; Seattle, Washington) have been descriptively compared for common elements (e.g., specialized team, separate court calendar, court supervision, interaction with the mental health system for treatment placement) as well as differences (Goldkamp & Irons-Guynn, 2000; Watson, Hanrahan, Luchins & Lurigo, 2001). Results of one Midwestern mental health court diversion program noted significant differences in population characteristics between those diverted and those not, and little difference between groups on outcomes at two months follow-up, with the exception of longer jail stays for non-diverted defendants. Conclusions supported the premise of criminal justice cost savings for diversion (Steadman, Cocozza, & Veysey, 1999). Studying the efficacy of different program components of these court-focused models and potential differences in the populations served is needed (Steadman, Davidson & Brown, 2001).

DIVERSION TO INTEGRATED TREATMENT FOR
CO-OCCURRING DISORDERS

Specialized diversion programs must not only keep people out of jail but also link clients into effective treatment services. Individuals with co-occurring mental illness and substance abuse problems, however, often do not respond well to traditional community mental health interventions. This population typically has multiple, complex problems that require specialized treatment planning for effective intervention. For example, the majority of people with co-occurring disorders have severe functional impairments in employment, interpersonal relationships, and physical health (Peters, Kearns, Murrin & Dolente 1992). They are often homeless (Osher et al., 1994); at increased risk for violence (Steadman et al., 1998; Monahan, 1995), and require hospitalization more frequently than other people with mental illness (Drake, Mercer-McFadden, Mueser, McHugo & Bond, 1998). Moreover, individuals with co-occurring illnesses have low rates of treatment compliance, more severe symptomatology, and higher relapse rates than those treated for a single disorder (Edens, Peters & Hills, 1997).

Traditional treatment approaches, which offer separate services and providers for mental health and substance abuse problems, are often ineffective for people with co-occurring disorders (Bowers, Mazure, Nelson & Jatlow, 1990; Drake, McLauglin, Pepper & Minkoff, 1991; Polcin, 1992; Ridgely, Goldman & Willenbring, 1990). Nevertheless, many programs which treat this population structure services in a sequential fashion in which individuals must complete the treatment for one diagnosis before they can enroll in treatment for the other. Osher and Kofoed (1989) refer to this model as "ping-pong" therapy. Research has shown that, when subjected to sequential treatment, individuals with co-occurring disorders are more likely to terminate treatment prematurely and to attend treatment less consistently (Hall, Popkin, DeVaul, & Stickney, 1977), and less likely to stay the course of extended treatment (Osher & Drake, 1996).

One alternative to sequential treatment is the parallel treatment model in which both treatments are offered simultaneously but by different providers. While the parallel model offers improvements over the sequential model, there are a number of difficulties created by having multiple, uncoordinated treatment providers (Weiss & Najavits, 1998). Services for this population are often divided by funding sources, admission criteria, treatment methods and philosophies, and staff training and qualifications (Sciacca, 1991).

The approach that appears to be most effective for people with co-occurring mental illness and substance abuse problems is "integrated treatment." Review of the principles and elements of integrated treatment, along with discussion of differing approaches, has been well described (e.g., Drake et al., 1998; Osher & Drake, 1996; Pepper & Hendrickson, 1998; Peters & Hills, 1999; RachBeisel et al., 1999; Ridgely, 1991; Sacks, 2000). The outcomes obtained from integrated treatment have been far superior to those obtained by either sequential or parallel methods. Mueser, Drake and Miles (1997) reported that the weight of the evidence for 30 studies of integrated treatment is overwhelmingly positive, indicating that mental health and substance abuse treatment that is coordinated and administered by the same person, organization or team and specialty integrated treatments (e.g., Weiss & Najavits, 1998) is more effective.

Jerrell and Ridgely (1995) studied three models of integrated treatment and discovered improvements in work, independent living, social relationships, perceived satisfaction, psychiatric symptoms, and decreased use of emergency room visits. Multiple studies have shown that integrated treatment significantly reduces hospital utilization (Bond, 1989; Kofoed et al., 1986; Hellerstein & Meehan, 1987). At least one study has reported an increase in drug/alcohol abstinence for inpatients enrolled in an integrated treatment approach (Ries & Ellingson, 1989). Drake, McHugo and Noordsy (1993) demonstrated that 60% of the patients who received integrated treatment remained abstinent during a four-year follow-up. Finally, in a review of 10 well-controlled studies, Drake et al. (1998) concluded that comprehensive, integrated treatment, "especially when delivered for 18 months or longer, resulted in significant reductions of substance abuse and, in some cases, in substantial rates of remission, as well as reductions in hospital use and/or improvements in other outcomes" (p. 601).

IMPLEMENTING DIVERSION: COMMON ELEMENTS

Once Steadman et al. (1994) operationalized diversion according to the three elements described above—screening, evaluation, and negotiation—he and his colleagues conducted a more detailed inquiry into 21 programs that did meet criteria for a jail diversion program (Steadman et al., 1995). All 21 identified programs served misdemeanor offenders, however, 15 of them served non-violent felons and 10 even included certain violent felons. Most of the jail diversion programs were based in mental health centers (75%), although less than half were funded by the local department of mental health. Most programs had at least one assigned staff member, although in one third of the programs the staff were part-time. In examining the factors that distinguished the effective programs, six central features emerged: integrated services, key agency meetings, boundary spanners, strong leadership, early identification, and distinctive case management.

Integrated services

Mentally ill offenders typically require services from multiple agencies such as mental health, substance abuse, social service, and housing authorities. When multiple services are coordinated within the auspices of a single entity, this degree of integration meets the offender's needs in a way that is more comprehensive and less redundant. Recent research evidence suggests that integrated mental health substance abuse treatment is particularly effective in improving outcomes for people with co-occurring disorders (e.g., RachBeisel et al., 1999).

Regular meetings of key agency representatives

The most effective programs were those that involved key stakeholders from multiple agencies early in the planning process and that maintained regular contact. Regularly scheduled meetings facilitate the sharing of information and concerns and foster a greater coordination of services.

In recent years, there has been increased attention to the development of collaborative multi-agency and multi-disciplinary infrastructures to support policy direction, individual program development, and a program's potential sustainability in a community (Broner, Franczak et al., 2001). Based on the premise that fragmented systems produce lack of continuity of care and negatively impact client outcomes, creating a mechanism for continuity of services through formal cooperative or collaborative agreement (i.e., memoranda of understanding) should theoretically directly impact clients' ability to receive the range and type of services they may need and thus improve desired outcomes. Further, projects that may ordinarily pose conflict between systems but whose implementation would support long-term coordination of services, such as management information systems, continuation of benefits and transportation from court or jail to the community service (National GAINS Center, 1999a, 1999b; Sherman & Taxman, 1998), may be more easily implemented within an ongoing collaborative meeting process.

Boundary spanners

Another key finding was that program effectiveness was highly reliant on the existence of one or more "boundary spanners"—individuals who serve as a formal link or liaison between the mental health/substance abuse service systems and the criminal justice/judicial systems. These designated individuals must have credibility and competence within both systems to manage critical aspects of ongoing inter-agency relationships and agreements and to facilitate the resolution of conflicts.

Strong leadership

The existence of a strong leader for the program was also important. The leader should possess strong communication skills, working knowledge of local criminal justice and mental health systems, and the ability to identify "key players" and formal/informal networks in both systems. This is particularly important in jurisdictions where there are not yet regular key stakeholder meetings and product-focused mechanisms to assist in program implementation, such as research practice collaborations, consensus panels or active local task forces (Broner, Franczak et al., 2001).

Early identification

The screening phase, to identify detainees with possible mental illness, should occur early in the process of criminal justice contact, ideally within the first 24 to 48 hours. This will typically occur in the jail but may also be conducted at the point of arraignment.

Early identification may be particularly complex in large urban areas with multiple courts and jails systems, each with somewhat different procedures for collecting and disseminating client responses to basic psychiatric questions regarding past treatment, medication, substance use, suicidality, and disorganized behavior. Thus, such communities may particularly benefit from key stakeholders meetings and a memorandum of agreement detailing confidentiality as well as a mechanism for transmitting basic information to the diversion programs in their jurisdiction. Detailed screening objectives, staff training, and tools for identification, screening, and assessment have been proposed and reviewed (e.g., Broner et al., Chap. 24; Peters & Peyton, 1998; Peters & Hills, 1999).

Distinctive case management services

Steadman et al. (1995) identify the case management effort as one of the most critical elements in creating an effective diversion program. Ideally, the case managers—like the boundary spanners—have an understanding of the mental health and criminal justice systems as well as an ability to closely monitor supervisees and maintain regular contact. They also argue that it is helpful if the case management staff is similar to the client population in cultural background and racial composition; detailed guidelines for developing culturally competent case management have been proposed (SAMHSA, 2000).

In addition to cross-training, Peters and Hills (1999) describe the need for case management to be model-driven and encompass a phase approach to support the client's integrated treatment work during the diversion program's monitoring phase. For example, Osher & Kofoed (1989) identify the stages of dual disorder treatment: engaging, persuading, active treatment and relapse prevention. Further, Peters and Hills (1999) recommend that case managers also be trained in the following areas: 1) recognition and understanding of psychiatric symptoms for mental illness and substance use, including when to refer for further evaluation; 2) mental status; 3) diagnostic classifications; 4) basic understanding of psychotropic medications, their classification, benefits, side effects, and interactions with psychoactive substances (with an ethno-cultural understanding of differential effects for ethnic and racial groups [SAMHSA, 2000]); 5) flexibility regarding non-compliance and supportive rather than confrontational supervision strategies; and 6) knowledge of and ability to access different treatment and services resources. We would add that staff should also be trained in how to describe clients' mental health problems accurately and from a strength's model for writing psycho-social reports and treatment and sanction plans.

SUMMARY

An interesting and pragmatic trend over the last decade in mental health diversion is the growing dialogue regarding systems and services integration through collaboration. This trend, combined with positive outcomes resulting from full-service drug courts, and the negative impact of growing arrest and incarceration rates of those with serious mental illness has shifted the discourse, in part, away from diversion—whose sole purpose is to remove an individual from criminal justice contact—to diversion as a mechanism to identify those in need of treatment, to broker treatment, housing, medical care, vocational and educational training, and often to remain involved with the individual through a monitoring or crisis intervention mechanism for a defined period of time in the community. The work of Steadman et al. (1994 & 1995), Peters and Hills (1999), and Drake et al. (1998), among others, highlight best practices in systems change, program implementation, and treatment. Their work impacts both jail and community policy by moving the discourse closer to issues which could have direct effect on client access to treatment and the quality of that treatment.

While many argue that it is not the diversion program's mandate to treat or to fix the community system, many programs, out of necessity, have turned to a collaborative process to share resources (funding, staff, sites, etc.). Consequently, each agency's outcomes become dependent on the functionality of the other. Through partnerships between criminal justice and mental health agencies as well as research universities, we may begin to see a broader change in the nature of what clients are receiving both in jail and in the community. First, systematic screening and assessment in jails and courts may increase access to services both for those who have previously been connected and for those who were unaware of having serious mental health problems. Second, the content of what a client receives once diverted into treatment systems that are part of a collaborative approach may be changing in a number of jurisdictions. For instance, both mental health and substance abuse treatment programs will interject a different understanding of their clients as their staff is cross-trained or new staff with multiple expertise is hired. Mental health programs are entertaining structures that they had not felt appropriate (bed checks, reporting, increased self-help, and phase-focused treatments). Substance abuse agencies are integrating professionals trained in both mental health and substance abuse, and modifying their milieu approach (e.g., Sachs, 2000). Criminal justice agencies, schooled now in substance abuse programs and steps of recovery, are entering the discourse of mandated services and sanctions which may be notably more intrusive, as well as potentially deleterious, for those with mental illness than for those with sole substance use disorders. Systems research on these trends and their effects would be productive.

A review of the literature emphasizes that the co-occurring mentally ill substance using population, while only a subset of the mentally ill population, is in great need of intervention due to the host of potential costly outcomes associated with this particular combination of classes of disorders. Current attempts to develop interventions to address this problem were highlighted through descriptions of several recent New York City post-booking programs that have adapted and modified models in an attempt to develop efficacious intervention strategies for this target population. These efforts, along with the diversion model features described, require additional research (such as that by Steadman et al., 1999) to clarify the differential effect of discrete models and differential value for population subsets.

REFERENCES

Abram, K.M. & Teplin, L.A. (1991). Co-occurring disorders among mentally ill jail detainees: Implications for public policy. *American Psychologist* *46*(10), 1036–1045.

American Bar Association. (1986). *Criminal justice mental health standards.* Chicago: Author.

Anglin, M.D., Longshore, D. & Turner, S. (1999). Treatment alternatives to street crime: An evaluation of five programs. *Criminal Justice and Behavior, 26*(2), 168–195.

Bahn, C. & Davis, J.R. (1997). An alternative to incarceration: The Fortune Society of New York. *Journal of Offender Rehabilitation, 24*(3/4), 163–181.

Banks, S.M., Stone, J.L., Pandiani, J.A., Cox, J.F. & Morschauser, P.C. (2000). Utilization of local jails and general hospitals by state psychiatric center patients. *Journal of Behavioral Health Services and Research, 27*(4), 454–459.

Barnes, P.G. (1998). Safer streets at what cost? *ABA Journal, 84,* 25.

Barr, H. (1999). *Prisons and jails: Hospitals of last resort.* New York: Correctional Association of New York and the Urban Justice Center.

Belenko, S. (1998). *Research on drug courts: A critical review.* New York: The National Center on Addiction and Substance Abuse (CASA) at Columbia University.

Belenko, S. & Dumanovsky, T. (1993). *Special drug courts: Program brief.* Washington, D.C.: U.S. Department of Justice, Bureau of Justice Assistance, Office of Justice Programs.

Berman, G. & Andersen, D. (1999). *Drugs, courts and neighborhoods.* New York: Center for Court Innovation.

Bond, G.R. (1989). Assertive community treatment of the severely mentally ill: Recent research findings. In K.E. Davis, R. Harris, R. Farmer, J. Reeves & F. Segal (Eds.), *Strengthening the scientific base of social work education for services to the long-term seriously mentally ill* (pp. 411–418). Richmond, VA: Virginia Commonwealth University.

Borum, R. (1999). *Jail diversion strategies for misdemeanor offenders with mental illness: Preliminary report.* Tampa, Florida: Department of Mental Health & Policy, Louis de la Parte Florida Mental Health Institute, University of South Florida.

Borum, R., Swanson, J., Swartz, M. & Hiday, V. (1997). Substance abuse, violent behavior and police encounters among persons with severe mental disorder. *Journal of Contemporary Criminal Justice, 13,* 236–250.

Bowers, M.B., Mazure, C.M., Nelson, J.C. & Jatlow, P.I. (1990). Psychotogenic drug use and neuroleptic response. *Schizophrenia Bulletin, 16*(1), 81–85.

Braun, E.J., Flanagan, T.J. & McLeod, M. (1983). *Sourcebook of criminal justice statistics.* Washington, DC: US Department of Justice, Bureau of Justice Statistics.

Broner, N., Borum, R., Whitmire, L. & Gawley, K. (in press). A review of screening instruments for co-occurring mental illness and substance use in criminal justice programs. In G. Landsberg, M. Rock, L. Berg & A. Smiley (Eds.). *Serving mentally ill offenders: Challenges and opportunities for mental health professionals.* New York: Springer.

Broner, N., Franczak, M., Dye, C. & McAllister, W. (2001). Knowledge transfer, policymaking and community empowerment: A consensus model approach for providing public mental health and substance abuse services. *Psychiatric Quarterly,* 72(1), 79–102.

Broner, Rock, & Landsberg, 1998; New York City Department of Mental Health, Mental Retardation and Alcoholism Services, 1998.

Broner, N., Rock, M. & Landsberg, G. (May, 1998). *Psychosocial and case management issues in services' linkage: A six-month follow-up of a jail diversion program for the mentally ill.* University of Pennsylvania, Mental Health and Public Policy Research Department Rounds.

Brown, J.R. (1997). Drug diversion courts: Are they needed and will they succeed in breaking the cycle of drug-related crime? *Criminal and Civil Confinement, 23,* 63–99.

Bureau of Justice Statistics (1998). *Prison and jail inmates at midyear 1997.* Washington, DC: Office of Justice Programs.

C.A.S.E.S. (2000). *The Nathaniel Project: A new alternative to incarceration program for mentally ill felony offenders in Manhattan* [agency brochure]. New York.

Center for the Study of Issues in Public Mental Health. (1998). Substance use and mental illness. *Center Update, (5)*1, 1.

Center on Crime, Communities & Culture (1996). *Mental illness in US jails: Diverting the nonviolent, low-level offender.* Open Society Institute Occasional Paper Series, 11:1.

Cote, G. & Hodgins, S. (1990). Co-occurring mental disorders among criminal offenders. *Bulletin of the American Academy of Psychiatry and Law, 18,* 271–281.

Deane, M., Steadman, H., Borum, R., Veysey, B. & Morrissey, J. (1998). Police/mental health system interactions: Program types and needed research. *Psychiatric Services, 50,* 99–101.

Ditton, P.M. (July, 1999). *Mental health and treatment of inmates and probationers.* Bureau of Justice Statistics Special Report, NCJ 174463. Washington, DC: U.S. Department of Justice.

Draine, J. & Solomon, P. (1999). Describing and evaluating jail diversion services for persons with serious mental illness. *Psychiatric Services,* 50(1), 56–61.

Drake, R.E., Alterman, A.I. & Rosenberg, S.R. (1993). Detection of substance use disorders in severely mentally ill patients. *Community Mental Health Journal,* 29(2), 175–192.

Drake, R.E., Bartels, S.J., Teague, G.B., Noordsy, D.L. & Clark, R.E. (1993). Treatment of substance abuse in severely mentally ill patients. *Journal of Nervous and Mental Disease,* 181(10), 606–611.

Drake, R.E., McHugo, G.J. & Noordsy, D.L. (1993). Treatment of alcoholism among schizophrenic patients: Four-year-outcomes. *American Journal of Psychiatry,* 150(2), 328–329.

Drake, R.E., McLaughlin, P., Pepper, B. & Minkoff, K. (1991). Dual diagnosis of major mental illness and substance use disorder: An overview. *New Directions for Mental Health Services, 50,* 3–12.

Drake, R.E., Mercer-McFadden, C., Mueser, K.T., McHugo, G.J. & Bond, G.R. (1998). Review of integrated mental health and substance abuse treatment for patients with dual disorders. *Schizophrenia Bulletin, 24*(4), 589–608.

Edens, J.F., Peters, R.H. & Hills, H.A. (1997). Treating prison inmates with co-occurring disorders: An integrative review of existing programs. *Behavioral Sciences and the Law, 15,* 439–457.

El-Bassel, N., Gilbert, L., Schilling, R.F., Ivanoff, A. & Borne, D. (1996). Correlates of crack abuse among drug-using incarcerated women: Psychological trauma, social support and coping behavior. *American Journal of Drug and Alcohol Abuse, 22*(1), 41–56.

Fabrega, H., Mezzich, J. & Ullrich, R.F. (1988). Black-white differences in psychopathology in an urban psychiatric population. *Comprehensive Psychiatry, 29,* 285–297.

Fiander, M. & Bartlett, A.E.A. (1997). Missed "psychiatric" cases? The effectiveness of a court diversion scheme. *Alcohol and Alcoholism, 32*(6), 715–723.

Freidberg, A. (1997). Court specialization in mental health cases opens. Judge hopes to stop offenders from "revolving through the system." *Sun-sentinel,* June 17, 1997: 1b.

Fullilove, M.T., Fullilove, R.E., Smith, M., Winkler, K., Michael, C., Panzer, P.G. & Wallace, R. (1993). Violence, trauma, and post-traumatic stress disorder among women drug users. *Journal of Traumatic Stress, 6,* 533–543.

Gelles, R.J. & Harrop, J.W. (1989). Violence, battering, and psychological distress among women. *Journal of Interpersonal Violence, 4,* 400–420.

Goldkamp, J. & Irons-Guynn, C. (2000). *Emerging judicial strategies for the mentally ill in the criminal caseload: Mental health courts in Fort Lauderdale, Seattle, San Bernardino, and Anchorage.* Philadelphia: Crime and Justice Research Institute.

Gordon, M. (1994). 54th Street: Midtown Community Court. *New York Magazine,* December 5, 1994.

Hall, R.C., Popkin, M.K., Devaul, R. & Stickney, S.K. (1977). The effect of unrecognized drug abuse on diagnosis and therapeutic outcome. *American Journal of Drug and Alcohol Abuse, 4*(4), 455–465.

Haywood, T.W., Kravitz, H.M., Goldman, L.B. & Freeman, A. (2000). Characteristics of women in jail and treatment orientations. *Behavior Modification, 24*(3), 307–324.

Hellerstein, D.J. & Meehan, B. (1987). Outpatient group therapy for schizophrenic substance abusers. *American Journal of Psychiatry, 144,* 1337–1339.

Henderson, D.J. (1997). Drug abuse and incarcerated women: A research review. *Journal of Substance Abuse Treatment, 15*(6), 579–587.

Hiller, M.L., Knight, K., Broome, K.M. & Simpson D.D. (1996). Compulsory community-based substance abuse treatment and the mentally ill criminal offender. *The Prison Journal, 76*(2), 180–191.

Hoff, R.A., Baranosky, M.V., Buchanan, J., Zonana, H. & Rosenheck, R.A. (1999). The effects of a jail diversion program on incarceration: A retrospective cohort study. *Journal of American Academy of Psychiatry and Law, 27*(3), 377–386.

Holden, P., Rann, J. & Van Drasek, L. (1993). *Unheard voices: A report on women in Michigan Jails.* Lansing, MI: Michigan Women's Commission.

Inciardi, J.A., McBride, D.C. & Rivers, J.E. (1996). *Drug control and the courts.* Thousand Oaks, CA: Sage.

Jacobson, A. & Herald, C. (1990). The relevance of childhood sexual abuse to adult psychiatric inpatient care. *Hospital and Community Psychiatry, 41*, 154–158.

Jerrell, J.M. & Ridgely, M.S. (1995). Comparative effectiveness of three approaches to serving people with severe mental illness and substance abuse disorders. *Journal of Nervous and Mental Disease, 183*(9), 566–576.

Jordan, B.K., Schlenger, W.E., Fairbank, J.A. & Caddell, J.M. (1996). Prevalence of psychiatric disorders among incarcerated women. *Archives of General Psychiatry, 53*(6), 513–519.

Kofoed, L., Kania, J., Walsh, T. & Atkinson, R.M. (1986). Outpatient treatment of patients with substance abuse and coexisting psychiatric disorders. *American Journal of Psychiatry, 143*(7), 867–872.

Lamb, H.R., & Weinberger, L.E. (1998). Persons with severe mental illness in jails and prisons: A review. *Psychiatric Services, 49*(4), 483–492.

Lamon, S.S., Cohen, N.L. & Broner, N. (in press). New York City's system of criminal justice mental health services. In G. Landsberg, M. Rock, L. Berg & A. Smiley (Eds.). *Serving mentally ill offenders: Challenges and opportunities for mental health professionals.* New York: Springer.

McBride, D.C. (1978). In J.A. Inciardi & K.C. Haas (Eds.), *Criminal justice diversion crime and the criminal justice process* (pp. 246–259). Dubuque, IA: Kendall/Hunt.

McFarland, B. Faulkner, L., Bloom, & J., Hallaux, R. (1989). Chronic mental illness and the criminal justice system. *Hospital and Community Psychiatry, 41*, 718–723.

Michaels, D., Zoloth, S.R., Alchabes, P., Braslow, C.A., & Safyer, S. (1992). Homelessness and indicators of mental illness among inmates in New York City's correctional system. *Hospital and Community Psychiatry, 43*(2), 150–154.

Miller, N.S. & Ries, R.K. (1991). Drug and alcohol dependence and psychiatric populations: The need for diagnosis, intervention, and training. *Comprehensive Psychiatry, 32*, 268–276.

Monahan, J. (1995). Clinical and actuarial predictions of violence. In D. Faigman (Ed.), *Modern science evidence: The law and science of expert witness testimony, Vol. 1.* St. Paul: West Publishing.

Mueser, K.T., Drake, R.E., & Miles, K.M. (1997). The course and treatment of substance use disorder in persons with severe mental illness. In L.S. Onken, J.D. Blaine, S.Genser, & A.M. Horton (Eds.), *Treatment of drug-dependent individuals with comorbid mental disorders* (pp. 86–109). Rockville, MD: National Institute on Drug Abuse.

Myers, J. K., Weissman, M. M., Tischler, G. L., Holzer, C. E. III, Leaf, P. J., Orvaschel, H., Anthony, J. C., Boyd, J. H., Burke, J. D., Kramer, M. & Stoltzman, R. (1984). Six-month prevalence of psychiatric disorders in three communities: 1980–1982. *Archives of General Psychiatry, 41*(10), 959–967.

National GAINS Center (Summer, 1999a). *Maintaining Medicaid benefits for jail detainees with co-occurring mental health and substance use disorders.* Delmar, New York.

National GAINS Center (Summer, 1999b). *Using management information systems to locate people with serious mental illness and co-occurring substance use disorders in the criminal justice system.* Delmar, New York: Author.

National GAINS Center (July, 1999c). *The courage to change: A guide for communities to create integrated services for people with co-occurring disorders in the justice system.* Delmar, New York: Author.

National Institute of Justice, U.S. Department of Justice. (1992). *Searching for Answers: Annual evaluation report on drugs and crime.* Washington, DC: Author.

New York City Department of Mental Health, Mental Retardation and Alcoholism Services (1996). *Local government plan: Adult mental health services.* New York.

New York City Department of Mental Health, Mental Retardation and Alcoholism Services (1998). *Local government plan: Adult mental health services 1998–2003.* New York: Author.

Osher, F.C. & Drake, R.E. (1996). Revising a history of unmet needs: Approaches to care of persons with co-occurring addictive and mental disorders. *American Journal of Orthopsychiatry, 66*(1), 4–11.

Osher, F.C., Drake, R.E., Noorsdy, D.L., Teague, G.B., Hurlbut, S.C. & Paskus, T.J. (1994). Correlates and outcomes of alcohol use disorder among rural schizophrenic outpatients. *Journal of Clinical Psychiatry, 55,* 109–113.

Osher, F.C. & Kofoed, L.L. (1989). Treatment of patients with psychiatric and psychoactive substance abuse disorders. *Hospital and Community Psychiatry, 40*(10), 1025–1030.

Paradis, C.M., Horn, L., Yang, C. M. & O'Rourke, T. (1999). Ethnic differences in assessment and treatment of affective disorders in a jail population. *Journal of Offender Rehabilitation, 28*(3–4), 23–32.

Pepper, B., & Hendrickson, E.L. (1998). *Developing a cross training project for substance abuse, mental health and criminal justice professionals working with offenders with co-existing disorders (substance abuse/mental illness).* www.monumental.com/arcturus/dd/ddhome.htm

Peters, R.H. & Hills, H.A. (1999). Community treatment and supervision strategies for offenders with co-occurring disorders: What works? In E. Latessa (Ed.), *Strategic solutions: The International Community Corrections Association examines substance abuse* (pp. 81–137). Lanham, MD: American Correctional Association.

Peters, R.H. & Hills, H.A. (1997). *Intervention strategies for offenders with co-occurring disorders: What works?* Delmar, NY: The National GAINS Center.

Peters, R.H., Kearns, W.D., Murrin, M.R. & Dolente, A.S. (1992). Psychopathology and mental health needs among drug-involved inmates. *Journal of Prison and Jail Health, 11,* 3–25.

Peters, R.H. & Murrin, M.R. (2000). Effectiveness of treatment-based drug courts in reducing criminal recidivism. *Criminal Justice and Behavior, 27*(1), 72–96.

Peters, R.H. & Peyton, E. (1998). *Guideline for drug courts on screening and assessment.* Washington, DC: U.S. Department of Justice, Office of Justice Programs, Drug Courts Program Office.

Polcin, D.L. (1992). Issues in the treatment of dual diagnosis clients who have chronic mental illness. *Professional Psychological Research and Practice, 23,* 30–37.

RachBeisel, J., Scott, J. & Dixon, L. (1999). Co-occurring severe mental illness and substance use disorders: A review of recent research. *Psychiatric Services, 50*(11), 1427–1434.

Rayburn, T.M. & Stonecypher, J.F. (1996). Diagnostic differences related to age and race of involuntarily committed psychiatric patients. *Psychological Reports, 73,* 881–882.

Richie, B.E. & Johnsen, C. (1996). Abuse histories among newly incarcerated women in a New York City jail. *Journal of the Medical Women's Association, 51*(3), 111–114.

Ridgely, S.M., Goldman, H.H. & Willenbring, M. (1990). Barriers to the care of persons with dual diagnosis: Organizational and financing issues. *Schizophrenia Bulletin, 16,* 123–132.

Ries, R. & Ellingson, T. (1989). A pilot assessment at one month of 17 dual diagnosis patients. *Hospital and Community Psychiatry, 41,* 1230–1233.

Rock, M. & Landsberg, G. (1998). County mental health directors' perspective on forensic mental health developments in New York State. *Administration and Policy in Mental Health, 25*(2), 327–332.

Rosenheck, R.A., Banks, S., Pandiani, J. & Hoff, R. (2000). Bed closures and incarceration rates among users of veterans affairs mental health services. *Psychiatric Services, 51*(10), 1282–1287.

Sacks, S. (2000). Co-occurring mental and substance abuse disorders:

Promising approaches and research issues. *Journal of Substance Use & Misuse, 35*(12–14), 2061–2093.

Sciacca, K. (1991). An integrated treatment approach for severely mentally ill individuals with substance abuse disorders. *New Directions for Mental Health Services, 50,* 69–84.

Shenson, D., Dubler, N. & Michaels, D. (1990). Jails and prisons: The new asylums. *American Journal of Public Health, 80*(6), 655–656.

Sherman, S.A. & Taxman, F.S. (1998). What is the status of my client? Automation in a seamless case management system for substance abusing offenders. *The Journal of Offender Monitoring, 31,* 25–27.

Spence, C.N. (1997). The impact of the deinstitutionalization movement upon the criminal justice system: A Georgia case study. *Prison Litigation and Inmates Rights.* Roxbury Publishing.

Steadman, H.J., Barbera, S.S. & Dennis, D.L. (1994). A national survey of jail diversion programs for mentally ill detainees. *Hospital and Community Psychiatry, 45*(11), 1109–1113.

Steadman, H.J., Cocozza, J.J. & Veysey, B.M. (1999). Comparing outcomes for diverted and nondiverted jail detainees with mental illness. *Law and Human Behavior, 23*(6), 615–627.

Steadman, H.J., Deane, M.W., Morrissey, J.P., Westcott, M.L., Salasin, S. & Shapiro, S. (1999). A SAMHSA research initiative assessing the effectiveness of jail diversion programs for mentally ill persons. *Psychiatric Services, 50*(12) 1620–1623.

Steadman, H.J., Morris, S.M. & Dennis, D.L. (1995). The diversion of mentally ill persons from jails to community-based services: A profile of programs. *American Journal of Public Health 85*(12), 1630–1635.

Steadman H.J., Mulvey, E.P., Monahan, J., Robbins, P.C., Appelbaum, P.S., Grisson, T., Roth, L.H. & Silver, E. (1998). Violence by people discharged from acute psychiatric inpatient facilities and by others in the same neighborhoods. *Archives of General Psychiatry, 55,* 339–401.

Steadman, H.J., Davidson, S. & Brown, C. (2001). Law and psychiatry: Mental health courts: Their promise and unanswered questions. *Psychiatric Services, 52*(4), 457–458.

Substance Abuse Mental Health Services Administration (SAMHSA) (2000). *Cultural Competence Standards.* Rockville, MD: U.S. Department of Health and Human Services, SAMHSA.

Substance Abuse Mental Health Services Administration, Office of Applied Studies. (1997). Unpublished data from the 1996 National Household Survey on Drug Abuse. In B.A. Rouse (Ed.) *Substance abuse and mental health statistics source book.* Rockville, MD: U.S. Department of Health and Human Services, SAMHSA.

Sung, H.E., Tabachnick, C. & Feng, L. (1999). *DTAP ninth annual report.* New York: District Attorney's Office, Kings County.

Swartz, M., Swanson, J., Hiday, V., Borum, R. & Wagner, R. (1998). Violence and severe mental illness: The effects of substance abuse and nonadherence to medication. *American Journal of Psychiatry, 155,* 226–231.

Swartz, M., Swanson, J., Wagner, R., Burns, B., Hiday, V. & Borum, R. (1999). Can voluntary outpatient commitment reduce hospital recidivism? Findings from a randomized controlled trail in severely mentally ill individuals. *American Journal of Psychiatry, 156*(12).

Tabachnick, C. (1999). *Treatment alternatives for the dually diagnosed quarterly report.* New York: New York State Division of Criminal Justice Services.

Teplin, L.A. (1994). Psychiatric and substance abuse disorders among male urban jail detainees. *American Journal of Public Health, 84,* 292–293.

Teplin, L.A., Abram, K.M. & McClelland, G.M. (1996). Prevalence of psychiatric disorders among incarcerated women. *Archives of General Psychiatry, 53,* 505–512.

Timler, S. & Linn, K. (1999). *An examination of treatment placements, January 1998–December 1998: New York City TASC.* New York: Education and Assistance Corporation (EAC), Criminal Justice Division.

Torrey, E.F., Steiber, J., Ezekiel, J., Wolfe, S.M., Sharfstein, J. & Flynn, L.M. (1993). Criminalizing the mentally ill: The abuse of jails as mental hospitals. *Innovations & Research, 2,* 11–14. Washington, DC: Public Citizen's Health Research Group.

U.S. Department of Justice Statistics (1997). *Correctional populations in the United States.* NCJ-163916.

Watson, A. Hanrahan, P., Luchins, D. & Lurigio, A. (2001). Mental health courts and the complex issues of mentally ill offenders. *Psychiatric Services, 52*(4), 477–481.

Weiss, R.D. & Najavits, L.M. (1998). Overview of treatment modalities for dual diagnosis patients: Pharmacology, psychotherapy, and 12–step programs. In H.R. Kranzler & B.J. Rousaville (Eds.), *Dual diagnosis and treatment: Substance abuse and comorbid medical and psychiatric disorders.* New York: Marcel Dekker.

Wexler, H.K. & Graham, W.F. (August, 1993). *Prison-based therapeutic community for substance abusers: Six month evaluation findings.* American Psychological Association, Toronto, Canada.

Winerip, M. (1999). After eight years drift, treatment in jail; advocates seek another change for a schizophrenic inmate. New York Times, June 3, 1999.

Young, A.M. & Boyd, C. (2000). Sexual trauma, substance abuse and treatment success in a sample of African-American women who smoke crack cocaine. *Substance Abuse, 21*(10), 9–19.

8

Jail Diversion in a Managed Care Environment: The Arizona Experience

Michael Franczak and Michael S. Shafer

By its very nature, the process of providing diversionary alternatives to jail for persons with co-occurring disorders requires extensive collaboration and cooperation. A whole host of agencies and organizations, including local law enforcement, courts, prosecuting and public defender offices, community behavioral health and substance abuse providers, and payor organizations, often approach this issue with different orientations, philosophies, and missions. As noted by Steadman (1992) & Steadman, Morris & Dennis (1995), an effective and comprehensive approach to providing jail diversion alternatives to persons with psychiatric disabilities is not possible without a number of critical preliminary activities that set the stage for the trust and cooperation that is necessary to create a successful program. In addition to an informed and enlightened criminal justice system, effective jail diversion programs are predicated on the presence of a comprehensive, responsive, and accountable behavioral health system. Without such a community-based behavioral health system, diversion efforts result in individuals being diverted "FROM" jail without the infrastructure of programs and services that allow the individual to be diverted "TO" effective community-based treatment. Such poorly organized programs

Preparation of this manuscript was supported in part by Grant No. 6 UIG SM52160-03-1 from the U.S. Department of Health and Human Services, Substance Abuse and Mental Health Services Administration. The opinions expressed in this manuscript are strictly those of the authors and no endorsement by the funding agency is to be inferred. Address correspondence to Dr. Michael S. Shafer, University of Arizona School of Public Administration & Policy, PO Box 210299, Tucson, AZ 85721 or shafer@u.arizona.edu.

may produce very short-term results that may eventually prove harmful to the person and the community.

Complicating the development of jail diversion alternatives is the increasing reliance of state agencies upon managed care contracting systems (Edmunds, Frank, Hogan, McCarty, Beale & Weisner, 1997) to control their publicly funded behavioral health care delivery systems. Driven by the concepts of capitated funding and risk-based contracting, managed care contracting forces service delivery systems to carefully assess their service systems response to high-cost clients, such as individuals with criminal justice involvement. In order to maximize the responsiveness of managed care systems to the needs of individuals with criminal justice involvement, it is essential that state agencies implement appropriate contractual specifications, licensing standards, and practice guidelines that provide meaningful incentives for managed care systems to address the needs of this critical population.

This chapter describes the development, structure, and operation of jail diversion and other criminal justice initiatives that have been developed in the state of Arizona to meet the needs of its behavioral health care population. This chapter will provide an overview to the structure of the behavioral health care system in the state, identify and describe a number of initiatives in place, and provide recommendations for creating responsive behavioral health care systems for addressing the needs of persons with criminal justice involvement within managed care contracting systems.

THE STRUCTURE OF THE ARIZONA BEHAVIORAL HEALTH CARE SYSTEM

The state agency responsible for the delivery of public health and behavioral health services (including both mental health and substance abuse) is the Arizona Department of Health Services (ADHS), Division of Behavioral Health Services (DBHS) which is responsible for planning, administering, and monitoring a comprehensive system of services for adults with a serious mental illness (SMI) and seriously emotionally disturbed (SED) children. DBHS is also mandated to administer a unified behavioral health service system that includes substance abuse services, prevention services and inpatient psychiatric care through the Arizona State Hospital. In 1999, the state-funded behavioral health system had an enrolled population of 71,634 individuals—approximately 19,635 individuals with a serious mental illness, 19,422 children, 14,534 individuals with general mental health issues, and 17,135 individuals with a substance abuse disorders.

The trend toward managed behavioral health care has taken hold in the public sector as more states adopt a variety of models of managed care service delivery. As resources become increasingly limited, managed care offers the capacity for greater value for all stakeholders through the use of cost controls and increased emphasis on quality assurance and quality control functions. Arizona's history in delivering managed behavioral health care began in the early 1990s, but the roots of managed care concepts began in primary health care in 1982. At that time, the Health Care Financing Administration (HCFA) granted approval for an 1115 waiver to the Arizona Health Care Cost Containment System (AHCCCS), Arizona's state Medicaid agency. The program was based on a managed care principles of a pre-paid, capitated system of care. Under the 1115 waiver, Arizona received permission to delay implementation of the Medicaid behavioral health services. The passage of legislation in 1990 established the mandate to provide a program of behavioral health services for Medicaid-eligible children. DBHS worked closely with AHCCCS to implement Medicaid-covered behavioral health services which eventually covered all eligible populations. With the advent of Medicaid funding, Arizona initially developed a fee-for-service model of service delivery. However, in just two short years the decision was made to move to a capitated, managed care service delivery system. While the new environment challenged the operational paradigms of the status quo, the system has introduced mechanisms intended to enhance service arrays taking the form of a defined package of services, financial viability and efforts of continuous quality improvement, and accountability. The current fiscal basis for behavioral health services includes federal Medicaid dollars distributed on a capitated basis, funds appropriated each year by the Arizona Legislature, and the federal substance abuse and mental health block grant funds distributed on a monthly basis (Arizona Department of Health, Division of Behavioral Health, 1999).

THE REGIONAL BEHAVIORAL HEALTH SYSTEM

Community-based behavioral health services in Arizona are delivered through contracts with Regional Behavioral Health Authorities (RBHAs). The RBHAs are private organizations that function in a similar fashion to a health maintenance organization (HMO). RBHAs are responsible for assessing the service needs in their region and developing a plan to meet those needs. The RBHA system has been integrated for a number of years, making one system responsible for coordinating alcohol, drug, and behavioral health services for all populations. The RBHAs develop a network of providers to deliver a full range of behavioral health care services, including prevention programs for adults and children, and a full continuum of services for adults with substance abuse and general mental health disorders, adults with serious mental illness, and children with serious emotional disturbance. The RBHAs are required to ensure that services are physically, geographically, and culturally accessible to all eligible persons in their geographic service area. Medicaid-eligible clients, both adults and children, are entitled to all medically necessary services to meet their behavioral health needs. Services are provided to the rest of the population based upon a sliding fee scale once they are screened and determined to meet diagnostic criteria.

The RBHAs act as the referral resource for individuals in need of behavioral health services. These individuals may be referred to the system, either through self-referral or referral by a primary care physician, provider or any other community source. Individuals referred for services are assessed for immediate and ongoing needs.

There are three contract areas that are critical in order to set the stage for the development of effective jail diversion efforts. ADHS/DBHS requires that RBHAs participate in collaboration with other agencies and develop comprehensive crisis systems and outreach services. ADHS/DBHS monitors contract requirements on an ongoing basis, through both formal and informal mechanisms. In addition to directly participating in many of the collaborative efforts, ADHS/DBHS formally monitors collaborative efforts, the crisis system, and outreach during annual operational/financial reviews. Each of these requirements is described below.

(1) Collaboration with other State and Local Agencies

As part of their contract with ADHS/DBHS the RBHAs are required to engage in collaborative efforts with fire, police, EMS, hospital emergency departments, and other providers of public health and safety services to: a) coordinate dispatch, assessment, transportation, and crisis interventions with local community crisis providers (police, fire, ambulance, county health departments, hospitals); b) develop protocols for and education on the appropriate use of the RBHA's crisis services vs. hospital emergency departments; and c) meet regularly with representatives of fire, police, EMS, and hospital emergency departments to coordinate services and to assess and improve the RBHA's crisis response services.

The RBHAs also collaborate with community and government agencies to coordinate the delivery of covered services with other services and supports needed by enrolled persons and their families, including: general medical care; education; probation; parole; court services; services to the homeless; services for persons with developmental disabilities; services for the elderly; emergency medical services; child welfare; parks and recreation; supports from religious institutions; housing and urban development; and vocational services.

In addition to collaboration, coordination with other state agencies is a significant activity of the Regional Behavioral Health Authorities. In Arizona these agencies include the Arizona Department of Corrections (ADC), Arizona Department of Juvenile Corrections (ADJC), Administrative Offices of the Court (AOC), and the Juvenile and Superior Courts. The Regional Behavioral Health Authority is required to ensure that: a) information and recommendations contained in the probation or parole case plan are considered in the development of service plans for enrolled persons, and that probation or parole personnel involved with enrolled persons are invited to participate in development of the behavioral health service plan and all subsequent planning meetings; b) detention centers are informed of the availability of behavioral health services and of procedures to refer enrolled or eligible persons for services; and c) upon referral or request, the RBHA or its providers evaluate and participate in transition planning prior to the release of eligible children and adolescents from public institutions back into the community.

With respect to coordination with the county jail systems, the RBHAs are required to conduct screening and assessment services for individuals who are in jail and are suspected to have a serious mental illness and to provide continuity of care, discharge planning, and timely sharing of information for enrolled persons with a serious mental illness who are in or are leaving the jail.

One specific example of collaboration is the requirement that RBHAs participate in the Arizona Council on Offenders with Mental Impairments (ACOMI). In 1992, the Arizona Legislature established the ACOMI. This 21-member council recommends state policy for the identification, diversion, and treatment of individuals with mental impairments (including persons with mental illness and persons with mental retardation) who are involved with, or at risk of becoming involved with, the criminal justice system (Arizona Council on Offenders with Mental Impairments, 1999). The council meets on a monthly basis throughout the state, touring local jails, correctional facilities, law enforcement units, and behavioral health agencies. In addition to the state-wide council, there are local interagency councils, providing coordinating and communication among the RBHAs, local treatment providers, law enforcement, corrections, and justice-related systems. The accompanying table delineates the mandates of the council.

(2) Crisis Services

An adequate array of responsive crisis services provides an alternative to incarceration. When police officers have an array of options to incarceration and have received training in using the options, inappropriate

Table 8.1 Mandates of the Arizona Council on Offenders with Mental Impairments

1. Protecting the rights of persons with mental impairments who are involved in or at risk of involvement in the criminal justice
2. Ensuring the safety of the general public while preserving the well-being of persons with mental impairments who are involved in or at risk of involvement in the criminal justice system
3. Determining the status of offenders with mental impairments who are in the state criminal justice system
4. Identifying the needed services for offenders with mental impairments
5. Developing a plan for meeting the treatment, rehabilitative, and educational needs of offenders with mental impairments that include the development of community-based alternatives to incarceration
6. Coordinating the delivery of services to offenders with mental impairments
7. Tracking programs both in this state and other states for offenders with mental impairments and recommending methods of improving programs to the directors of state agencies
8. Collecting and disseminating information about available programs to judicial officers, probation and parole officers, and the general public
9. Providing technical assistance to agencies and organizations in the development of appropriate training programs
10. Establishing a psychiatric security review board
11. Establishing computer linkages of psychiatric units and the intake and treatment areas of hospitals so that case-managed patients can be quickly and easily identified and, if appropriate, released to case managers or to community agencies
12. Securing additional services for persons with serious mental illness who are incarcerated
13. Establishing increased levels of case management available to mentally ill persons who are released from incarceration
14. Expanding transition programs to assist incarcerated mentally ill persons who are released from incarceration
15. Developing a statewide forensic psychiatric data information system that would monitor service efforts and provide basic statistics on prevalence and incidence rates of mentally disordered persons being processed throughout the state's criminal justice system

---

Table 8.1 *(continued)*

---

16. Establishing requirements to ensure that the training of law enforcement officers includes instruction to recognize mentally ill persons, procedures to detain and commit the mentally ill to a psychiatric facility, and procedures to obtain court ordered custodial evaluations
17. Changing the current law in order to allow law enforcement officers to place individuals who are subject to arrest and who display obvious signs of psychosis in a secure evaluation center for 72 hours before charges are filed against that person
18. Developing a plan for a front-end jail diversion program for offenders with mental impairments that would place these persons in a treatment program before they are prosecuted
19. Allowing law enforcement officers and certain providers of health care to temporarily place persons who display obvious signs of psychosis in a secure setting

---

incarcerations are avoided. RBHA crisis services are designed for crisis prevention, intervention and resolution, triage, and transfer, and must be provided in the least restrictive setting possible, consistent with need and community safety. Each urban Regional Behavioral Health Authority is required to maintain a 24-hour, seven-day-a-week crisis response service for eligible and enrolled persons that meets all of the following requirements: a) crisis telephone number; b) face-to-face mobile crisis services within one hour of referral; and c) 24-hour crisis walk-in services in at least one location. The RBHAs are required to ensure effective coordination among and between these systems, as delineated in the accompanying table.

(3) Outreach

Another alternative to incarceration is an effective behavioral health outreach program. When individuals who are at risk of incarceration are actively identified and engaged in services, their chance of inappropriate involvement in the criminal justice system is minimized. The RBHAs are required to conduct ongoing outreach efforts to ensure that they are identifying persons in need of behavioral health services. These outreach activities are aimed at populations who are traditionally hard to reach, such as the homeless and individuals who are involved in the criminal justice.

**Regional Behavioral Health Authorities' Responsibilities
Related to Mental Health Crisis Services Coordination**

- Coordinate dispatch, assessment, transportation, and crisis interventions with local community crisis providers (police, fire, ambulance, county health departments, hospitals).
- Develop protocols for and education of EMS, fire, and law enforcement personnel on: identifying and handling psychiatric crises, familiarity with the RBHA network of service providers, and the appropriate use of the RBHA's crisis services vs. hospital emergency departments.
- Meet regularly with representatives of fire, police, EMS, and hospital emergency departments to coordinate services and to assess and improve the RBHA's crisis response services.

The RBHAs are required to design and implement outreach tailored to the special characteristics of the population, including: a) geographic or social isolation; b) serious and persistent mental illness; c) homelessness; d) language barrier; e) adult or juvenile criminal justice involvement; f) poverty; g) injection drug use; h) pregnancy and/or presence of dependent children; and i) involvement with child protective services.

ARIZONA CRIMINAL JUSTICE SYSTEM

During an average year, nearly 110,000 individuals are booked into the Maricopa County Jail System serving metropolitan Phoenix, and an additional 26,000 individuals are booked into Tucson's Pima County Detention Center. The Maricopa County Jail has an average daily census of 6,600 prisoners. In 1978, a psychiatric unit was established in the Maricopa County Jail. A second unit was added to the Madison Street Jail in 1985. These two licensed facilities serve approximately 110 inmates on a daily basis. The Pima County Jail has an average daily census of 1,325. In Pima County, a Mental Health Unit (MHU) was added to the Pima County Detention Center in 1986 and has the capacity to house 49 individuals. During the past year, the average daily attendance in the MHU was 40 individuals.

RBHA-BASED JAIL DIVERSION EFFORTS

At this time, formalized programs of diverting individuals with mental illness and/or co-occurring disorders are in place in Tucson and Phoenix. Combined, these two communities represent a general population of 2.7

million, representing 81% of the population of the state. Phoenix and Tucson are served by two Regional Behavioral Health Authorities (RBHAs) contracted by the state to manage the provision of publicly funded behavioral health services. In 1999, the state reported a total of 19,625 individuals statewide meeting legislative criteria as seriously mentally ill. Of these individuals, ValueOptions (VO) in Phoenix served 11,200 while 4,284 were served in Tucson by the Community Partnership of Southern Arizona (CPSA). Combined, these two agencies serve approximately 80% of all individuals identified as seriously mentally ill in the state of Arizona. Using a conservative prevalence estimate of 50% (Drake, Rosenberg & Mueser, 1996) ADHS/DBHS projected that nearly 7,750 individuals served by ValueOptions and CPSA have had or will experience a co-occurring substance abuse disorder at some point in their lives.

ARIZONA'S THREE-TIERED MODEL OF JAIL DIVERSION

After extensive study, consultation with national experts, and numerous public hearings, the Arizona Council on Offenders with Mental Impairments (ACOMI) endorsed a three-tiered model of jail diversion for persons with serious mental illness. This model is described in the accompanying table. While the two participating RBHAs serving Phoenix and Tucson have implemented diversion alternatives that are consistent with the three-tier model, minor variations in implementation warrant discussion.

ValueOptions (VO)

ValueOptions, which serves the greater metropolitan community of Phoenix, provides a vast array of resources devoted to diverting individuals with serious mental illness from the criminal justice system. Front-end diversions occur through the ValueOptions Crisis network which includes Mobile teams and Urgent Care Centers. Police officers have priority status for crisis response. The Forensic Team of ValueOptions performs the remaining program tiers. This team is comprised of a forensic clinical specialist, a clinical court liaison, a team leader, seven case managers, one half-time RN, one half-time psychiatrist, a team secretary, an office manager, and a community support worker. The forensic clinical specialist and court liaison work in the county jail Monday through Friday from 7:00a.m. to 4:00p.m. to help identify potential clients for diversion and to assist the jail staff in dealing with mentally disordered offenders. There are also many other clients receiving the assistance of the forensic clinical specialist and court liaison that may not end up on the forensic team for case management; these account for many tier 2 and tier 3 diversions. Approximately 30 clients per month are diverted through these three tiers.

Table 8.2 Arizona's Four-Tiered Diversion Program

Tier 1: Post-Booking: Release from Jail with Conditions	As the first tier of post-booking diversion, individuals who are identified as seriously mentally ill may be released from jail with special conditions related to their need for further evaluation and/or treatment. Individuals currently served by ValueOptions or CPSA are interviewed by the jail diversion team of each agency (VO or CPSA), with subsequent contact with the individual's case management team. Based upon the jail team's interview, a recommendation for release with special conditions may be developed and made to the Initial Appearance (IA) court judge. If the client is released, the case manager is notified and provided with the specifications regarding the special conditions that the individual must follow. In Maricopa County, supervision of the individual regarding these special conditions remains the responsibility of the case manager. In contrast, in Pima County, supervision responsibilities remain the function of the Pre-Trial Services Unit of the Court.
Tier 2: Post-Booking: Deferred Prosecution	Deferred prosecution can occur at any time during Deferred Prosecution the court process as a follow-up to individuals issued field citations, individuals released from jail with special conditions, and individuals booked and detained prior to adjudication. This method of diversion involves an agreement between the RBHA and the prosecutor's office specifying special treatment/intervention conditions that the individual must follow. Time frames for these types of programs are usually four to six months. If the individual complies with the treatment requirements, the charges are dismissed at the end of the specified time frame. If the individual fails to adhere to the requirements, the prosecutor's office may, at its discretion, resume prosecution and incarceration.

Table 8.2 *(continued)*

Tier 3: Post-Booking: Summary Probation	Summary probation involves agreement between the RBHA and prosecutor's office to specific conditions that the individual must meet in order to avoid incarceration. However, the Summary Probation Grant does not result in the dismissal of criminal prosecution, only criminal incarceration.

Community Partnership of Southern Arizona (CPSA)

CPSA also provides a three-tiered diversion model. However, since CPSA does not provide mental health services directly, these diversion alternatives are provided through CPSA's network of four Comprehensive Service Providers (CSPs) which are fully capitated, at-risk community mental health providers and the court's pretrial services. There are no specialty Forensic Case Management Teams in CPSA's region. Rather, the RBHA works closely with Pretrial Services that provides supervision and monitoring of those individuals released from jail with conditions as well as those receiving deferred prosecution. CPSA employs two criminal justice specialists to develop, implement, and coordinate diversion programs throughout the community. Duties include monitoring the population of the Pima County Adult Detention Center for RBHA members who may become incarcerated, encouraging CSPs to ensure continuity of care for their incarcerated clients, and working as a liaison with local criminal justice system components to address the treatment needs of the CPSA members. Front-end diversion is provided through a combination of hot lines, warm-lines, crisis centers, and mobile crisis response teams. The Pre-Trial Services Unit of the Superior Court provides third party supervision to program participants and monitors compliance with conditions of release.

RBHA RESPONSIBILITIES RELATED TO PROBATION AND PAROLE

Special provisions have been put in place to ensure effective coordination between the Regional Behavioral Health Authorities and the various agencies responsible for the incarceration and supervision of individuals with psychiatric disabilities who are under criminal justice supervision. In Arizona these agencies include the Arizona Department of Corrections

(ADC), Arizona Department of Juvenile Corrections (ADJC), Administrative Offices of the Court (AOC), and the Juvenile and Superior Courts. The Regional Behavioral Health Authority is required to ensure that:

1. information and recommendations contained in the probation or parole case plan are considered in the development of service plans for enrolled persons, and that probation or parole personnel involved with enrolled persons are invited to participate in development of the behavioral health service plan and all subsequent planning meetings;
2. detention centers are informed of the availability of behavioral health services and of procedures to refer enrolled or eligible persons for services; and
3. upon referral or request, the RBHA or its providers evaluate and participate in transition planning prior to the release of eligible children and adolescents from public institutions back into the community.

The result of collaborative efforts between the Division of Behavioral Health and the Arizona Department of Corrections, the Correctional Officer/Offender Liaison program has created liaison positions within the RBHAs to coordinate with local parole officers. These liaison positions facilitate appropriate service placement of offenders who are clients of the RBHA by:

1. making referrals for services based on availability and recommendations of the parole officer;
2. facilitating the collection of required authorization information (Referral Forms, Client Right, Appeals/Grievance, Confidentiality, Consent to Treatment);
3. coordinating the collection of progress reports to the client/offenders parole officer;
4. coordinating the reporting of all incidents of client/offender non-participation/ compliance within 48 hours of incident; and
5. maintaining a current roster of client/offender referrals and case status.

SUMMARY AND CONCLUSIONS

The Arizona experiment in providing jail diversion services is a study in process. Of particular note is the operations of these systems of outreach, assessment, linkage, and treatment within risk-based, capitated contracting systems. Promoting such a system of care has been achieved in part by identifying and responding to the needs and contingencies of the various stakeholders affected by such programs. Through the use of an overarching interagency body such as the Arizona Council on Offenders, the issues, needs, and restrictions of the various diverse organizational bodies could be heard and organized to create a viable "win-win" situation. Nonetheless, additional attention and efforts are needed to ensure that individuals with serious mental illness who are affected by these jail diversion programs are indeed receiving the services mandated by court, that these individuals are complying with the conditions of the court, and that, as a result of the services they are provided, their risk of re-offending and resulting risk to the public have been reduced. As such, developing, implementing, and sharing the results of common evaluation systems, unified information systems, and other cross-agency quality management and accountability systems is essential to ensuring the operation of effective systems of jail diversion and community-based mental health services.

REFERENCES

Arizona Department of Health, Division of Behavioral Health. (1999). *Managed Care in Arizona.*

Arizona Council on Offenders with Mental Impairments. (1999). *Annual Report 1999.*

Drake, R.E. Rosenberg, S.D. & Mueser, K.T. (1996). Assessing substance use disorder in persons with severe mental illness. In R.E. Drake and K.T. Mueser (Eds.). *Dual diagnosis of major mental illness and substance abuse,* Vol. 2: Recent and Clinical Implications (pp. 3–17). San Francisco: Jossey-Bass.

Steadman, H.J. (1992). Boundary Spanner: A key component for effective interactions of the justice and mental health systems. *Law And Behavior, 16*(1):75–87.

Steadman, H.J., Morris, S.M. & Dennis, D.L. (1995). The diversion of mentally ill persons from jails to community based services: A profile of programs. *American Journal of Public Health, 85*(12):1630–1635.

Edmunds, M., Frank, R., Hogan, M., McCarty, D., Beale, R. & Weisner, C. (1997). (Eds.) *Managing Managed Care: Quality Improvement in Behavioral Health.* National Academy Press, Washington, D.C.

9

Friends of Island Academy
Providing Youth with Positive
Opportunities After Jail

Beth Navon

BACKGROUND

Friends of Island Academy (FOIA) is a private non-profit, 501 (c)(3) organization which was originally established to provide support services to young males, primarily 16 to 18 years old, who had completed their jail sentences on Rikers Island. FOIA works in conjunction with The Island Academy, an alternative high school at this jail, run by the Board of Education. Since the organization's inception over 11 years ago, Friends has provided a crucial link back into the community for those youngsters leaving Rikers Island. The work has focused on assisting them to recognize that they have the choice to reject criminal behavior and can become productive citizens. This is accomplished by providing opportunities, guidance, and nurturing to these young people who are excluded from most avenues of support and who virtually always reside in environments where crime and violence are an accepted part of life. The work is unique and holistic in that it combines service delivery with the fundamental principles of youth development and leadership. Consistent with this approach is focusing on the youths' assets and empowering them in the decision to change their lives.

Although our population was originally designed to serve sentenced youth on Rikers Island, since 1998 we began to open our program to sentenced and detained females. The entry process into FOIA begins with one of its staff—a successful member of the program for seven years—who addresses groups of student inmates on Rikers Island, encouraging

---

Portions of this chapter appear in Friends of Island Academy documentation, co-authored with Barbara Grodd and Christine Pahigian.

them to join FOIA upon their release from jail. It is important to note that those who do join, do so on a voluntary basis. Our role is to assist them in identifying and selecting positive goals—education, employment, a drug free existence, a non-violent lifestyle, and the development of healthy interpersonal relationships—and to provide the necessary tools to achieve them. As these goals become a reality, we ask the participant to consider serving as a positive role model in the community where he or she once served in a negative capacity. Our purpose, therefore, is to engage these youth in actively transforming their lives and in redefining their relationship to the community.

The primary goals and objectives of FOIA are to provide services and options to these youngsters to help them overcome years of oppression and discrimination and to achieve their dreams of economic and social stability.

The young people who have joined Friends of Island Academy over the years have in common with the overall jail population the same demographic origins of New York City. Generally, they all come from the same neighborhoods: East New York, Bushwick, Bedford-Stuyvesant, the South Bronx, Harlem, Washington Heights, and Jamaica. Not surprisingly, these neighborhoods are among the most devastated in New York City with their high rates of poverty, unemployment, and violent crime.

With an awareness of these challenges posed by the home communities of our youth, and in response to the needs expressed to us by the participants themselves, FOIA has developed appropriate services that meet their practical and emotional needs. Unlike many organizations, our youth join FOIA as members who assume responsibilities both to the organization and to themselves. In return, and free of charge, they benefit from many of the support systems they have lacked throughout their lives, and which we will now describe in more detail.

TRADITIONAL PROGRAMS

The Progress Plan: Setting Goals

Youth who are nearing release from jail are often eager for help as they envision future plans. The youth leaving Rikers Island are not required to participate in the program. However, as mentioned above, they are made aware of FOIA and encouraged to take advantage of it through presentations at the jail and discharge planning meetings. All interested youth are given an appointment to visit FOIA when they complete their sentences, and participants agree to abide by Friends program rules, essentially embodying a commitment to respect themselves and others.

As they return home from jail, we encourage the youth to focus first on personal responsibility and accountability. Each participant is then asked to consider and complete a Progress Plan which charts previous and future life directions. The Progress Plan assists youth in identifying problem areas prior to arrest and to set their primary goals. Friends' role is to assist them in establishing these goals as well as facilitating their attainment. All goals and objectives are reviewed monthly by staff and participant and modified when appropriate.

Friends of Island Academy provides critical services tailored to meet the youths' needs, including counseling, vocational training, one-on-one mentoring, leadership training, job readiness skills, job placement, educational services, crisis intervention, exposure to cultural and recreational activities, and scholarship assistance. In addition, FOIA serves as an invaluable drop-in center for participants who are seeking nurturing, guidance, and support on how best to address social and familial pressures.

The Mentoring Project: One-on-One Role Models

Increasingly, the power of one-on-one relationships with adults is regarded as an effective method for helping youth stay out of jail. In 1991, FOIA, in recognition of this valuable resource, established the Mentoring Program. Its goal is to enable adolescent offenders to successfully make the transition from jail into the community by providing the consistent emotional and practical support they need to become independent adults. To this end, FOIA recruits and intensively trains community volunteers; it then pairs them with young people released from Rikers Island. Mentor and mentee meet on at least a biweekly basis. They are supported by a FOIA staff member who monitors the progress of the pairing. As positive role models, they provide the mentees with moral support as well as an opportunity for positive social interaction. As an adult connection to a more stable environment, FOIA's mentors are an invaluable resource to their mentees. Importantly, many mentors have helped FOIA youth find employment. It is for all of these reasons that youth with mentors have a higher rate of success.

Supported Learning: FOIA Education Initiatives

At FOIA, emphasis is placed on education as a necessary route to successful employment. Currently there is an on-site FOIA classroom for ex-offender youth to work toward passing their General Educational Development (GED) exam. Additionally, FOIA has established a community linkage in two alternative schools in Harlem and the South Bronx. There, classrooms have been created to receive youth released from jail on an ongoing basis. The Board of Education will provide teachers but FOIA will have case managers to transition and support these youth in their re-entry.

Also, 1998 FOIA is providing its own on-site pre-GED or literacy program. According to statistics from the jail population, 75% of incarcerated youth read below an eighth grade level. FOIA thus felt that it was imperative to offer this literacy program to its youth.

FOIA hired an education director in August, 1999 who has developed a strong network of referrals to educational programs outside of FOIA such as the CUNY system, the alternative high school system, and other literacy programs. Friends also offers modest scholarship assistance to members in need who are moving on to higher education and vocational training. Currently, the agency has 10 members in college.

Looking to the Future: Employment Preparation and Placement

When asked what goal they most wanted help in achieving, the majority of youth at Island Academy indicated jobs. Because of FOIA's assistance in obtaining even temporary or part-time employment, participants are more inclined to consider upgrading educational skills or enrolling in training programs.

Upon arrival at FOIA, as part of the intake process, new members participate in a job readiness course based on role-playing and workshop instruction; it hones skills in preparing a résumé, personal appearance, and interviewing.

Since 1993, FOIA has had a full-time job developer/employment coordinator who places more than 80 members in part- and full-time jobs per year. In February, 1999, Friends received funds to add an assistant employment coordinator to the staff, thus offering intensive Job Readiness training for our youth, many of whom had not held jobs prior to incarceration.

Counseling Services Department

All of the services mentioned above are augmented by group and individual counseling sessions with licensed clinicians. In these sessions, the youth deal with issues such as interpersonal, family, and peer relations; rage; conflict resolution; stress and harm reduction; bereavement; sexuality; health care; and chemical dependency. Many members have abused alcohol and illegal addictive substances as have many of their friends, partners, and family members. It is estimated that 75% of the New York City inmate population are substance abusers; addiction among the adolescent population is less significant than among adult offenders because they are more amenable to appropriate education and recovery.

Friends has also seen an increase in youth who are severely depressed. This is consistent with the national upward trend in suicide rates among adolescents. FOIA has therefore expanded to partnering with community psychiatrists, outpatient treatment centers, and some psychiatric inpatient facilities. Additionally, FOIA has recognized in the female population a high percentage of histories of sexual, physical, and/or emotional abuse. Therefore, it has become imperative to tailor an on-site therapeutic program which addresses these very significant issues.

NEW PROGRAMS:

Preventative Intervention: Adolescent Link

Based on Friends' visible success with young adults from Rikers Island, the agency was awarded a contract in February, 1998. In conjunction with the Department of Mental Health of the City of New York, FOIA provides services to a younger and equally neglected population: young people (10 to 17 years of age) involved in the juvenile or criminal justice system. The specific task is to focus on young people with mental health problems who, without intervention, would have serious difficulty reintegrating into their communities. Statistically, it is estimated that between 60–80% of youth in the juvenile justice system suffer from mental illness.

Currently, Friends is providing case management and referral services to 125 youth upon release. FOIA is contracted to monitor and support their progress over a two-year period. Because these young people return to their families and communities (unlike many of the agency's older adolescents who live independently) we have increased our knowledge of community resources. In addition, Friends now offers support to a growing number of parents.

Friends of Island Academy Rosewood Program for Adolescent Females

More than 128,000 women are incarcerated in the United States. Women are the most rapidly growing segment of the jail and prison population. The number of females in prison has quadrupled in the last 10 years. As a reflection of this trend, there are now female members at Friends of Island Academy. Friends is quite proud of its newest sibling, the Rosewood program, which works in conjunction with the Rosewood High School in the

Rose M. Singer correctional facility at Rikers Island. On November 16, 1998, the program accepted its first member.

Like the Friends and LINK programs, Rosewood provides continuity of care by making initial contact within the jail. A Friend's staff member meets with individuals and small groups of young women to recruit them. Upon release, these women participate in intake, further comprehensive assessment, and the development of a Progress Plan Chart. Members are provided with intensive case management services. They will be assisted in the pursuit of their educational goals through access to the Friends GED and literacy programs and will participate in the employment preparation and placement program with FOIA's job developer. As noted previously, Friends' counseling services are of great importance in the Rosewood program since the majority of these young women have experienced abuse during or throughout their lives. They are often in domestic violence situations and have children with whom they want to be reunited. Friends has had to intensify its clinical services to address these gender-specific issues.

Youth Leadership and the GIIFT Pack: The Core Program

Youth released from jail must make two critical and difficult transitions, one from a criminal to a productive lifestyle, the other from youth to adulthood. It is well-documented that minority youth feel a tremendous sense of alienation from the community at large and, given their lack of experience with success, face adulthood with an acute sense of hopelessness. Their pursuit of a positive plan of action is made even more difficult by the intense negative peer pressure they experience on a daily basis.

The Youth Leadership program at FOIA provides members with the opportunity to meet together through group and peer counseling and recreational and educational activities, instilling these adolescents with a new sense of purpose and the chance to transform their identities as they relinquish some of their former behaviors.

Participants attend weekly meetings and workshops devoted to pertinent issues. Periodically, Friends organizes special events and field trips with the intention of broadening the horizons of the participants and providing them with cultural enrichment and non-violent social activity. Speakers from the youths' communities who act as role models are brought in periodically to offer inspiration and knowledge.

As young people at FOIA begin achieving the goals they have set out in their Progress Plan, they are asked to return to their community of origin—where they once behaved in a negative capacity—to serve as a positive role model. These youth leaders, trained by FOIA staff, form the core of the "GIIFT Pack" (Guys and Girls Insight on Imprisonment for Teens). The GIIFT Pack was developed (and named) by youth members as a vehicle through which they would share their experiences and insights on how to reverse a cycle of negative behavior, crime, and violence in order to become productive citizens. Members of the GIIFT Pack travel to public schools, group homes, juvenile justice facilities, and community centers where they describe their experiences and deliver their very compelling message. GIIFT Pack leaders attend meetings in which staff assist them in organizing workshops and developing communication and leadership skills. GIIFT Pack presenters have a profound impact on their audiences; they are asked back again and again to talk to children at risk. The GIIFT Pack reaches about 2,000 youth per year at over 30 sites.

This prevention program inspires change in individuals. Some examples of its effectiveness range from youngsters turning in their guns to showing up at Friends offices seeking services. Several schools have requested that FOIA youth leaders become a permanent part of their guidance department. For the past four years, we have served in one school in the South Bronx, the Paul Laurence Dunbar Junior High School. Our outcome data indicates that both teachers and students have benefited from FOIA's program in this school. We have also developed a comprehensive Violence Prevention school curriculum to address these problems facing adolescents. This curriculum will now be affected in two more neighbourhood schools, highlighting the philosophy that these youth must prevent their younger brothers and sisters from following in these paths.

CONCLUSION

What makes Friends unique is that its programs are based on a prevention model that focuses on the empowerment of the individual realized through goal setting and community involvement. In a nurturing, stable, safe environment, FOIA is able to break down social isolation and build peer support networks to help these youth eventually attain independence. Its positive results inspired New York State Attorney General Dennis Vacco in 1997 to cite Friends of Island Academy as "one of the ten best programs in the state dealing with crime prevention." Friends' mission to help young people make the transition from jail to a positive life style in their home community not only saves lives but also saves the city an enormous amount of money. It costs approximately $60,000 to house one adolescent on Rikers Island for one year and $80,000 a year for a youth to be detained in the Juvenile Justice system. FOIA services cost approximately $4,500 per youth per year, making Friends one of the most cost-effective programs in the city.

Friends' original concept as a voluntary support system to prevent recidivism has proven to be an effective violence prevention and Youth Leadership model. In expanding its population to include adolescent females and younger children, Friends has taken an important step in its development. Friends of Island Academy is convinced that with the assistance of new supporters it will be able to: 1) institutionalize its programming, 2) conduct more research documenting FOIA's effectiveness, and 3) reach out to more organizations to help train them in Friends' Youth Development Model. Friends was recently awarded a grant from the Department of Labor as a model demonstration project for youth re-entering the community from incarceration. Thus, Friends is now in the position to be a national leader in representing best practices for this often neglected and most vulnerable population of Children.

10

Broward's Mental Health Court: An Innovative Approach to the Mentally Disabled in the Criminal Justice System

Ginger Lerner-Wren

An ever-increasing trend throughout our nation is that jails have become mental institutions of last resort. According to a special report published in July, 1999 by the U.S. Department of Justice, an estimated 283,8000 mentally ill offenders were incarcerated in our nation's jails and prisons.[1] This trend, known as the criminalization of the mentally ill, is the result of a number of precipitating social, legal, and political factors.

While the area of Mental Disability law is growing and evolving at a rapid pace, local jails and state prisons have, in effect, replaced long-term psychiatric institutions.[2] As a result of "The Civil Rights Revolution" and its expansion to include mentally disabled persons, particularly those residing in dangerous living conditions in both state hospitals and state schools for the mentally retarded, the U.S. Supreme Court and Federal Courts have expanded the rights of the mentally disabled, resulting in a well-intentioned and theoretically sound policy of deinstitutionalization.[3] The expansion of legal rights, both through litigation and legislation, together with changes in clinical treatment approaches, new and more effective antipsychotic medications have made recovery and community-based living possible. Yet, it remains tragically out of reach for the majority of Americans who suffer from severe and chronic mental disabilities.

The paradox, however, has been that the expansion of legal rights has come without adequate funding of community-based treatment, services, and housing. Restrictions on managed care, shrinking state and local budgets and the privitization of government-run mental health programs have led to a narrowing of the population receiving publicly funded mental health services. The targeting of specific populations has created wider gaps in the mental health system, causing more individuals to have less or no services. In the years following the movement to deinstitutionalize the mentally ill, the nation's streets, jails, and prisons have increasingly become the residence of persons with serious mental disorders, co-occurring substance disorders and related challenges rather than community-based treatment programs and facilities as intended. Untreated mental illness in our communities has a direct relationship to homelessness, increased substance abuse, quality of life offenses, and, at times, more serious crime. Often, law enforcement officers with little training to identify those in psychiatric crisis vs. those committing some type of volitional offense find jail to be the least burdensome repository for persons acting out bizarrely in public. With no mechanism to help distinguish true violators from those who are simply in the throes of mental illness, the cycle of decompensation in jails, stabilization, and release onto the streets with no treatment perpetuates a vicious revolving door in and out of the criminal justice system.

According to the U.S. Department of Justice, mentally ill defendants are expected to serve 15 months longer than non-disabled inmates in prison. For the mentally ill non-violent offender without appropriate treatment and supports, life is reduced to the endless revolving between jail cells and local psychiatric crisis units. It is a life filled with alienation, hopelessness, humiliation, and suffering.

A COMMUNITY READY FOR CHANGE

In 1994, a high-profile criminal case in Broward County involving a mentally disabled young man, a scathing grand jury report relating to severe shortfalls in Broward's community mental health system, and tragic deaths in the county jail led to the creation of a local *ad hoc* criminal justice task force led by Circuit Judge Mark A. Speiser. Major stakeholders in the criminal justice system, law enforcement, and the consumer and mental health provider community came together as a working group to identify points in the criminal justice system which could be streamlined to improve the administration of justice for defendants who suffer from major mental disorders and related disabilities. Participants on the task force included the Broward Public Defender's Office, State Attorney's Office, Broward Sheriff's Office, Broward county Governmental staff, and local members of the National Alliance for the Mentally Ill (NAMI), and community mental health and substance abuse providers, including Henderson Mental Health Center and Nova Southeastern University.

BROWARD'S MENTAL HEALTH COURT

Through ongoing meetings of the task force, Assistant Chief Public Defender Howard Finkelstein advocated for the creation of a specialized court to target this population. In what was described by Howard as a "leap of faith," Chief Circuit Judge, Dale Ross entered an Administrative Order in May, 1997 creating the nation's first Mental Health Court as a specialized subdivision of the County Criminal Court. The mission of the Mental Health Court is to better address the unique and complex needs of the mentally disabled misdemeanant defendant arrested on non-violent offenses. The Court is uniquely designed to rapidly intercept and divert those defendants arrested with non-violent petty misdemeanant charges from the jail and into appropriate treatment facilities/hospitals wherever possible without compromising public safety.

Goals of the Court

- To create a courtroom with a high degree of sensitivity to the specialized needs of this population.
- To expedite the mentally ill defendant through the criminal justice system without compromise.
- To assure that the mentally disabled defendant does not languish in jail because of his illness and, if in need of emergency psychiatric treatment, that the individual is able to obtain it without compromise of individual substantive legal rights.
- To balance the defendant's individual rights, treatment considerations, and public safety.
- To apply a therapeutic approach to the processing of offenders to better assist them and family in the recovery process and assuming personal responsibility for their comprehensive health needs and to help reduce the stigma of mental illness..
- To better ensure and oversee the coordination, effectiveness, and accountability of both the delivery of community-based treatment and services and compliance with treatment by the individual defendant.
- To reduce the contact of the mentally ill with the criminal justice system by creating a bridge between the community system and jail system.

Unique and Innovative Features of the Court:

1.   The Court is a voluntary, part-time court which convenes on a daily, "as needed" basis with referrals from various sources, including family members, lawyers, jail staff, magistrate judges, and other county criminal court judges.
2.   The Court wholly adopts and applies the principles of Therapeutic Jurisprudence, a legal construct which advances the court's role as an active therapeutic agent in the recovery process.
3.   The Court acts as a coordinator and integrator of treatment, services, and housing through a multidisciplinary approach, with clinical and treatment recommendations being made on an ongoing basis for those working with the court.
4.   The Court makes every effort to promote the assumption of personal responsibility and personal empowerment of the court participant. The goal, of course, is to create safer and more secure communities, reduce or eliminate recidivism, and promote the quality of life of the participant and public at large.

THE MENTAL HEALTH COURT TEAM

The success of the operations of Broward's Mental Health Court is directly linked to the support and tireless efforts of both the internal court staff and the external supportive services provided by a wide array of community-related agencies and treatment facilities. The strength of the operations of the court and the swift response time in the ability to assess cases each day and to divert defendants to treatment facilities is due to the dedicated and shared vision of the collaborative spirit of community and criminal justice system partners. However, it should be noted that this innovation is not without limitation. The court is not a substitute for desperately needed community resources but does represent an effective albeit limited diversion strategy for a targeted population of defendants.

Since its inception, Broward's Mental Health Court has seen over 1,400 defendants. In 1998, the Florida Legislature appropriated funds to establish a transitional, residential dual diagnosis treatment facility, "The Cottages in the Pines," to house and treat homeless and at-risk of homelessness defendants participating in the court. The Department of Justice, Bureau of Justice Assistance has funded a trauma-based, gender-specific program through Nova Southeastern University dedicated to treating women with co-occurring disorders. The court, with its therapeutic approach, has become a national model for jurisdictions across the nation as well as a venue for visitors from all over the world who come to observe the proceedings.

Broward's Mental Health Court received the 1999 Florida Circuit Conference of Judges award for innovation and has been featured on National Public Radio and Good Morning America. Judge Lerner-Wren and the Mental Health Court were showcased at the White House Conference on the Mentally Ill. Currently, Federal Legislation is pending to proliferate the development of diversionary mental health courts throughout the country.

Notes

1. U.S. Department of Justice Bureau of Justice Statistics Special Report, "Mental Health and Treatment of Inmates and Probationers," July 1999.
2. Perlin, Mental Disability Law, Civil and Criminal, 1989, 1998.
3. Perlin, Mental Disability Law, Criminal and Civil, 1989, 1998.

11

Preventing Incarceration of Adults With Severe Mental Illness: Project Link

J. Steven Lamberti and Robert L. Weisman

Project Link is designed to prevent arrest and incarceration of adults with severe mental illness who have histories of involvement with the criminal justice system. Located in Rochester, New York, the project consists of a university-led consortium of community agencies that spans health care, social service, and criminal justice systems. Project Link provides comprehensive, community-based services through a mobile treatment team with a forensic psychiatrist, a mental illness and chemical abuse treatment residence, culturally competent staff, and integration with the criminal justice system. This chapter will provide an overview of the development and operation of Project Link.

BACKGROUND

Deinstitutionalization of the mentally ill has posed many challenges for communities across America. Between 1955 and 1994, the number of mentally ill persons residing in public psychiatric hospitals was reduced by almost one-half million (Torrey, 1997). Conditions inside of public hospitals were sometimes poor, but these institutions did provide psychiatric, medical, and residential care. In the wake of their demise, a major challenge has been developing adequate community-based services for deinstitutionalized patients and for a new generation of never-institutionalized patients. Although the Community Mental Health Center Act of 1963

Supported by a grant from the Robert Wood Johnson Foundation's Local Initiative Funding Partner's Program.

sparked the development of community mental health centers nation-wide, these centers were ill equipped to address the comprehensive needs of the severely mentally ill. Many individuals failed to engage in services as a result, often becoming isolated, homeless, and drug addicted. Of the 5.6 million individuals with severe mental illness currently living in the United States, an estimated 2.2 million are not receiving treatment (Torrey, 1997).

The development of adequate outpatient services for the severely mentally ill has been particularly challenging for communities in New York State. New York has historically had the highest utilization rate of inpatient psychiatric beds in the nation (New York State Office of Mental Health, 1997). Its hospitals have also deinstitutionalized the largest number of patients. The total inpatient census in New York public hospitals was reduced by over 80,000 individuals between 1955 and 1996, leaving an inpatient census of approximately 9,000 (New York State Office of Mental Health, 1998). While the number of psychiatric hospital beds has declined, the number of jail and prison beds in New York State has increased rapidly. Between 1976 and 1996, the total number of available jail and prison beds rose from approximately 28,000 to 101,000 (New York State Commission of Corrections, 1999). This growth is consistent with the rapid growth of correctional facilities that has been occurring across the nation (U.S. Department of Justice, 1999). As jails and prisons have expanded nationally, persons with severe mental illness have become over-represented among those incarcerated. The prevalence of individuals with severe mental illness residing in correctional facilities has recently been estimated to range as high as 15% (Lamb & Weinberger, 1998). Given this prevalence rate, there may now be more severely mentally ill persons residing in state prisons than in state hospitals in New York.

Several factors have probably contributed to the overrepresentation of mentally ill persons in correctional facilities in New York and across the nation. In addition to deinstitutionalization and the rapid growth of correctional facilities, these include lack of access to community-based care, fragmentation of health care services, restrictive civil commitment laws, and the stigmatizing effects of mental illness. Considering the magnitude of these combined factors, it is perhaps not surprising that this phenomenon has occurred. What is surprising, however, is that it has even occurred in communities with the best systems of health care in place. One example of such a community is Rochester, New York.

THE ROCHESTER EXPERIENCE

Rochester is located on the south shore of Lake Ontario in Monroe County, New York. Including the Rochester metropolitan area, Monroe County spans an area of approximately 700 square miles and has a population of

750,000. As the home of Eastman Kodak and Bausch & Lomb corporations, and of manufacturing facilities for Xerox, General Motors, and IT&T Automotive, Rochester has enjoyed considerable economic prosperity. The University of Rochester Medical Center and five area hospitals have provided excellent health care to area residents. Rochester Psychiatric Center (RPC) is the regional state hospital and has provided long-term inpatient psychiatric care to county residents since 1891. Originally known as Rochester State Hospital, the facility held over 3,000 inpatients at its peak capacity during the mid 1960s. Deinstitutionalization began at that time and has continued until the present day, with RPC now providing psychiatric treatment to less than 200 inpatients.

As part of the deinstitutionalization process, RPC was the primary site of the innovative Monroe Livingston demonstration project (Reed & Babigian, 1994; Reed et al., 1994; Cole et al., 1994). Conducted between 1987 and 1993, the project was designed to ensure that funding followed deinstitutionalized patients as they left RPC and entered the surrounding community. The Monroe-Livingston Project accomplished this task by establishing the nation's first large capitated payment program for the severely mentally ill. It also led to the creation of a community corporation to facilitate coordination and planning of care and to monitor and evaluate programs. Capitated funding was allocated to cover deinstitutionalized patients' psychiatric, medical, and dental care in addition to medications, sustenance, lodging, and transportation (Marshall, 1992). As a result, Rochester became host to a broad and comprehensive array of community-based services for the severely mentally ill. Existing programs were enhanced through the infusion of capitated funding, and new services were created. The array of available programs included clinics, continuing day treatment programs, day hospitals, psycho-social rehabilitation clubhouses, case management programs, and a mobile crisis program. In addition to psychiatric services, a wide variety of residential services ranging from group homes to independent apartments were provided by three local residential rehabilitation agencies. Throughout the late 1980s and early 1990s, it appeared that Rochester had developed a system of care that was truly seamless and comprehensive. Despite this wide array of services, however, problems eventually began to surface in Rochester's mental health system.

The Monroe County Jail is Rochester's largest correctional facility, serving a total of 1,000 inmates. Mental health services have been provided to inmates in the jail through the Monroe County Clinic for Socio-Legal Services in collaboration with the University of Rochester Department of Psychiatry since the mid 1970s. During the early 1990s, county clinic staff began to notice growing numbers of mentally ill persons residing in the jail. Driven by concern for these individuals and for rising costs associated with their care in jail, the Monroe County Office of Mental Health con-

ducted a survey of the jail in 1993. The survey identified a group of mentally ill inmates that had experienced multiple incarcerations during the
previous three years. In addition, it revealed several demographic factors
that appeared to be associated with jail recidivism. These included being
male, having psychotic symptoms, using illegal drugs or alcohol, having
residential instability, and failing to engage in outpatient mental health
services. African-American and Hispanic persons were found to be highly
over represented among this group of individuals.

   In response to these findings, the Monroe County Office of Mental
Health issued a request for proposals to develop case advocacy services.
The target population of these services was defined as multicultural populations with severe mental illness at risk for involvement with the criminal justice system. The primary goal was to prevent arrest and incarceration
within the target population, with additional goals that included preventing
hospitalization and promoting community re-integration. The request for
proposals involved development of a culturally diverse team of bachelor's-
level case advocates to engage previously unengaged individuals and to
connect them to existing services in the community. County officials used
the term "case advocacy" instead of the more traditional case management designation to enable the team to achieve flexibility by functioning
independently of case management regulatory requirements. The spirit
of advocacy was also felt to be consistent with meeting the needs of a target population that represented underserved minority groups. In essence,
the plan called for a culturally competent "brokerage" model of intervention whereby staff would engage clients and link them to community-
based mental health services rather than providing the services directly.

DEVELOPMENT OF PROJECT LINK

Strong Ties Community Support Program of the University of Rochester
Department of Psychiatry responded to the request for proposals by forming Project Link in partnership with five local community agencies. The
agencies provide health care, social services and criminal justice services.
They were selected in order to span boundaries between these systems of
care. With Strong Ties as the lead agency, Project Link's community partners are Action for a Better Community, the Ibero-American Action League,
the Urban League of Rochester, Unity Health System, and the Monroe
County Clinic for Socio-Legal Services. In addition, consultation is provided to Project Link by the university's Psychiatry and the Law Program.
A director from each community partner agency sits on Project Link's
Collaborative Management Team to oversee the project.

   A total of five bachelor's-level case advocates were hired and employed by Project Link's community partner agencies. Case advocates carry a case-load of 20 clients each, giving Project Link a total capacity of 100. The case advocate team is available to assist clients seven days a week, 24 hours a day. Each case advocate is supervised by the Project Link coordinator, a master's-level nurse with mental health and chemical dependency treatment experience. The coordinator also directs public awareness efforts and represents the case advocates on Project Link's Collaborative Management Team.

Project Link places a special emphasis on engaging clients who are members of minority groups. In order to bridge barriers related to differences in culture, ethnicity, and language, Project Link features a diverse staff including African-American and Hispanic case advocates. In addition, all administrative and clinical staff of Project Link received cultural competence training at the initiation of the program.

With community partnerships and a team of case advocates in place, Project Link became operational on April 1, 1996. Referrals were received from a variety of places, with jails and prisons quickly becoming the largest referral sources. Although the case advocates were effective at engaging the clients, two serious operational problems arose within six months of program initiation. First, case advocates were unable to secure housing for many clients. Those with histories of felony crimes, homelessness, and active drug or alcohol abuse were rarely accepted into supervised housing facilities. The supervised facilities were geared toward managing clients who were likely to succeed in existing rehabilitation programs. Some clients presented the additional challenge of having "burned their bridges" at many local residences including churches and emergency shelters. In the absence of residential support, case advocates had to house the clients in low priced hotels that were typically located in drug-infested neighborhoods. In addition to this problem, the case advocates had difficulty gaining access to outpatient mental health and primary medical care programs. These programs typically lacked the outreach necessary to engage severely mentally ill individuals, and they often closed clients' cases after missed appointments. Taken together, these barriers left the case advocates to manage their most highly impaired clients with little direct support, despite the abundant presence of services in the community.

In order to address these problems, the director of Project Link applied for development funding through the Robert Wood Johnson Foundation's Local Initiative Funding Partner's Program. Grant funding was obtained in 1997 and was used to initiate new services, including a mobile treatment team that is integrated with a mental illness/chemical abuse (MICA) treatment residence. As a result of these developments, Project Link currently offers an array of services described in the following section.

PROJECT LINK SERVICES AND OPERATION

Admission Criteria

Project Link serves clients who have a severe mental illness, difficulty engaging with outpatient mental health services, and previous involvement with the criminal justice system. While substance abuse is not an admission requirement, the vast majority of clients referred to Project Link have histories of substance abuse or dependence. Referrals are accepted from multiple sources, including area jails and prisons, police departments, hospitals, settlement houses, emergency shelters, and churches. In order to raise public awareness of Project Link services, staff members frequently visit agencies in the community that are likely to have contact with the target population. Basic information about mental illness and about Project Link is provided during these visits along with referral forms. The Project Link coordinator processes all referrals and assigns each newly enrolled client to a case advocate. Estimated average length of stay for all services in Project Link is approximately two years.

Case Advocacy Services

Case advocates are responsible for engaging clients and linking them to existing healthcare, social, and residential services in the community. When an incarcerated or hospitalized client is referred to Project Link, case advocates will meet with the client in the jail or hospital prior to discharge into the community. Case advocates see new clients on a frequent and sometimes daily basis in order to promote engagement. This intensive level of contact also enables the case advocates to become familiar with each client's clinical, residential, financial, and social needs. Once engaged, case advocates continue to meet with clients regularly to assess their needs, plan their services, and provide support. Case advocates have access to emergency funds totaling $600 per client annually in order to provide urgently needed goods and services including clothing, groceries, housing, and transportation. Although case advocates successfully link many clients to existing services, some need a higher level of care in order to engage in treatment. These clients usually have histories of multiple arrests and incarcerations, untreated addictions, and active resistance to engagement. Clients who require more intensive levels of intervention are assigned to Project Link's mobile treatment team.

Mobile Treatment Team Services

The mobile treatment team consists of a forensic psychiatrist (0.6 full-time equivalent) and a full-time nurse practitioner who work with case advocates to serve the most highly impaired clients in Project Link. Clients are assigned to the mobile treatment team by the Project Link coordinator following discussion with the case advocates and mobile team clinicians. The mobile treatment team is designed to ensure the delivery of comprehensive health care services to 40 of the 100 total clients in Project Link. Mental health services are provided directly by the forensic psychiatrist and nurse who work closely with representatives of the criminal justice system in order to promote integration and continuity of services. The mobile treatment team incorporates the basic principles of assertive community treatment (ACT), including a high staff to client ratio, multidisciplinary staffing, around-the-clock availability, *in vivo* service delivery, and assertive outreach. Modifications to the model include the involvement of a forensic psychiatrist, and integration of clinical services with criminal justice services and residential addiction treatment services. Given the forensic nature of the target population and the goals of reducing arrest and incarceration, this approach may be viewed as representing a new forensic assertive community treatment (FACT) model of care.

Clients enrolled in the mobile treatment team receive primary medical care through the Medicine in Psychiatry Service (MIPS). MIPS is a program of the University of Rochester Department of Psychiatry that provides medical care to adults with severe mental illness. MIPS and Project Link's mobile treatment team are both based at the Strong Ties Community Support Program. Strong Ties specializes in providing comprehensive health services for adults with severe mental illness, including outpatient psychiatric, medical, pharmacy, day treatment, and rehabilitation services. To promote continuity of care, all mobile treatment team clients are eventually transferred to Strong Ties following treatment and stabilization. The average anticipated length of stay in Project Link's mobile treatment team is approximately two years.

Mental Illness/Chemical Addiction (MICA) Residential Services

The MICA treatment residence is a 10-bed, supervised apartment facility that is operated in conjunction with a DePaul Residential Services, a local mental health housing provider. Clients must have co-occurring mental illness and substance abuse and be willing to enter the facility voluntarily in order to qualify for admission. All clients in the MICA treatment residence are served by Project Link's mobile treatment team. Grant funding was used to increase the existing level of staffing in the residence, including the addition of a certified substance abuse counselor. Staff supervision is present around the clock at the residence. The goals of the MICA treatment residence are to promote abstinence, reduce psychiatric symptoms, and improve community living skills. The MICA treatment residence is based on the modified therapeutic community model of care (Carroll & McGinley, 1998; Sacks et al., 1999). Consistent with the model, the residence utilizes structured step-wise programming and peer modeling and support. Staff encourage client participation in therapeutic groups, work assignments, and recreational activities as tolerated. Participation in off-site Alcoholics Anonymous and Narcotics Anonymous meetings is also encouraged. In addition, staff at the MICA residence work to promote utilization of social services and development of shopping, cooking, basic hygiene, and transportation skills. The average expected length of stay in the MICA treatment residence is approximately two years. Depending upon their level of progress and individual preferences, clients are subsequently offered supervised or unsupervised housing options within the community.

Service Integration

Clients in Project Link have multiple needs that span the health care, social service, and criminal justice systems. Project Link represents a step towards integration of these service systems. One important aspect of integration involves health care and criminal justice services. Project Link staff members work with clients in courtroom and jail settings where they have frequent contact with judges, public defenders, and jail staff. They also work closely with parole and probation officers whenever the officers are involved. This accessibility of Project Link staff members facilitates the disposition of clients into Project Link as a condition of release or as an alternative to incarceration. In addition, the resulting dialogue between Project Link and criminal justice staff enables the generation of therapeutic leverage to promote client participation in essential clinical and social services when necessary.

To promote integration of clinical and residential services, Project Link's mobile treatment team visits clients at the MICA residence on a regular basis. These visits provide an opportunity for clinical and residential staff to work together in developing individualized treatment plans. To promote integration with social services, liaison persons have been established within each local Department of Social Services (DSS) office. The DSS liaisons function as single points of contact for all Project Link clients, reducing the complexities and delays commonly involved in obtaining public assistance, medical assistance, and food stamps. An additional aspect of integration in Project Link involves the delivery of both psychiatric and medical services which is achieved through the combined efforts of the mobile treatment team and MIPS.

Efforts to integrate health care, criminal justice, and social services at an operational level are reinforced on an administrative level by Project Link's Collaborative Management Team. As noted above, Project Link's partner agencies were chosen to represent each of the three primary service systems. Director-level members represent each agency so that the team has the authority necessary to make systems changes when needed. In addition, local and state mental health officials have supported the funding and development of Project Link. Their involvement has promoted ongoing dialogue between service system representatives at a health care policy level in New York State.

PROGRAM EFFECTIVENESS

To examine the effectiveness of Project Link's mobile treatment team at engaging the target population, data was gathered on the first 46 clients admitted for treatment. All clients were admitted between October 1, 1997 and December 1, 1998, and their average length of stay in Project Link at the time of data collection was 278 days. Thirty percent of clients were referred from area jails and prisons, 28% from the local state hospital, and the remainder from community mental health centers, emergency rooms, and other sources. Eighty percent of clients were male, and average age at admission was 34 years. Seventy-two percent were African-American, 15% were Caucasian, 7% were Hispanic and 6% were other. Approximately one-quarter of all clients were homeless at the time of admission, and 80% had failed to graduate from high school. Forty-six percent of clients met DSM-IV criteria for schizophrenia, 26% for psychotic disorder NOS, 13% for schizoaffective disorder, 9% for bipolar disorder, and 6% for other diagnoses. Eighty-three percent of clients were actively abusing substances at the time of admission. Mean admission score on the Global Assessment of Functioning Scale was 39. Fifty percent of clients were on either probation or parole, and 43% were noted to have previous felony convictions at the time of admission.

During the year prior to enrollment in Project Link, the group spent an average of 9.1 days in jail per client per month and an average of 8.3 days in the hospital per client per month. Multiplying these service frequencies by local service costs, the combined pre-treatment costs of jail and hospital services averaged $4,975 dollars per client per month. While this data indicates that Project Link has succeeded in engaging the intended target population, the effectiveness of the program remains to be established. Prospective studies are currently underway to determine whether this model represents a cost-effective approach to preventing jail and hospital recidivism, reducing substance use, and improving community adjustment in this challenging population.

SUMMARY

Project Link represents a promising new approach to prevention of jail and hospital recidivism among adults with severe mental illness and histories of involvement with the criminal justice system. By involving elements of health care, criminal justice, and social service systems, Project Link provides an integrated and comprehensive array of services. The development of integrated services is an important goal for programs seeking to achieve optimal efficiency and effectiveness in serving persons with severe mental illness. This goal is especially important for programs that serve individuals with histories of arrest and incarceration, addiction, homelessness, and failure to engage in traditional outpatient services. Project Link has taken significant steps towards integration and has been recognized by the American Psychiatric Association as a model for prevention of criminal justice involvement among the severely mentally ill (Gold Award, 1999). Controlled research is needed to examine the effectiveness of Project Link, and to determine whether this model can be replicated in other urban communities.

REFERENCES

Carroll, J.F. & McGinley, J.J. (1998). Managing MICA clients in a modified therapeutic community with enhanced staffing. *Journal of Substance Abuse Treatment, 15*(6), 565–577.

Cole, R.E., Reed, S.K., Babigian, H.M,. Brown, S.W. & Fray, J. (1994). A mental health capitation program: I. Patient outcomes. *Hospital and Community Psychiatry, 45*(11), 1090–1096.

Gold Award (1999). Prevention of jail and hospital recidivism among persons with severe mental illness. Project Link, Department of Psychiatry, University of Rochester, Rochester, New York. *Psychiatric Services, 50*(11), 1477–1480.

Lamb, R.H., & Weinberger, L.E. (1998). Persons with severe mental illness in jails and prisons: A review. *Psychiatric Services, 49*(4), 483–492.

Marshall, P.E. (1992). The mental health HMO: Capitation funding for the chronically mentally ill. Why an HMO? *Community Mental Health Journal, 28*(2), 111–120.

New York State Commission of Corrections. (1999). www.scoc.state.ny.us/
  pop.htm. Additional data on file.
New York State Office of Mental Health. (1997). Statewide Comprehensive
  Plan for Mental Health Services 1997–2001.
New York State Office of Mental Health. (1998). NYS Chartbook of Mental
  Health Information. www.omh.state.ny.us/chartbk/SeriesE/e3.htm.
Reed, S.K., & Babigian, H.M. (1994). Postmortem of the Rochester capi-
  tation experiment. *Hospital and Community Psychiatry, 45*(8), 761–764.
Reed, S.K., Hennessy, K.D., Mitchell, O.S., & Babigian, HM. (1994). A
  mental health capitation program: II. Cost–benefit analysis. *Hospital
  and Community Psychiatry, 45*(11), 1097–1103.
Sacks, S., Sacks, J.Y. & DeLeon, G. (1999). Treatment for MICAs: Design
  and implementation of the modified TC. *Journal of Psychoactive Drugs,
  31*(1), 19–30.
Torrey, E.F. (1997). *Out of the Shadows. Confronting America's Mental Illness
  Crisis.* New York: Wiley.
United States Department of Justice. (1999). Bureau of Justice Statistics.
  www.ojp.usdoj.gov/bjs/correct.htm.

12

New York City's System of Criminal Justice Mental Health Services

Stacy S. Lamon, Neal L. Cohen, and Nahama Broner

As New York City has moved from a system of institutionalized care to community-based services for seriously mentally ill patients, it has had to confront the issue of treating people involved in the criminal justice system. The reason is that large numbers of mentally ill people have come into contact with the police, court and correctional systems. The data suggest that jails have replaced psychiatric hospitals for a significant segment of the overall mentally ill population.

The problems created by this phenomenon have been particularly challenging. The number of mentally ill people in the court and correctional systems is significant. Addressing the needs of this population requires cooperation between city agencies in areas where none existed before. Finally, this population is challenging because it is difficult to track and manage in a complex urban environment.

New York, like other large municipalities, has experienced difficulty in creating services for the forensic mentally ill population. In recent years, however, both New York City and State have become more aggressive about developing a network of services for this group. Among the most important are diversion, jail-based treatment, discharge planning, linkage and transition (LINK) services, case management, and housing. These services have done much to ease a difficult problem. However, much remains to be done. Existing programs need to be expanded and new initiatives started.

This chapter will discuss how the city is serving people with serious mental illness who become involved in the criminal justice system and will

The authors would like to thank Frederick Patrick, M.P.A., Deputy Criminal Justice Coordinator of the City of New York, and the Hon. Martin G. Karopkin, Judge of the Criminal Court of New York, for their review of this chapter.

examine the existing network of services for them. In addition, it will look at service delivery problems and suggest recommendations on how they can be addressed.

SCOPE OF THE PROBLEM

It is estimated that 15,000 mentally ill people are released to the community each year from New York City jails (New York City Department of Mental Health, Mental Retardation and Alcoholism Services [DMH], 1998). In addition, approximately 1,500 return to New York City annually from state and federal prisons, and an undetermined number are released directly from arraignment courts (Broner, Owen, Lamon, & Karopkin, 2000). In New York City more than one third of mentally ill people leaving jail are homeless (Martell, Rosner & Harmon, 1995; Michaels, Zoloth, Alcabes, Braslow & Safyer, 1992), and most have drug and alcohol abuse problems (Broner, Rock & Landsberg, 1998; cf. Abram & Teplin, 1991; Peters & Hills, 1993). Many also have no means to pay for treatment or medication (DMH, 1998).

In addition, the city confronts the issue of "transinstitutionalization" (Barr, 1999; Shenson, Dubler & Michaels, 1990; Torrey et al., 1992) in which mentally ill people are confined to jails rather than hospitals. The result is that jails have become providers of a broad spectrum of treatment services (New York City Board of Correction, 1984). While some may question the wisdom of treating this population in the community, transinstitutionalization has created a major problem in providing treatment that extends beyond jail-based services. It has made accessing services in the community more difficult for many forensic clients after their release from jail (Griffin, 1991; Veysey, Steadman, Morrissey & Johnson, 1997). According to Solomon and Drain (1995), "A clear link with aftercare services is vital to ensuring continuity of care after release from jail" (p. 27). But they note that jail-based services are "grossly separate" from community services.

A decade ago it was difficult to connect people released from jail with community mental health services, and there were few community programs targeted to them. To address the complexity of these problems, New York City has worked to develop a network of services to ensure that people with mental health problems remain in the community with adequate treatment and support and do not return to the criminal justice system (DMH, 2000).

DEVELOPMENT OF THE SYSTEM

The major problem confronting the system as it set out to address the needs of the mentally ill client was the need for coordination. It was necessary for the mental health and criminal justice systems to work in tandem. While services were available in the community for people with serious mental illness, there was no mechanism to ensure that people leaving the criminal justice system could get them, and there was no way of ensuring that this population would remain in treatment. That produced a "revolving door" of criminal justice and mental health for this population (Cohen, 1998). Repeatedly, these individuals went from the streets, to arrest, to court, to confinement. When released, they returned to the streets to start the cycle again.

By the 1990s, New York had developed models for delivering mental health services in prisons (Dovskin, Smith & Broaddus, 1993) and jails (e.g., Landsberg, 1992). However, in New York City too many people returning from jails and prisons never entered the community mental health system. Ensuring continuity of care imposed some daunting challenges. Most important was the need to coordinate efforts between centralized court and correctional systems and a highly decentralized mental health system characterized by a large number of small community-based providers.

New York City began exploring more effective ways to ensure continuity of care by examining forensic service models, enlisting planning efforts among city agencies and consulting with mental health providers and consumers. What emerged was a pilot project designed to provide discharge planning in jail and case management in the community. The project demonstrated that case managers could connect clients to community services. It also identified important service needs including housing, peer support, and creating a practical method to provide medication to people immediately upon release from jail. Initially, the project only provided discharge planning to people completing their jail sentence. However, it soon found that it could divert people from jail and provide discharge plans for them as well.

On the basis of this pilot project, a system of services for forensic clients began to grow (DMH, 1998). The pilot project itself first became the LINK program providing discharge planning, court diversion, and community case management for people leaving jail as well as medication and peer support. The LINK program, in turn, was divided into two initiatives, one providing discharge planning in jail and the other court diversion and case management in the community. A third LINK program was developed to provide case management for clients returning from State prisons.

Initially, LINK programs served only adults, but a large population of adolescents in the Juvenile Justice System also needed discharge planning and community case management. In 1997, a LINK program was established to provide services to adolescents. By 2000, LINK programs for adults had been established in each of the city's boroughs and a second program for adolescents had been implemented.

In addition to LINK services, programs for long-term case management were established specifically for forensic clients. A forensic Intensive Case Management (ICM) program assists forensic clients in complying with treatment, and an Assertive Community Treatment (ACT) team for forensic clients provides both case management and treatment (DMH, 1998). A specialized New York State Assisted Outpatient Treatment (AOT) team identifies clients in jail who have histories of treatment non-compliance and connects them with case management and community treatment (Cohen, Lamon & Katz, Chapter 23). Recently, a service was developed to divert mentally ill defendants from arraignment court, and specialized mental health courts are being planned (Center for Court Innovation, personal communication, 2000; Linn, Broner & Rotter, 2000).

In addition to these governmental initiatives, other institutions began to take a more active role in forensic services. New York University and Long Island Jewish Medical Center both began forensic institutes. The federal government became more involved as the Substance Abuse and Mental Health Service Administration funded both a nation-wide study of diversion which included New York City (Steadman, Barbera & Dennis, 1994; Landsberg, Rock & Broner, 1999) and a mental health court diversion project (Broner, Franczak, Dye & McCallister, 2001). The Mayor's Office of the Criminal Justice Coordinator, with the John Jay College of Criminal Justice, started a planning team to investigate the management of sex offenders in the community. New York University began to conduct forensic conferences.

THE SYSTEM

All of this activity resulted in a network of services for mentally ill people who have become involved in the criminal justice system. Table 1 lists the programs involved in this network. The key components are diversion from incarceration, services in jail, discharge planning, linkage to community services and case management.

Diversion

Diversion provides treatment as an alternative to adjudication and incarceration for people with mental illness (cf. Steadman, Morris & Dennis, 1995; Steadman et al., 1994). It can occur at a number of points in the

Table 12.1 Programs and Services in New York City's System of Criminal Justice Mental Health Services

1. Jail-based Services
2. Hospital-based Correctional Wards
3. Jail-based Discharge Planning
4. Community-based Discharge Planning (SPAN)
5. Brooklyn/Staten Island LINK
6. Bronx LINK
7. Manhattan LINK
8. Queens LINK
9. State LINK (prison released clients)
10. Adolescent LINK (City-wide)
11. Brooklyn Adolescent LINK
12. LINK Prescription Medication Service
13. LINK Peer Support Groups
14. LINK Outreach
15. Forensic ACT Team
16. Forensic/MICA ICM
17. Arraignment Court Mental Health Diversion
18. Nathaniel Felony Diversion
19. Bronx Mental Health Felony Court Diversion
20. Brooklyn Mental Health Court Planning
21. Court Mental Health Evaluation Clinics
22. Forensic AOT Team
23. Police Mental Health Training
24. Project Fresh Start (legal advocacy)
25. Bronx Clinic Forensic Specialist
26. Queens Clinic Forensic Specialists
27. Forensic Housing
28. Sex Offender Treatment Planning
29. NYU Evaluation Research
30. NYU Forensic Conferences

Note: Included are programs and services sponsored by the City of New York and cooperating programs sponsored by other organizations. Not all programs are city-wide.

criminal justice system. When New York City police officers encounter a person in need of mental health or substance abuse services, if arrest is not necessary, the person is given a "LifeNet" card and may be escorted to a hospital or treatment provider. The cards provide information about the city's LifeNet hotlines operated by the Mental Health Association of

New York in conjunction with the Department of Mental Health. These 24-hour hotlines, staffed by English and Spanish speaking professionals, connect the caller to services, and, when needed, to one of the city's 22 mobile crises teams (DMH, 1998).

Diversion can occur early in the judicial process, at arraignment. Diversion at this point provides an opportunity to avoid both trial and incarceration. In 2000, New York City started its first Arraignment Court Mental Health Diversion Service based on a needs assessment study which found that many defendants had severe psychiatric disorders and histories of homelessness (Broner et al., 2000). It also identified procedures to make a diversion program effective which include police, correctional and court personnel, as well as mental health professionals. As a result, the Arraignment Court Diversion Service has the ability to evaluate people in court, present treatment alternatives to a judge and prosecutor, provide residential placement, develop treatment plans, and link clients to services.

A final opportunity for diversion occurs after arraignment and the LINK programs also offer services at this juncture. Working with discharge planners in the jails, LINK diversion staff evaluate detentioners and develop treatment plans which are presented to a judge and prosecutor as an alternative to incarceration. With judicial approval, clients are connected to community services and provided case management. While LINK diversion is designed primarily for misdemeanor offenders, the Nathaniel Project (Center for Alternative Sentencing and Employment Services, 2000) has been developed to provide diversion services to felony offenders. Together, LINK and Nathaniel provide diversion in all post-arraignment settings.

Jail Mental Health Services

Individuals not released from court are taken to one of New York City's 16 jails. There, psychiatric screenings and examinations are conducted and, when necessary, individuals are referred for mental health services. Jail-based mental health services include medication management, counseling, drug and alcohol treatment, specialized housing, crisis management, and suicide prevention (New York City Board of Correction, 1984). However, half or more of the individuals who are determined to need mental health services are confined for less than two weeks, many for only a few days. Consequently, one of the most useful services provided in jails is discharge planning which connects people with community services.

Discharge Planning

Jail-based discharge planning identifies a person's mental health needs, finds services in the community, and when possible arranges appointments for treatment (Griffin, 1991). In addition, discharge planners link clients to social and income support services. In New York City jails, discharge planners are available to every client who remains in jail long enough for a discharge plan to be completed. For those who leave jail quickly, a program is being developed to provide discharge planning in the community.

LINK Transition Services

LINK programs provide transition case management which makes it easier for a forensic client to move from a jail or court to the community. When possible, LINK transition staff meet clients prior to release, accompany them to community service providers, and assist in completing applications for entitlements. LINK continues to provide case management until clients are connected to community services.

Another significant component of LINK is a prescription medication service. Many people who leave city jails have no means of paying for medication. They did not have Medicaid when they entered jail or it was terminated while they were in jail. In order to ensure that clients get needed medication, participating pharmacies are asked to fill prescriptions with the assurance that LINK will pay the bill if the client is not enrolled in Medicaid (DMH, 1998).

LINK also provides peer support groups (DMH, 1998). These groups allow clients to express concerns and see how others overcome similar difficulties. They provide support consistent with clients' culture and ethnicity, and they foster relationships with community organizations, such as churches and civic groups.

Community Case Management

Case management significantly increases the treatment compliance of severely mentally ill clients (Rubin, 1992) by escorting clients to appointments and ensuring that they take medication. Because LINK provides case management, it has been able to reduce the concerns of many mental health providers who believed forensic clients were non-compliant and resisted accepting this population into community-based programs. In addition, the Department of Mental Health assigns forensic specialists to mental health care providers in the community. They counsel forensic clients and train agency staff.

System Integration and Coordination

Ensuring that mental health clients in the criminal justice system get appropriate services ultimately rests on the ability of many agencies and programs to work together. Positive outcomes depend largely on a coordinated and integrated effort. This can be illustrated by understanding how the court-based diversion services link clients to community-based providers. The diversion services connect clients to case management programs. Once that is achieved, case managers make referrals to all needed services in the community. However, the obligations of the diversion services and case management programs extend beyond referrals. Both must track clients and ensure that they remain in treatment. All agencies and programs work together to ensure that clients receive treatment in the community. Figure 1 provides a diagram of the interaction of programs and agencies.

RECOMMENDATIONS

This network of services has done much to provide for the needs of forensic clients. Yet, more remains to be done. Below are recommendations for further improvements in the system.

1. Housing

Appropriate housing provides the structured environment that allows mentally ill clients to develop more organized life styles. This results in greater compliance with treatment. While additional housing for the forensic population is becoming available, three categories of beds are still needed. The first is "immediate placement beds" for individuals released directly from court. The second are "transitional beds" for people with a planned release from confinement or from immediate placement beds. Finally, "permanent housing" is needed for the chronic mentally ill.

2. Hospitalization of the mentally ill by police

Better procedures are needed to facilitate police taking people with mental illness to hospitals, when appropriate, rather than arresting them. Diversion at this point is clinically appropriate and cost-effective. Police need to better understand the behavior of mentally ill people, and this can be achieved through additional in-service training. In addition, police should not be penalized for taking people to the hospital. At present, the

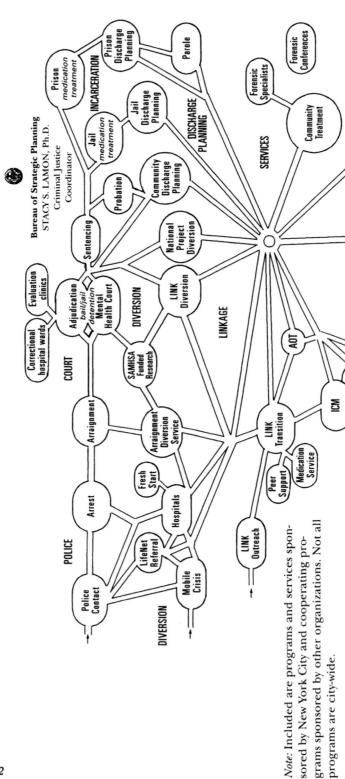

The City of New York
Department of Mental Health, Mental Restoration and Alcoholism Services
NEAL L. COHEN. M.D.
COMMISSIONER

Bureau of Strategic Planning
STACY S. LAMON, Ph.D.
Criminal Justice
Coordinator

Note: Included are programs and services sponsored by New York City and cooperating programs sponsored by other organizations. Not all programs are city-wide.

Sources: City of New York Department of Mental Health, Mental Retardation and Alcoholism Services, Bureau of Strategic Planning.

FIGURE 12.1 Network and flow of New York City's Criminal Justice Mental Health Services.

police have no incentive to choose hospitalization over arrest. In fact, they are penalized for choosing hospitalization because they have to wait for extended time periods while people are admitted.

The waiting time needs to be reduced, and a model for doing so already exists. Several years ago, an effort to reduce waiting time for police officers was initiated in cooperation with the city's Comprehensive Psychiatric Emergency Programs (CPEP), (DMH, 1998). In this model a police officer simply completed a release form and gave it to the CPEP psychiatric staff. The hospital then accepted custody for the person. Consideration should be given to fully implementing this procedure.

3. Police crisis response

During the past two decades, the New York City Police Department has made significant strides in dealing with mentally ill individuals. Yet, police continuously find themselves in difficult situations. Models for police mental health crisis intervention have been developed throughout the country (Borum, Deane, Steadman & Morrissey, 1998; Dupont & Cochran, 1996; Finn & Sullivan, 1988, 1989; Deane, Steadman, Borum & Morrissey, 1998) and components of these models may be useful in New York. The New York City Police Department has asked the Department of Mental Health and other agencies for advice on this issue. Every effort should be made to assist them.

CONCLUSION

Treatment of mentally ill New Yorkers who come into contact with the criminal justice system has improved markedly in the past 10 years. During this period a network of programs specifically targeted to this population has been developed. In addition, forensic clients have benefitted from the growth of the larger community mental health system and from the fact that services for those with chronic mental illness have become more assertive. Finally, forensic clients have profited as New York State and City made a concerted effort to better coordinate the mental health system with the criminal justice system.

Yet, for all that has been achieved, much remains to be done. Forensic mentally ill clients live with a particularly heavy burden of stigma. Society remains wary of them because they have committed crimes and because they are mentally ill. Their involvement with the criminal justice system has made it more difficult to ensure that they can be integrated into the community mental health system. For these reasons, this disorganized, fragile population has frequently been the last to benefit from improvements in mental health care. Sufficient resources have not been targeted to address their needs, and too little pressure has been put on government agencies to overcome barriers to coordinate service delivery. Mental health advocates, public policy researchers, and government administrators need to pay more attention to the clinical needs of the forensic mentally ill population.

There is also a pressing need for society to more completely understand the benefit of improving services to the forensic mentally ill population. This can be achieved through more public education efforts by the City and other concerned organizations. The public needs to be aware that improved treatment and services reduce recidivism and minimize the need for police intervention. Moreover, specialized services reduce criminal justice expenditures and the need for expensive, hospital-based mental health care. Finally, more adequate services for this population result in a better quality of life for many mentally ill forensic clients and a more liveable, safer city.

REFERENCES

Abram, K.M. & Teplin, L.A. (1991). Co-occurring disorders among mentally ill jail detainees: Implications for public policy. *American Psychologist, 40*(10), 1036–1045.

Barr, H. (1999). *Prisons and jails: Hospitals of last resort.* New York: Correctional Association of New York and Urban Justice Center.

Borum, R., Deane, M.W., Steadman, H.J. & Morrissey, J. (1998). Police perspectives on responding to mentally ill people in crisis: Perceptions of program effectiveness. *Behavioral Science and the Law, 16,* 393–405.

Broner, N., Franczak, M., Dye, C. & McCallister, W. (2001). Knowledge transfer, policymaking and community empowerment: A consensus model approach for providing public mental health and substance abuse services. *Psychiatric Quarterly, 72*(1), 79–102.

Broner, N., Owen, E., Lamon, S. & Karopkin, M.G. (March, 2000). *Mental illness and substance use of pre-arraignment detainees: Population characteristics and service needs.* Paper presented at the biannual meeting of the American Psychological Association's American Psychology Law Society (APLS), New Orleans, LA.

Broner, N., Rock, M. & Landsberg, G. (May, 1998). *Psychosocial and case management issues in services' linkage: A six-month follow-up of a jail diversion program for the mentally ill.* Paper presented at grand rounds of the Mental Health and Public Policy Research Department, University of Pennsylvania, Philadelphia, PA.

Center for Alternative Sentencing and Employment Services. (2000). *The Nathaniel Project: A new alternative to incarceration program for mentally ill felony offenders in Manhattan* [agency brochure]. New York: Author.

Cohen, N.L. (1998, April). *Commissioner of Mental Health testimony to the New York City Council Subcommittee on Mental Health* [subcommittee transcript]. New York: Author.

Cohen, N.L., Lamon, S.S. & Katz, N. (in press) Implementing Kendra's Law. In G. Landsberg, M. Rock, L. Berg & A. Smiley (Eds.), *Serving mentally ill offenders: Challenges and opportunities for mental health professionals.* New York: Springer Publishing.

Deane, M., Steadman, H., Borum, R., Veysey, B. & Morrissey, J. (1998). Police-mental health system interactions: Program types and needed research. *Psychiatric Services, 50,* 99–101.

Dvoskin, J.A., Smith, H. & Broaddus, R. (1993). Creating a mental health care model. *Corrections Today,* 114–119.

Dupont, R. & Cochran, S. (1996).*Crisis Intervention Team training manual* [departmental manual]. Memphis, TN: Memphis Police Department.

Finn, P. & Sullivan, M. (1988, January). Police response to special populations: Handling the mentally ill, public inebriation, and the homeless. *Research in Action, National Institute of Justice,* 1–6.

Finn, P. & Sullivan, M. (1989). Police handling of the mentally ill: Sharing responsibility with the mental health system. *Journal of Criminal Justice, 17,* 1–14.

Griffin, P. (1991). The back door of the jail: Linking mentally ill offenders to community mental health services. In H.J. Steadman (Ed.), *Jail Diversion for the mentally ill: Breaking the barriers* (Chapter 5). Washington, DC: U.S. Department of Justice.

Linn, K., Broner, N. & Rotter, M. (2000). Quarterly reports (1st, 2nd & 3rd quarters). *SAMHSA Community action grant for planning comprehensive court-based diversion for individuals with co-occurring mental illness and substance use disorders.* New York: Educational Assistance Corporation—TASC.

Landsberg, G. (1992). Developing comprehensive mental health services in local jails and police lockups. In S. Cooper & T.H. Lentner (Eds.), *Innovations in Community Mental Health.* Sarasota, FL; Professional Resources Press.

Landsberg, G., Rock, M. & Broner, N. (1999). *Pathways of the mentally ill into criminal justice systems: Initial findings and recommendations* [institute report]. New York: New York University, Ehrenkranz School of Social Work, Institute Against Violence.

Martell, D.A., Rosner, R. & Harmon, R.B. (1995). Base-rate estimates of criminal behavior by homeless mentally ill persons in New York City. *Psychiatric Services, 46*(6), 596.

Michaels, D., Zoloth, S.R., Alcabes, P., Braslow, C.A. & Safyer, S. (1992). Homelessness and indicators of mental illness among inmates in New York City's correctional system. *Hospital and Community Psychiatry, 43*(2), 150–155.

New York City Department of Mental Health, Mental Retardation and Alcoholism Services. (1998). *Local government plan: Adult mental health services 1998–2003.* New York: Author.

New York City Department of Mental Health, Mental Retardation and Alcoholism Services. (2000). *The New York City system of criminal justice—mental health services* [departmental brochure]. New York: Author.

New York City Board of Correction. (1984). *Mental health minimum standards for New York City correctional facilities.* New York: Author.

Peters, R.H. & Hills, H.A. (1993). Inmates with co-occurring substance abuse and mental disorders. In H.J. Steadman & J.J. Coczza (Eds.), *Mental illness in America's prisons.* Seattle: National Coalition for the Mentally Ill in the Criminal Justice System.

Rubin, A. (1992). Is case management effective for people with serious mental illness? A research review. *Health and Social Work, 17*(2), 138–150.

Solomon, J. & Draine, J. (1995). Issues in serving the forensic client. *Social Work, 40*(1), 25–33.

Steadman, H., Barbera, S. & Dennis, D. (1994). A national survey of jail mental health diversion programs. *Hospital & Community Psychiatry, 45*, 1109–1112.

Steadman, H.J., Morris, S.M., & Dennis, D.L. (1995). The diversion of mentally ill persons from jails to community-based services: A profile of programs. *American Journal of Public Health 85*(12), 1630–1635.

Shenson, D., Dubler, N. & Michaels, D. (1990). Jails and prisons: The new asylums. *American Journal of Public Health, 80*(6), 655–656.

Torrey, E.F., Steiber, J., Ezekiel, J., Wolfe, S.M., Sharfstein, J., Noble, J.H. & Flynn, L.M. (1992). *Criminalizing the seriously mentally ill: The abuse of jails as mental hospitals.* Washington, DC: Public Citizen's Health Research Group.

Veysey, B.M., Steadman, H.J. Morrissey, J.P. & Johnson, M. (1997). In search of the missing linkages: Continuity of care in U.S. jails. *Behavioral Sciences and the Law, 15*, 383–397.

SECTION III
Serving Emotionally Disturbed Women

13

Overview:
Working With Women in Jails:
Developing A Gender-Based
Network of Services for
Strengthening Women and
Their Families

Susan Salasin

BACKGROUND

Developing an overview that highlights the unique program development goals for in-jail programs for women in Massachusetts and Maryland is an exciting challenge. These two programs that are presented are firmly grounded in the most up-to-date information and gender-based thinking about what appears to best serve women in jail. However, it is the translation of these emerging guidelines into actual programs that illustrates the synergy of cutting-edge innovation that make them such attractive models to help in the development of other new and emerging jails programs for women.

In the mid-1990s at the Center for Mental Health Services, Substance Abuse and Mental Health Services Administration, DHHS, a new Congressional mandate in the criminal justice arena led us to begin to develop, as one of our initiatives, a project of services development for women in jails and prisons. Prisons, as we learned, already served as sites for some modest, gender-based program development for female inmates. Jails, however, had not served as sites for offering these types of services.

At that time, our Federal agency had become accustomed to pressures from specialized advocacy groups demanding services for every population in every type of setting for which we had an agency responsibility.

Thus, it came as no small surprise to learn that, although such advocacy groups did exist to press for improved services for women in prison, no such advocacy group had existed for women in jail.

This was an important "finding." It suggested that intensive efforts would be needed to raise consciousness about the dilemmas and challenges for women in jails. Jails, which are a local community-based institution, potentially have the best opportunity to provide shorter-term interventions, linked to community resources, that can play a critical role in preparing women for re-entering the community as contributing members. Even if some of these women go on to serve time in prisons, an early gender-based program intervention can play a strong role in preparing them to effectively cope with the rigors of prison life. With this goal in mind, our next steps were to learn what we could about the background and facts of these women's lives and to develop a gender-based program model that maximized their strengths and coping capacity while in jail and also provided a better, more lasting transition into the community.

We learned that, at the present time, over a million women are booked into jail annually. Women account for over 12% of jail inmates, and this percentage is growing at a faster rate than males. From surveys, research, case studies, and program descriptions such as those presented in this section we have acquired specialized knowledge about who these women are, their histories prior to incarceration, and their profile of needs and life circumstances that determine the parameters of what can and must be accomplished to develop coping capacities and build constructive passages into the community. A summary of our specialized knowledge on the background, characteristics, and life themes of these women and the services delivery challenges they present is outlined below.

SUMMARY: CURRENT KNOWLEDGE BASE REGARDING WOMEN IN JAILS

1. Why Are These Women in Jail?

Typically, they are booked in jail due to drug or property crimes when they are picked up as a "mule" acting to support a male partner's lifestyle and to provide income for support of their children. Rarely are alternatives such as community treatment and other alternative community sanctions available and so these woman proceed right to jail. (For a description of one of the few alternative programs, see Chapter 14 on Maryland's Phoenix project.). Once in jail, they serve longer sentences than their male counterparts picked up for drug crimes. This is because, in their role as "mule," they are not in charge of the overall drug operation and have no information with which to plea-bargain for lighter sentences.

2. Who Are These Women?

Women currently incarcerated in jails or detention centers are, to a large extent, poor, of color, and have histories of physical and/or sexual abuse. Many are diagnosed with serious mental illness and serious substance abuse habits, and 8 out of 10 of them are mothers. A large number, estimated at over 60% to 70%, have lost primary custody of their children.

3. What Are the Most Common Themes in These Women's Lives?

The majority of these women have described growing up in a family where one or both parents suffered from mental illness and/or alcohol and drug abuse. Almost all of them talk about early childhood sexual abuse by fathers, other family members including stepfathers, or foster care fathers or family members. Most of these women experienced early signs of mental illness or substance abuse problems and suicide attempts when they were young.

4. Who Cares for Her Children Following A Woman's Arrest?

At the present time, there appears to be no consistently authorized or appointed authority responsible for the immediate placement of children, which frequently occurs on an almost "ad hoc" basis at the time of arrest. Relatives and/or close friends or temporary and/or permanent foster care are the common first lines of response. These children are deeply affected by their mother's incarceration with all of its unknowns, uncertainties, and accompanying life changes, and there are no resources available to help them address these needs. Reunification with their children is the most important goal for most women and often serves as a core motivation for gaining release into the community.

5. What Helps Women to Change and Recover?

Interpersonal Necessities

An important foundation for thinking about how women change and recover is the centrality of relationships with others in their development and maturation. To feel able to communicate feelings and experience reciprocity, to feel free from harm so that communication is possible, and to see in others, i.e., "role models," what a woman hopes to learn for herself are all fundamental.

a) *A woman's first imperative, by all accounts, is safety.* Until a feeling of safety is assured, it is difficult for any other recovery to take place. An important aspect of this is the planned and actual reduction of retraumatization/victimization within the jail itself. This retraumatization/victimization often occurs not only from staff and other inmates but also from use, by staff, of policies of actual restraint and seclusion to subdue agitated or aggressive behavior which can recreate the actual conditions of the original abuse in a woman's life history.

b) *A second key component is the time and space to develop relationships* with other inmates and female staff who care, listen, and can be trusted. This involves planning for time to be spent together, often in special areas that afford privacy and circumstances more conducive to building personal rapport.

c) *A third, and described by many as a "without-which-not" component, is the availability of other inmates and staff who can serve as role models.* This is described as having other women in the milieu who "look like me," "dress and eat as I do," and whose "philosophies, attitudes, and ability to move forward *show* me that I can make it."

Skills and Resource Building

Themes running throughout many of the case studies that have been conducted suggest that women particularly value programs that offer the following resources and opportunities from which they can grow.

a) *Proper assessment/classification of problems and proper corresponding medication.* Many accounts exist of lost opportunity and stagnation and regression due to improper screening for ALL relevant problem areas, mis-diagnosis, and mis-use of prescribed medications that have short-circuited services interventions.

b) *Programs that offer grief counseling and mental health, substance abuse, and parenting skills development.* Also important are programs that offer educational and vocational skills development.

c) *Planned events to visit with their children.* Examples would be in-residence programs, frequent contact visits, and co-counseling mother and children sessions.

d) *Planning for re-entry into the community.* This includes establishing prerelease contacts and relationships with a range of relevant community care providers, arranging for housing, transportation and child care support (if appropriate), etc.

IN FOCUS: VOICES PROGRAM IN MASSACHUSETTS AND TAMAR PROGRAM IN MARYLAND

A comparison of the Massachusetts and Maryland in-jail programs for women offers two excellent examples of the manner in which the above principles may be tailored and put into practice according to the needs and resources of the local community. Some fundamental planning steps were critical to begin the process or program development at both sites. These were undertaken to: 1) capitalize on the existing and emerging motivation of old and new staff to develop truly women-sensitive programs that were steeped in the latest knowledge; 2) maximize motivation and broaden insight of planning undertaken by staff through a series of focus groups with all relevant stakeholders for the new program (primarily, of course, with the women inmates themselves); and 3) undertake program planning linked conceptually and practically to the local communities that were homes to these women. In the case of both of these sites, planning for the new programs was participatory and progress in the program was individually assessed and based on incremental steps of accomplishment.

Not surprisingly, as is so often true for programs developed to serve women, those that were developed by these two sites were given names that reflected their overall goals: VOICES in Hampden County, Massachusetts, which is an acronym for *V*alidation, *O*pportunity, *I*nspiration, *C*ommunication, *E*mpowerment, and *S*afety; and TAMAR in the Maryland counties of Dorchester, Calvert, and Frederick which is an acronym for *T*rauma, *A*ddictions, *M*ental *H*ealth, and *R*ecovery. In the case of VOICES, the acronym represents a program developed and implemented in a single county jail, while the Maryland TAMAR program represents a federal/state/county collaborative effort for three counties in Maryland following the same model that will eventually be expanded to all of the counties of that state.

FEATURES COMMON TO THE VOICES AND TAMAR PROGRAMS

Pointed differences in VOICES and TAMAR can be seen in means of entry into the program; formal program structure and length; emphasis on some services as primary and others as companion services; and how linkage to the community is accomplished. In addition to their differences, however, there are several notable features common to both.

1. Both programs are voluntary at the woman's request for inclusion.
2. Both are group programs—each session is a group session.
3. Each program includes a range of important services which address mental health and substance abuse; trauma issues related to physical and sexual abuse; impaired independent living skills (including parenting); and problem-solving skills in addition to identifying and planning for women's connections with new and ongoing resources in the community.

EVALUATION PLANNING FOR VOICES AND TAMAR

Since both programs are in early developmental stages, formal program evaluation has not yet been instituted. Planning for strategies to summarize the formal, traditional measures such as numbers of women served, for what time periods, with what characteristics, etc. is beginning to take place. In addition to these traditional methods of accountability, each program is planning to use unique measures that will hopefully capture the accomplishments tailored to the uniqueness of their specific approaches.

To this end, VOICES is planning for testing pre- and post-mastery levels for the contents of the program, evaluating satisfaction upon program completion, and identifying change in areas related to the ability to make effective choices and avoid past mistakes. TAMAR is developing a cross-site evaluation approach for participating counties that will include some of these same measures in addition to examining changes in a woman's learning history. Each sees evaluation as a progressive activity to use in program improvement.

EMERGING OPPORTUNITIES FOR PROFESSIONAL DEVELOPMENT

The challenges and opportunities for professionals to learn to apply their expertise in settings new to most professionals emerging from today's training programs are self-evident. Fundamental to the transition to work in jails and with the criminal justice system is both the willingness and motivation to engage in cross-training with criminal justice and allied professionals regarding the philosophy, structure, and operating principles of these systems. Collaboration is the key to success, as is grounded knowledge about women in jail and how new skills needed for self-development in their roles as women, mothers, and community members can be acquired. Given the backgrounds and life experiences that these women bring to the jail setting, there are many issues that need careful and sustained attention. Most of these women have already known frustration, rejection, abuse, and failed opportunities in many areas of their lives, and skillful in-jail interventions can serve as a first positive step forward.

14

Maryland's Programs for Incarcerated Women With Mental Illness and Substance Abuse Disorders

Joan Gillece and Betty G. Russell

The Division of Special Populations of the Mental Hygiene Administration of the Maryland Department of Health and Mental Hygiene oversees programs for individuals with mental illness who may also have co-occurring substance abuse disorders, and/or HIV/AIDS, and are homeless, and/or deaf, and in the criminal justice system. As the number of women in jails has increased nationwide, there has also been a corresponding increase in female inmates in the detention centers in Maryland. While Maryland detention centers have been providing mental health services to inmates of both genders since 1992, their female inmates have not been the focus of specialized treatment until recently.

The Division of Special Populations of the Mental Hygiene Administration began the Maryland Community Criminal Justice Treatment Program (MCCJTP) as a pilot program in four counties in 1992. Since that initial program, the Division has developed the program in 22 of Maryland's 23 counties. In 1995, the Division began a focus on treatment programs for women in response to the concerns of wardens about the special problems incarcerated women presented to correctional staffs. These problems included increased suicidal threats; reclusive behaviors (i.e., women's refusal to be involved in activities) resulting in a lack of concern for personal hygiene and medical care; and the lack of ability to cope with their situations as inmates. In many cases, these behaviors resulted in institutional infractions. In response to the wardens concerns, the Division and its partner, the Center for Mental Health Services Research

(CMHSR) of the University of Maryland School of Medicine (Department of Psychiatry), applied for two grants from federal agencies that would address these and related issues.

THE PHOENIX PROJECT

Background

In 1997, the Substance Abuse Mental Health Services Administration (SAMHSA) of the United States Department of Health and Human Services requested grant applicants for demonstration sites that would divert individuals from jail to the community. The Division of Special Populations applied for and received funding of $1,575,442 for a gender-specific grant for females with co-occurring serious mental illness and substance abuse disorders in rural Wicomico County on the Eastern Shore of Maryland. Wicomico County has an estimated population of approximately 79,000. The major urban center is the city of Salisbury (population 21,8827). This county was one of the original pilot counties in 1993. The local detention center holds approximately 600 to 700 inmates on any given day.

Women eligible for the services of the Phoenix Project must be 18 or older and have a severe mental illness as evidenced by a DSM-IV Axis I clinical diagnosis and a substance abuse disorder. The woman must also face arrest for a misdemeanor or a non-violent felony.

Before writing the grant, staff from the division and CMHSR conducted a focus group with five women in the Wicomico County, Maryland Community Criminal Justice Treatment Program. The women were inmates in the detention center at the time of the interviews when they were asked what services could have helped them and their children. Each of the women had extensive substance abuse problems, and all suffered from serious mental illnesses. The women spoke of their shame and desperation at the time of and following their arrest.

When determining the services and procedures that would be implemented in the Phoenix Project, the responses of the focus group were given great consideration. The police and mental health staff have been trained in recognizing symptoms of mental illnesses and substance abuse disorders and works with the Mobile Crisis Unit (MCU) which is available 24 hours a day. The MCU consists of a case manager, a sheriff's deputy, and a mental health professional. When police respond to a complaint, the MCU is called if a woman exhibits signs or symptoms of mental illness or a substance abuse disorder. The disposition of the case is a joint effort between the MCU and the police, contingent on multiple factors including the nature and severity of the offense, the mental status of the woman, her criminal history, and her behavior and conduct. If she is eligible, she is diverted into the Phoenix Project and is not arrested.

Diversion

A woman who is eligible for Phoenix and agrees to participate in the project will at that point be diverted into emergency crisis housing where she will be further evaluated and stabilized, or she will receive intensive case management and clinical interventions in her home. Her children will also remain with her. She and the children will be moved to transitional housing as soon as she is ready. In addition to transitional housing, she will be eligible to access the Shelter Plus Care rental assistance available through the Division of Special Populations' HUD grant if she is homeless. A key component of the services available to a woman is a case manager who specializes in mental health and substance abuse. The case manager provides direct mental health/substance abuse treatment services and brokers other community services for the woman and her children as needed. With Maryland's entry into a managed public mental health fee for service care system, community services are most often reimbursable.

Evaluation

The evaluation of the Phoenix Project to be conducted by CMHSR features two major focuses. One is the compilation of a *Learning History* that will explore how the various "communities of practice" within the Wicomico County mental health, substance abuse, and criminal justice systems learn to work with a jail diversion program. The learning history is a special type of case study that employs a narrative approach to tell the story of the development of the program in the words of the participants who made it happen.

A second focus of the local evaluation is the use of *Lifelines* of the women in the Phoenix Project. The client reviews her life through the time of the interview by means of a chart that maps changes in life satisfaction to the present. The lifeline will reflect "peaks" and "valleys." For each of these "turning points," the client is asked a series of questions. The answers reflect the interviewee's views of herself, others, and the events of her life. The lifeline interview is administered at the time of admission to the project and again in 12 months.

In addition to these primary studies, the evaluation will also focus on several secondary studies. These include the impacts on the children of these women and a study of the costs associated with developing and operating a jail diversion program. The evaluative component of the grant includes the director of the research project, three assistants, and various consultants.

The Phoenix Project had a late start-up due to issues at other sites involved in the SAMHSA grant. Wicomico County had its first woman enter the Phoenix Project in September, 1998. Since October, 1998, 33 women have been served. The grant ends on September 30, 2000. With the development of pre-booking diversion, women with co-occurring disorders and their children should be able to rejoin their communities and look to brighter futures.

THE TAMAR PROJECT

Background

Women with histories of violence are not uncommon in local jails. A woman in one of the jails told a staff member: " I was raped when I was six by my mother's boyfriend and he kept on for the next two years until my mother threw him out. I thought I was just a bad person and deserved all of that. When I was 14, I started smoking grass and then ended up a heroin addict. I stole from everybody, passed bad checks and worked the streets. No one told me that that stuff from the past was eating me up until I talked to another woman in here who had some of the same background but had gotten some help about it."

The Division of Special Populations became concerned about trauma issues when staff members visited a substance abuse group in one of the detention centers in the MCCJTP program and listened to all of the women in the group describe the physical and sexual abuse they had suffered. When SAMHSA announced funding for a Women and Violence study in February,1998, the Division once again collaborated with the Center for Mental Health Services Research at the University of Maryland at Baltimore to apply for funding. The TAMAR Project funded by SAMHSA provides services for women who have histories of sexual and physical abuse, mental illnesses, and substance abuse disorders and who are in the criminal justice system. The project brings together agencies such as social services, mental hygiene, substance abuse, domestic violence, and parole and probation in a collaboration to serve these women in more efficient and beneficial ways.

The three counties selected for the project represent various areas of Maryland. Dorchester County is a rural county on the Eastern Shore. Calvert

County is in the southern part of the state and is rural as well as a bedroom community for upper management who work in the Washington, D.C. Frederick County is also a bedroom community for the district but with a more middle-class population. There are still some rural areas in this county. The majority of women inmates in these three counties' jails may have received mental health and substance abuse treatment in the past, but this project allows the state to create an integrated system of services in each jurisdiction to serve this population more comprehensively.

Members of the Division and CMHSR once again went to the women who would be served by this project and asked them what services would have been of help to them. They were especially concerned about the importance of being able to discuss their difficulties with someone. They were concerned about their children and their inadequacies as mothers; they did not want to abuse their children. They admitted that they needed help both in the detention center and in the community upon release.

The Division of Special Populations was notified that, effective October 1, 1998, the Mental Hygiene Administration would be the only one of the 14 sites funded by SAMHSA for the Women and Violence study to serve women in correctional settings. Building on the Maryland Community Criminal Justice Treatment Program, the Division has developed an integrated system to provide services for these women. Each of the three counties involved in TAMAR offered letters of support from numerous agencies that have a stake in the project. Meetings are held in each jurisdiction with agency representatives on a regular basis. The goal is to build a system that not only meets the needs of the women and their children but also reflects that county's uniqueness such as suburban vs. rural, available housing, and seriousness of crimes committed. This may produce three models with major commonalties but some variations that would be replicable by other similar jurisdictions.

Phase I of the grant, a two-year period, provided $1,139,430 and allowed each site to establish the programmatic services that would be provided. Although building on the existing MCCJTP, sites had to begin partnering with other agencies as a requirement of the grant. This necessitated the building of relationships that may have been perfunctory in the past. Many agency heads had never been in the same room together. Because of the time it took to build these networks, many months passed before the actual services were in place and women could begin to receive treatment.

Services

The women being served in this project are women with any mental illness and/or substance abuse disorder who have experienced violence at any time in their lives and who are or have been in the criminal justice system. Women in the detention center are assessed and diagnosed after arrest. A woman's condition may be identified either through the mental health or substance abuse counselor or through the medical personnel in the detention center. The trauma specialist will focus on safety and containment issues of symptom management through treatment groups within the detention center. Participation in the psycho-educational groups is voluntary. The trauma specialists, medical officer, mental health and substance abuse counselors, and classification officer of the detention center meet weekly to discuss providing the coordinated services these women need.

Upon release, these women will continue to meet in each county treatment groups that are developed by the trauma specialist. Women also may be referred to the trauma specialist for community groups through parole and probation. A community team consisting of representatives from mental health, substance abuse, domestic violence, parole and probation, and social services and the trauma specialist meet weekly to coordinate community services.

An additional feature of the services is a community peer support group. Advocates from the Advocates Advisory Board are working in each of the counties to establish peer support groups that women can attend. The women in the groups will determine the groups' focuses. Funding is available to pay for transportation to the support groups as well as for child care while the groups meet so that the mothers will not be distracted from the meetings.

The trauma specialist will also ensure that, upon release, a woman and her children will be connected to a case manager and access any needed services. Services are available in Maryland to children but mothers are not included. The challenge is to expand services such as mental health and substance abuse to include the mothers as well. To facilitate this integration, the Division holds workshops and trainings on issues related to parenting and children's needs.

To facilitate the work of the trauma specialists, a clinical supervisor (a Ph.D. in psychology with vast experience in trauma therapy) has been hired as a consultant. When the specialist is faced with a dilemma, the clinician is available to offer assistance. The clinician also meets with the three trauma specialists weekly to analyze specific cases. The clinician and the three trauma specialists designed the 12-week, three-hours-a-week, curriculum that is being used in the groups. The curriculum includes journal writing and art therapy.

The Division of Special Populations is also using grant funding to develop and implement training related to trauma. The Sidran Foundation, a private nonprofit publishing house that focuses on trauma issues, has conducted the training. All correctional officers within the detention center have received training in symptoms and trauma. A curriculum specifically tailored to the needs of correctional staff has been developed after consultation with the wardens of each county. The Maryland Correctional Officers Training Academy credits this as in-service training. The Academy will also be including a course in trauma as a part of training for new officers. In addition to training those within the jails, there has also been training for representatives of the various agencies in the community that are providing services to the women in the TAMAR Project including social services, parole and probation, mental health, substance abuse, domestic violence and children's services. Training is developed and delivered as needs and issues arise.

A unique feature of the grant is the inclusion of a Director of Trauma Services at the state level who works in the Division of Special Populations. There are very few state level positions such as this nationally. The Division will be providing the expansion of trauma services to male offenders beginning the summer of 2000, thanks to funding from the Mental Hygiene Administration.

Evaluation

Maryland's local evaluation will use life stories and learning histories to determine the effectiveness of the integrated systems approach to treatment as well as the process of integrating various systems around the issues of trauma.

From September 1, 1999 until March 1, 2000, the first six months of the actual provision of services, 82 women had been served in the detention centers. Treatment groups in the community began on January 1, 2000, and 20 women had been served in the community by March 1, 2000. Peer support groups have recently been developed in each community. Preliminary interviews with 12 women indicate that the women are very enthusiastic about the provision of trauma services in the detention centers and the communities. All of the women currently incarcerated have stated that they will continue in the community treatment groups. There has been no formal evaluation of recidivism to detention centers or psychiatric hospitals in Phase I.

The Mental Hygiene Administration recently approved funding to provide trauma treatment for women and men in eight other detention centers in Maryland. Clearly, the issue of trauma is of paramount importance in serving individuals in the criminal justice system.

15

A Gender-Specific Intervention Model for Incarcerated Women: Women's V.O.I.C.E.S. (Validation Opportunity Inspiration Communication Empowerment Safety)

Kate DeCou with Sally Van Wright

INTRODUCTION

The majority of female offenders come to jail with complex problems which are related to long-standing histories of physical and sexual abuse. While jail may seem to be an unlikely setting to begin a therapeutic journey, it can provide the opportunity to introduce the possibility of healing. For most of these women, the future looks bleak; they feel destined for more deprivation, addiction, violence, pain, and crime. A model which incorporates the understanding of women's unique experiences of injury, growth, and identity and which offers the elements of education, skill building, and treatment can instill a sense of hope, choice, and mastery for female inmates. An effective treatment program needs to be relational, comprehensive, multi-dimensional, and tailored to these unique experiences of women. It must give women the tools for empowerment, provide them with addictions and trauma treatment and link their concrete problems to resources in the community.

The need for such specialized intervention for women in corrections will be explored here. In point of fact, nearly all programming in county corrections (i.e., jail settings) has been oriented toward the male offender (Gray, Mays & Stohr, 1995; Jackson & Stearns, 1995). Recent research has demonstrated that women's pathways to criminal behavior are tied to their earlier experiences of sexual and physical abuse and addictions (Covington, 1998, 1999; Kerr, 1998; Owen, 1998). New gender-specific treatment models are being discussed and utilized in community settings (Brown,1997; Covington,1998; Finkelstein et al.,1997; Harris, 1998). However, comprehensive gender-specific program models have rarely been implemented in corrections, and virtually none of these have been included in jail settings. In one jail in Hampden County, Massachusetts, a gender-specific program for women is integrated into the correctional jail environment; it will be the focus of this discussion.

THE TARGET POPULATION: WOMEN IN JAILS

Jails are locally administered confinement facilities with a legislated authorization for the sheriff or local administrator to house pre-trial detainees and inmates with short sentences that are generally one year or less (Bureau of Justice Statistics, 1998). On June 30, 1998, there were 664,847 people being held or supervised in the 3,328 U.S. jails (Bureau of Justice Statistics,1998). This number nearly triples the 1986 jail population of 222,619. Because of the frequent shorts stays of people in jails, there were 9.8 million inmates booked into U.S. jails in 1995 (Bureau of Justice Statistics, 1996). Ten percent of this figure—about 980,000—represents the number of women booked into jails that same year. In 1998, women in jail accounted for almost 12% of the nation's jail inmates (Bureau of Justice Statistics, 1998). The number of women in jail is growing at a faster rate than that of males: in 1983, only 7.1% of jail populations were female. For the most part, this rise in the number of females arrested and incarcerated in the last 15 years is due to the war on drugs and the "tough-on-crime" legislation which has affected females even more than male offenders (Bloom, Chesney-Lind & Owen, 1994; Chesney-Lind, 1998; Owen,1998).

There is very little research done on females in jail settings (Bergsman, 1989; Connolly, 1983; Jalbert, 1987). Most research on jails is gender-neutral or assumes that conditions are similar for male and female inmates (e.g., Zupan, 1991). However, a few studies on women in jails indicate that women have access to fewer resources and that programs designed specifically for women in the mostly co-ed settings are rare (Austin, Bloom & Donohue, 1992; Flanagan, 1995; Jackson & Stearns, 1995; Glick & Neto, 1982; Gray et al., 1995; Jalbert, 1987; Morash, Bynum & Koons, 1998; Neto, 1981; Veysey, 1998). In their research study of 1995, Gray, Mays and Stohr concluded that even in the 18 all-female jails in the country, with the exception of self-help provided by community groups such as Alcoholics

Anonymous and Narcotics Anonymous, programming for women was "woe-fully inadequate. . . . Few programs were directed at repairing the damage done by victimization, including programs aimed at building self-esteem, improving communication skills, or managing stress and anger" (Gray et al., 1995). Programming for women offenders which does exist inside jails is usually fragmented and unstable; moreover, it is provided by groups outside the corrections environment (Weisheit, 1998).

PROFILE OF FEMALE OFFENDERS

Numerous research studies have attempted to document and understand the characteristics of this female population from which the following profile has emerged. Female offenders commit crimes which are largely non-violent. These include such crimes as shoplifting, larceny, passing bad checks, drug possession and drug sales, prostitution, and other sex charges (all of which comprise about 80% of total charges). These crimes are frequently committed to get money to sustain expensive drug addictions (Immarigeon & Chesney-Lind, 1992; Pollack-Byrne, 1990; Wellisch, Anglin & Prendergast, 1993). Research further reveals that 75% to 90% of women offenders are addicted to drugs and alcohol (Bloom, Chesney-Lind & Owen, 1994; Browne, 1998; Covington, 1998; DeCou , Haven & Vivian, 1998). Most female offenders, 75% to 85%, are mothers of whom over 90% are single caretakers (Bloom & Steinhart, 1993; Bureau of Justice Statistics, 1991; Buccia-Notaro, 1996; DeCou et al., 1998; Finkelstein, 1997; Gray et al., 1995). Histories of multiple, chronic experiences of sexual and physical abuse are present in 78% to 85% of these women (Bill, 1998; Browne, 1998; Bureau of Justice Statistics, 1999; DeCou et al, 1998; Kerr, 1998, Owen, 1998). Diagnosed severe mental illnesses are present in 18.5% of the population (Teplin, Abram & McClelland, 1996), with another 55% showing PTSD (Post Traumatic Stress Disorder) symptoms (DeCou et al., 1998). Other problems include health issues and a rate of HIV infection twice as high as in male offenders, inadequate or no housing and financial difficulties upon release, poor education and limited employment experience (DeCou et al., 1998; Galbraith, 1998; Gray et al., 1995; Singer, Bussey, Song & Lunghofer, 1995). In two recent jail studies, women inmates were found to leave home during early adolescence and most had their first child between the ages of 12 and 16 years (DeCou et al., 1998; Norton-Hawk, 1999).

In summary, the histories of trauma, leaving home at an early age, early parenthood, the presence of addictions, and histories of violent, unstable relationships are shared by most female offenders. These problems are therefore multiple, complex, and interrelated. These early life problems have contributed to deficits in practical life and problem-solving skills (Wolfe & Gentile, 1992) which, in turn, have led to poor education and employment histories and subsequently to a high degree of poverty. Also, consequences of early and repeated trauma include insecurity, fear, low self-esteem, and an inability to imagine an alternative healthier lifestyle.

CONSEQUENCES OF ABUSE: DEVELOPMENTAL IMPLICATIONS AND CO-OCCURRING DISORDERS

Based on the above female offender profile, between 75% and 90% of female offenders in a jail setting appear to have co-occurring substance abuse disorders and mental health problems. Often these same women face child custody problems and have health and other concerns (Owen, 1998). This profile suggests that just as these problem areas are multiple and complex, the need for intervention must similarly address developmental deficits, impaired independent living skills, addictions, trauma histories, and mental health. If one area alone is addressed, such as addictions, the neglected problem area, such as mental health, will likely sabotage progress (Alexander, 1996; Alexander & Muenzenmaier, 1998).

In 1998, in a project for the National Institute of Corrections (DeCou, et al., 1998), a survey of 156 Hampden County Correctional Center female offenders was conducted in conjunction with policy team members from several Massachussets criminal justice departments. The purpose of the project was to determine a detailed profile of Hampden County female offenders in order to consider policy implications regarding intermediate sanctions. The survey was administered by a team of trained researchers. Participation of inmates was voluntary and anonymous. Their responses to the survey regarding their mental health problems and trauma histories were significant. The results point to the connection between patterns of abuse originating at an early age and current, complex abuse problems. The survey listed seven categories of trauma and abuse—physical, sexual, severe neglect, accident, death or loss of parent before age 16, serious illness, natural disaster, and ritual abuse. The women were asked to report their abuse as a child and as an adult. The findings were as follows:

- 68 % reported histories of sexual abuse as an adult or child.
- 76% reported histories of physical abuse as an adult or child.
- 88% reported some type of abuse as a child.
- *51% reported 3 or more types of abuse* as a child.
- *55% reported 3 or more types of abuse* as an adult.
- 7% reported ritual abuse as a child and as an adult.
- 32% *witnessed* sexual abuse of another person as a child.
- 67% *witnessed* physical abuse as a child.

Regarding their self-reported mental health considerations:

- 68% were depressed at the time of the survey.
- 21.9% reported having some suicidal thoughts in the past 30 days.
- 7% had attempted suicide in the past six months.
- 37.6% reported a history of suicide attempts.
- 19.5% reported phobias.
- 10.2% reported auditory hallucinations.
- 48.4% reported anxiety.
- 18.4% reported violent outbursts.
- 35.2 %reported memory impairment.

In addition, 39.3 % stated they had lost one or more of their children.

When the researchers analyzed data according to specific mental health symptoms and connections to the criminal justice system, the results were as follows:

Of those women who had histories of sexual and/or physical abuse:

- 84% reported attempted suicide (compared to 16% with no history of abuse).
- 82% reported a history of depression (compared to 21% with no abuse history).
- 86% reported a history of hallucinations(compared to 14% with no abuse history).
- 88% reported a history of memory impairment (compared to 12% with no abuse).
- 25% reported a history of phobias (compared to 3% with no abuse history).
- 42% reported a history of anxiety (compared to 24% with no history of abuse).
- 36% reported a history of violent outbursts (compared to 14% with no abuse).

Criminal Justice Correlation:

- 89% have current sex-related charges (compared to 11% with no abuse history).
- 68% have drug-related charges (compared to 47% with no abuse history).
- 35% have 3 or more incarcerations (compared to 12% with no abuse history).
- 33% were arrested before the age of 16 (compared to 10% with no abuse history).

These findings mirror the effects of childhood and chronic trauma in studies of non-incarcerated women. Extremely high levels of guilt and shame and low levels of confidence and self-esteem are cited by most researchers in the field of trauma as common results of early childhood abuse (Barnett, Miller-Perrin & Perrin, 1997; Blume, 1990; Briere, 1989; Conte & Berliner, 1988; Courtois, 1992; Herman, 1992; Terr, 1991). Lenore Walker, a specialist in adult partner violence, applied Beck's concept of "learned helplessness" which is associated with a tendency to inaction or hesitation to effect life change as a direct consequence of chronic abuse (Walker, 1984). Terr noted a similar characteristic in childhood trauma survivors. She described the concept of "foreshortened future," a tendency to limit planning for the future due to the terror of facing the possibility of repeated trauma (Terr, 1990). Most theorists agree that other common effects of abuse are dissociations of memory and affect, over- or under-sexualization, hyper-vigilance, hallucinations, and tendencies to self-harm (mutilation, suicidal ideation or attempts, eating disorders), fears, phobias, and somatization. Other psychological symptoms include mistrust, depression, bi-polar disorders, and poor boundary definitions (Barnett et al., 1997; Bass & Davis, 1988; Blume, 1990; Briere, 1989; Evans & Sullivan, 1995; Herman, 1992; Terr, 1991; Zetlin, 1989). It is not surprising that with such profound injury in childhood, female offenders frequently leave home at early ages, often as runaways (Prescott, 1997).

A summary of research findings on the possible problematic effects of childhood neglect on adults include social difficulties, such as disturbed parent-child interactions and disturbed peer relations; intellectual deficits and intellectual delays; less creative, flexible problem-solving; deficits in language comprehension and verbal abilities; and emotional and behavioral problems such as low self-esteem and physical aggression and outbursts (Barnett et al., 1997).

Another way in which women are impacted by adult violence relates to domestic violence and its correlation to substance abuse in both female offenders and their partners. In the Hampden County Survey, 73.2% of the women offenders reported that their partner had a substance abuse history (DeCou, et al., 1998). Researchers have found that one-fourth to one-half of all men who commit acts of domestic violence also have substance abuse problems (Gondolf, 1995; Kantor & Strauss, 1987; Leonard & Jacob, 1987). Other studies report that women who abuse alcohol and other drugs are more likely to be victims of domestic abuse (Miller, Downs & Gondoli, 1989). In a major epidemiological study of substance users, women were found to have nearly four times the rate of post traumatic stress disorder than men—43% for females and 12% for men (Cottler, Compton & Mager, 1993).

The effects of domestic violence are similar to that of other trauma.

The negative effects observed in domestic violence victims include recurrent fear, feelings of helplessness, and stress. Fear, anger, and frustration evoke a sense of helplessness followed by depression and anxiety (Shepherd, 1990). The learned helplessness concept described by Lenore Walker is associated with depression, intellectual impairment (i.e., confusion and poor problem-solving ability) and motivational impairment (passivity) (Barnett et al., 1998; Walker, 1984). In the 1985 National Re-Survey, Strauss and Smith found that suicide attempts were four times more likely in women who were assaulted than in those who were not assaulted (Barnett et al., 1998). Over 60% of battered women in two samples of women seeking treatment experienced PTSD symptoms (Saunders, 1994).

A key aspect in the treatment of substance abuse is *encouraging* the client to *assume responsibility* for her addiction. For a female abuse survivor, it is important to *dispel* the idea that she is responsible for her partner's behavior. She is only responsible for her own behavior. Also, poorly developed decision-making is a problem for substance abusers. When a female offender is also a victim of violence, that inadequacy may be compounded (American Medical Association, 1993).

In summary, the consequences of histories of physical and sexual abuse, compounded by serious chemical addictions, create a variety of problems in female offenders which are cognitive, affective, and behavioral. Developmental growth in these areas can also be impaired in women who suffer from abuse at an early age. These numerous traumatic events contribute to an overall sense of helplessness, hopelessness, and isolation for female offenders. Their problem-solving skills may be limited as a result of trauma, chaos, and poor role-modeling in families of origin. In the Hampden County Survey, the high incidence of substance abuse problems of family members suggests that female offenders may be further influenced by the environment of addiction. Almost half (48.6%) of female offenders reported a mother with a substance abuse problem; 60.6% a father with this problem and 63.8% siblings with this same problem (DeCou, et al., 1998).

One further social issue relevant to female offenders' addictions and related criminal path is the ambivalence, anguish, and stigma women experience in relation to their roles as mothers (Bloom & Steinhart, 1993; Clark, 1995). Women describe feeling guilty about choosing male partners who were injurious to their children. They also describe their guilt in relation to their own criminal activities, such as shoplifting to procure food and clothing for their children. Women frequently cite their motivation to be effective mothers as a reason to engage in substance abuse treatment in order to provide safe, nurturing homes for their children (Bloom & Steinhart, 1993). They experience extreme emotions of guilt and shame regarding their addictive and criminal behavior as these impact on their children.

WOMEN'S VOICES: THE HAMPDEN
COUNTY PROGRAM RESPONSE

To address the range and interrelatedness of the issues described above, staff at Hampden County Correctional Center created the following program which is open to all the female offenders. The program offers a mandatory 28-day women's addictions program followed by a series of eight-session, psycho-educational and treatment groups in developmentally appropriate sequences. Although much of the learning and healing takes place in structured program offerings, it is understood that support from an environment responsive to women's relational and behavioral needs is instrumental to the success of the program. This milieu depends largely on the quality of interaction with staff, a constant flow of communication, and the quality of role definitions and boundaries, consistent with systems theory. These interactions are designed to create maximum safety and meaningful connection among peers and staff. In this light, the Mission Statement of the women's unit has been articulated as follows:

> To house female inmates in a safe, orderly, and secure manner which acknowledges women's developmental, experiential, and physical realities; to create an opportunity for personal growth through the environment, education, gender-specific programs, and greater connection to community resources; and to empower women by discovering and restoring a basic sense of self-worth, dignity, behavioral options, and accountability.

THEORETICAL CONSTRUCT FOR A COMPREHENSIVE
GENDER-SENSITIVE PROGRAM

Stephanie Covington has defined addiction as a "chronic neglect of self in favor of something or someone else" (Covington, 1998). Approaches to changing the direction of female offender behavior toward healthy, non-criminal (i.e., non-addictive) choices need to address this problem of self-neglect. A treatment program must include elements of safety, connection, information, and empowerment to instill hope and confidence to effect change. Like other comprehensive, integrated treatment programs for women outside corrections, the Hampden County model utilizes a combination of Empowerment and Relational Models (Brown, 1997; Covington, 1998; Finkelstein, 1997; Garcia-Coll, et al., 1998; Harris, 1998).

Empowerment Model

An empowerment model (Payne, 1997) seeks to help clients gain the power of decision and action over their own lives. This model considers obstacles to exercising power which may include the need for information, for increased self-esteem and confidence, and for strategies for problem-solving and change. An empowerment model seeks to guide individuals away from a state of fear, confusion, limited self-awareness, and hesitation to take risks to change. It directs them toward a state of increased capacity to identify and select from a greater range of personal needs, action strategies, and resources.

An empowerment model can help women grow by:

- Identifying women's personal strengths, resources, and problem areas;
- Teaching problem-solving skills, independent living skills and information about women's issues;
- Assisting women to gain mastery over the skills by personalizing them and practicing their application; and
- Connecting women to new resources both in jail and in the community.

Relational Model

For empowerment for women to be effective, it must be grounded in women's sense of self, development, and psychology. For women, relationships are central to core identity, functioning, and growth. The relational model of women's development and growth has been most clearly articulated in the works of Jean Baker-Miller (*Towards a New Psychology of Women,* 1976) and Carol Gilligan (*In a Different Voice,* 1982) and further developed at Wellesley College's Stone Center for Women. According to this theory, women's development does not seek autonomy and separation as successful adult goals. Rather, women's primary motivation is to build a sense of connection with others. Women develop a sense of identity and self-worth when their actions emerge from, and lead back into, connection with others. The traditional "other connections" for women include parents, families, children, and partners. Also, according to the relational model, true connections involve relationships which are characterized as mutual, authentic, and empathic. Through these relationships women are more energized, creative, validated, and empowered. Their self-awareness expands (Covington, 1998; Gilligan, 1982; Jordan, Kaplan, Miller, Stiver & Surrey, 1991). Furthermore, women's psychological problems can be traced to disconnections or violations in relationships (Miller, 1976). Gilligan expands this relational concept to gender-specific forms of moral reasoning and decision-making (Gilligan, 1982) in that women take into consideration the effects of their actions on others more frequently than men.

With this theory in mind, an integrated addictions program for women must focus on women's roles with respect to others (i.e., parent, partner, etc.). This theoretical perspective suggests that cognitive change is best received when services are delivered by a "caring" staff member and through dynamic exchange with peers. The relational model emphasizes empathy and caring, which may provide an emotional and interactional basis for change (Jordan, 1994; Jordan et al., 1991).

CHALLENGES OF EMPOWERMENT AND RELATIONAL MODELS IN A CORRECTIONAL ENVIRONMENT

Although these theoretical constructs of empowerment and relational models have relevance for female learning, their basic tenets may cause a unique tension in the correctional environment. Value systems clash. For example, in corrections, security staff are always powerful. Inmates, in contrast, have very little free choice or power. Empowerment theory, however, encourages new choices and hence a greater sense of power on the part of the inmates. The challenge, then, is to provide maximum opportunity for inmates to exercise individual control within the constraints of necessary security imperatives. This reflects the need of all members of society to integrate personal needs with social responsibility.

For an empowerment and relational approach to be operationalized, the setting must acknowledge and permit the professional use of affective language—both verbal and non-verbal. The correctional culture strives for extreme neutrality in expression of staff and views staff-inmate relationships as potential security threats. This is especially true in the area of cross-gender supervision. It is critical therefore that staff be adept at balancing affective presence with professional detachment.

IMPLICATIONS FOR PROGRAM DESIGN: A PHASE-ORIENTED EMPOWERMENT APPROACH

To address the wide range of problems of female offenders, the scope of programming needs to be comprehensive, integrated, and multi-tiered. Programming must contain affective, cognitive, and behavioral elements. It must provide information, teach skills, permit an application of new information to inmates' own personal lives, and finally, for those who are ready, create the opportunity for more in-depth healing and treatment of trauma scars. Program elements need to be practical and concrete and refer women to community resources that match their particular personal needs (CSAT, 1994). In addition, groups must encourage attention to dynamics which promote meaningful affiliation and connection with others.

A major feature of programs is the need for women-only groups and classes. Research has concluded that women experience more growth in this format, share more feelings and issues about key relationships, explore identity issues more easily, and receive more validation (Aries, 1976; Covington, 1998; Martin & Shanahan, 1983; Priyadarsini, 1986). Staff running group sessions need training and knowledge in women's treatment issues. The conditions of confinement in the jail setting must be adapted to allow women to explore their vulnerable concerns in a safe, nurturing, relational, and self-esteem-building climate.

The Hampden County Program operates in phases which enable progressive depth and personalization. Inmates can learn the concept of containment and proper channels for their learning. The nature of the learning and increasing self-awareness is incremental and carefully guided. Emphasis is placed on pacing, management of intrusive symptoms and flooding, and building effective support systems. This concept has been used in psychological models of trauma treatment (Keane, 1995; van der Hart, 1993). In early phases, more emphasis is placed on an educational process. As women become more aware of both their own personal issues and of a broader understanding of women's issues and topics, more personal application and self-disclosure may emerge.

What follows is a description of the phases and tasks of the Hampden County Correctional Center's gender-specific women's change model. The Hampden County model, which is referred to as *women's V.O.I.C.E.S.*, contains four progressive phases. It was designed to address the needs of women inmates with an average stay of about nine months. At the end of each phase, inmates complete a personal growth plan called a MAP. This MAP permits them to clarify their needs with increasing specificity, reflected in their programming choices for the next phase.

Phase I—Exploration/Discovery This phase begins a series of initial explorations of the program itself, of one's own current needs and circumstances, and of general women's issues. In this phase, women begin to identify and prioritize their own problem areas and strengths. The goal is for women to acquire essential skills in problem-solving, which includes planning for safety and making effective choices.

Phase II—Information, Education, and More This second phase introduces a more detailed approach to the various topics discussed. The Intensive 28-Day Addictions component applies the addictions' informational content to inmates' personal lives. More intense group interactions encourage women to begin "telling their stories" within a supportive psycho-educational setting. Women's natural emotional expressiveness is understood, validated, and channeled to appropriate treatment venues. Other groups, such as domestic violence and parenting, offer information and education about skills or topics related to women.

Phase III—Treatment/Healing In this third phase participants are screened, and those who are motivated and ready for in-depth healing enter in treatment groups. These groups are led by trained treatment staff and are closed-membership groups with short-term contracts. Participants learn to identify earlier painful experiences and recognize how they can resurface in their adult life and distort emotional behavior.

Phase IV—Community Integration Inmates in all groups and classes receive training in skills and information. Moreover, they learn about specific community agency contacts and how to access them. In this final phase, inmates formalize a personalized action plan for the community.

women's VOICES Components

Exploration/Discovery

- My Journey Begins Here: Overview of *women's VOICES*
- Core Curriculum
- AIDS/HIV Peer Education
- Creating Safety
- Introduction to Family Services
- Staying Out of Jail Skills: Effective Choices

Information and More

- Beginner's Addiction Program
- Love and Violence I
- Anger Basics
- Mother-Child Connection
- Understanding Trauma
- Women's Health Issues
- Problem-solving Skills: New Options II
- Independent Living Skills for Women
- Women's Writing Workshop: Voices from the Inside

Healing and Treatment

- 28-Day Addiction Treatment Program
- Love and Violence II
- Channeling Your Anger (for women having committed violent crimes)
- PlayCare Project
- Breaking the Silence—Trauma Survivors
- Interpersonal Relations Group: Women with Voices

Community Integration

- Pulling It All Together—Release Planning
- Coping with Fear and Transition

PARTICIPANT SELECTION

Participants express their interest in program participation by submitting Request Slips. These are coordinated through a case plan and reviewed weekly by an interdisciplinary team. In keeping with the empowerment approach, participant selection honors client choice wherever possible. Our experience is that, early in the jail stay, inmates sense the extent of their learning and healing needs, but they often do so in a vague, undifferentiated manner. Perhaps the most frequent Request Slip received by orientation staff reads, "Sign me up for everything." Another common phenomenon is the new inmate who is experiencing near-debilitating shame, guilt, and depression, resulting in significant cognitive confusion. In response, program phases assist clients in identifying and unfolding content areas and levels of detail in tandem with their growing abilities and strengths.

STAFFING AND IMPLICATIONS FOR SOCIAL WORK

The Hampden County Correctional Center model employs staff with various levels of training. The women's unit director and the unit manager both have advanced social work degrees. Counselors with an MSW carry individual caseloads and conduct Level III Treatment and psycho-educational groups. Correctional case workers carry case management caseloads and conduct more cognitive-oriented groups. Each staff has a specialized area of expertise in one aspect of women's issues, such as parenting, domestic violence, addictions, anger management, or mental health.

Besides hiring staff with the above formalized credentials, student interns from the Graduate School of Social Work at Springfield College participate in a popular student unit. They carry caseloads and operate groups. Staff duties are consistent with the Generalist Approach and include a range of practical and treatment skills as well as advocacy. Staff interface with community resources frequently through the Release Planning efforts. Finally, all staff must participate in interdisciplinary case conferences and group supervision. All staff receive weekly individual supervision by licensed social workers. Most employees are sheriff's department staff, although volunteers and some contracted providers also offer services.

EVALUATION

Evaluation research and tools for measuring success of innovative women's programs have been found to be limited, especially in corrections. In the recent analysis of programming needs and promising approaches for women, Morash concluded that, although many corrections' administrators could identify innovative program characteristics for women, few outcome measurements had been conducted, and a mere six programs included recidivism measurements (Morash et al., 1998). An evaluation mechanism has not yet been designed to assess the effectiveness of comprehensive gender-specific programs or their specific outcomes in corrections (Covington, 1999, personal conversation). The Hampden County Correctional Center's program design may be used to begin this evaluation effort.

The Hampden County model uses pre-tests and post-tests to assess progress in mastery of content. In addition, client satisfaction surveys are administered upon group completion. A specific instrument is being developed to measure empowerment utilizing the MAPS developed by the inmates.

Ideally, outcome measures will examine areas related to participants' ability to make effective choices and avoid repeat offenses. Women need to be empowered to engage in ongoing addictions treatment, make improved choices about partners, select new positive social supports, utilize community resources, and create a stable home and financial base for themselves and their children. The tools offered in the program instill a sense of hope to create a more positive life.

REFERENCES

Alexander, M.J. (1996). Women with co-occurring addictive and mental disorders: An emerging profile of vulnerability. *Journal of American Orthopsychiatry, 66*, 61–70.

Alexander, M.J. & Muenzenmaier, K. (1998). Trauma, addiction, and recovery: Addressing public health epidemics among women with severe mental illness. Pp. 215–239 in Levin, B.L., Blanch, A.K. & Jennings, A. (Eds.) *Women's Mental Health Services: A Public Health Perspective.* Thousand Oaks, CA.: Sage. 215–239.

American Medical Association. (1994). *Diagnostic and treatment guidelines on domestic violence.* Chicago, Il. AMA.

Aries, E. (1976). Interaction patterns and themes of male, female, and mixed groups. *Small Group Behavior, 7*(1), 7–18.

Austin, J., Bloom, B. & Donahue, T. (1992). *Female offenders in the community: An analysis of innovative strategies and programs.* San Francisco, CA: National Council on Crime and Delinquency.

Baker-Miller, J. (1976). *Towards a New Psychology of Women.* Boston, Boston:Press.

Barnett, O.W., Miller-Perrin, C.L. & Perrin, R.D. (1997). *Family Violence Across the Lifespan.* Thousand Oaks, CA: Sage. Chapters 3, 4, 5, & 8.

Bass E. & Davis, L. (1988). *The Courage to Heal: A Guide for Women Survivors of Child Sexual Abuse.* New York: Harper & Row.

Bergsman, R. (1989). The forgotten few: Juvenile female offenders. *Federal Probation, 53* (1), 73–78.

Bill, L. (1998). The victimization and revictimization of female offenders: Prison administrators should be aware of ways in which security procedures perpetuate feelings of powerlessness. *Corrections Today, 60* (7), 106–114.

Bloom, B., Chesney-Lind, M. & Owen, B. (1994). *Women in prison in California: Hidden victims of the war on drugs.* San Francisco, CA: Center on Juvenile and Criminal Justice.

Bloom, B. & Steinhart, D. (1993). *Why punish the children?* San Francisco, CA: National Council on Crime and Delinquency.

Blume, E.S. (1990). Am I crazy? No, you're coping. Pp. 75–94 in *Secret Survivors: Uncovering Incest and Its Aftereffects in Women.* New York: John Wiley & Sons.

Briere, J. (1989). Chapters 1 & 2, pp. 5–50. in *Therapy for Adults Molested as Children.* New York: Springer Publishing.

Brown, V. (1997). *Gender-specific treatment: Effective components in women's treatment programs.* California: Prototypes Systems Change Center. Clinical Briefing Paper.

Browne, A., Miller, B. & Maguin, E. (1998). *Prevalence and severity of lifetime physical and sexual victimization among incarcerated women.* In press. Buffalo, N.Y.: Research Institute on Addictions.

Buccio-Notaro, P., Molla, B. & Stevenson, C. (1996). *Social justice for women creates alternative sentencing services for women involved in the criminal justice system.* Prepared for American Society for Criminology. Nov. 1996. Chicago, Il. Conference. Boston: Social Justice for Women.

Bureau of Justice Statistics. (1992). *Special Report: Women in Jail 1989.* Washington DC .: U.S. Department of Justice.

Bureau of Justice Statistics. (1994). Washington D.C.: U.S. Department of Justice.

Bureau of Justice Statistics. (1995). *Jail and Jail Inmates 1993–94.* Washington DC: U.S. Department of Justice.

Bureau of Justice Statistics. (1996). *Special Report: Profile of Jail Inmates 1996.* Washington DC: U.S. Department of Justice.

Bureau of Justice Statistics. (1998). *Prison and Jail Inmates at Midyear 1998.* Washington DC: U.S. Department of Justice.

Bureau of Justice Statistics. (1999). *Mental Health and Treatment of Inmates and Probationers.* Washington DC: U.S. Department of Justice.

Center for Substance Abuse Treatment, Substance Abuse prevention and Treatment Block Grant. (1994). *Assessment and treatment of patients with coexisting mental illness and alcohol and other drug abuse:* TIP9 (Treatment Improvement Protocol. DHHS Publication #SMA-24-9078. Washington DC: U.S. Government Printing Office.

Center for Substance Abuse Treatment (CSAT); Women's and Children's Branch (1994). *Practical approaches in the treatment of women who abuse alcohol and other drugs.* Rockville, MD.: U.S. Department of Health and Human Services.

Chesney-Lind, M. (1998). Women in prison: From partial justice to vengeful equity. *Corrections Today, 60* (7), 66–74.

Clark, J. (1995). The impact of the prison environment on mothers. *The Prison Journal, 75* (3), 306–329.

Connolly, J.E. (1983). Women in county jails: An invisible gender in an ill-defined institution. *The Prison Journal, 63*(2), 99–115.

Conte, J.R. & Berliner, L. (1988). The impact of sexual abuse on children: empirical findings. Pp. 72–93 in Walker, L.E. (Ed.) *Handbook on Sexual Abuse of Children.* New York: Springer Publishing.

Cottler, L.B., Compton, W. III, Mager, D., Spitznagel, E.L. & Janca, A. (1992). Posttraumatic stress disorder among substance abusers from the general population. *American Journal of Psychiatry, 149* (5), 664–670.

Courtois, C.A. (1992). The memory retrieval process in incest survivor therapy. *Journal of Child Sexual Abuse* Vol. 1 (1), 15–31.

Covington, S. (1998). Creating gender-specific treatment for substance-abusing women and girls in community corrections settings. Presentation to ICCA Conference, September 1998, Washington, DC LaJolla, CA: Institute for Relational Development.

Covington, S. (1999). *Helping Women Recover: A Program for Treating Addiction.* San Fransisco, CA.: Jossey-Bass Publishers.

DeCou, K., Haven, T. & Vivian, J. (1998). *Women involved in the criminal justice system in Hampden County: Who are they? Results of a Survey.* In press. Prepared for National Institute on Corrections. Technical Assistance Project on Intermediate Sanctions for Women. Ludlow, MA.: Hampden County Correctional Center.

Evans, K. & Sullivan, J.M. (1995). Chapters 1 & 2, Pp. 1–66 in *Treating Addicted Survivors of Trauma.* New York: The Guilford Press.

Flanagan, L.W. (1995). Meeting the special needs of women in custody: Maryland's unique approach. *Federal Probation, 59* (2), 49–53.

Finkelstein, N. (1991). Treatment issues for alcohol and drug dependent pregnant and parenting women. *Health and Social Work, 19* (1), 7–15.

Finkelstein, N., Kennedy, C., Thomas, K. & Kearns, M. (1997). *Gender-specific Substance Abuse Treatment.* Washington DC: Center for Substance Abuse prevention (CSAP). Research conducted for the National Women's Resource Center for the Prevention and Treatment of Alcohol, Tobacco, and other Drug Abuse and Mental Illness.

Galbraith, S. (1998). *And So I Began To Listen to Their Stories: Working with Women in the Criminal Justice System.* Delmar, NY: GAINS Center.

Garcia-Coll, C., Miller, J. & Mathews, B. (1998). The experience of women in prison: Implications for services and prevention. In Harden, J. & Hill, M. (Eds.) in *Breaking the Rules: Women in Prison and Feminist Therapy.* New York: Haworth.

Gilligan, C. (1982). *In a Different Voice.* Cambridge, MA.: Harvard University Press.

Glick, R. & Neto, V. (1977). *National Study of Women's Correctional Programs.* Washington DC: U.S. Government Printing Office.

Gondolf, I.W. (1995). Alcohol abuse, wife assault, and power needs. *Social Service Review, 69* (2), 274–284.

Gray, T., Mays, G.L. & Stohr, M.K. (1995). Inmate needs and programming in exclusively women's jails. *The Prison Journal, 75* (2), 186–202.

Grice, D.E., Brady, K.T. & Dustan, L.R. (1995). Sexual and physical assault history and posttraumatic stress disorder in substance-dependent individuals. *The American Journal on Addictions, 4* (4), 297–305.

Harris, M. (1998). *Trauma Recovery and Empowerment.* New York: The Free Press.

Herman, J. L. (1992). *Trauma and Recovery.* N.Y.: Basic Books.

Immarigeon, R. & Chesney-Lind, M. (1992). *Women's prisons: Overcrowded and over-used.* Madison, WI.: National Council on Crime and Delinquency.

Jackson, P. & Stearns, C.A. (1995). Gender issues in a new generation jail. *The Prison Journal, 75* (2), 203–221. Sage Publications.

Jalbert, A. (1987). *Holding patterns: A report on women, the forgotten offenders in the Nassau County jail.* Boulder, Co.: National Institute of Corrections Information Center.

Jordan, J. (1994). *A relational perspective on self-esteem.* Publication # 70. Wellesley, MA.: Stone Center, Wellesley College.

Jordan, J., Kaplan, A., Miller, J., Stiver, I. & Surrey, J. (1991). *Women's Growth in Connection: Writings from the Stone Center.* New York: The Guilford Press.

Kantor, G. & Straus, M.A. (1987). Substance abuse as a precipitant to wife abuse victimizations. *American Journal of Drug and Alcohol Abuse, 156,* 173–189.

Keane, T.M. (1995). Psychological and behavioral treatments for post-traumatic stress Disorder. Pp. 398–407 in *Psychological and Behavioral treatments of PTSD: A Guide to Treatments that Work.*

Kerr, D. (1998). Substance abuse among female offenders: Efforts to treat substance-abusing women must address underlying reasons for use. *Corrections Today, 60* (7), 114–122.

Leonard, K.E. & Jacob, T. (1987). Alcohol, alcoholism, and family violence. Pp. 383–406 in Van Hasselt, V.D., Morrison, R.L., Bellack, A.S. & Herson, M. (Eds.) *Handbook of Family Violence.* New York: Plenum.

Martin, P.Y. & Shanahan, K.A. (1983). Transcending the effects of sex composition in small groups. *Social Work with Groups, 6*(3/4), 19–32.

Miller, B.A., Downs, W.R. & Gondoli, D.M. (1989). Spousal violence among alcoholic women as compared to a random sample of household women. *Journal of Studies on Alcoholism, 50* (6), 533–540.

Morash, M., Bynum, T. & Koons, B. (1998). *Women offenders: Programming needs and promising approaches.* Washington DC: National Institute for Justice.

Neto, V.V. (1981). *Programming for women in the jail setting.* Boulder, CO.: National Institute of Corrections Information Center.

Norton-Hawk, M. (1999). *A harm reduction approach to prostitution.* Boston: Suffolk University. Research in press.

Owen, B. (1998). *In the Mix: Struggle and Survival in a Women's Prison.* Albany, NY: SUNY Press.

Owen, B. & Bloom, B. (1995). Profiling women offenders: Findings from the national surveys and a California sample. *The Prison Journal, 75* (2), 165–185. Sage.

Payne, M. (1997). *Modern Social Work Theory.* Chicago, Il: Lyceum Books.

Pollack-Byrne, J.M. (1990). *Women, Prison, and Crime.* Belmont, CA: Wadsworth.

Prescott, L. (1997). *Adolescent Girls with Co-occurring Disorders in the Juvenile Justice System.* Delmar, NY: Policy Research Associates.

Priyadarsini, S. (1986). Gender role dynamics in an alcohol therapy group in Strug, D.L., Priyadarsini, S.P., & Hyman, M.M. (Eds.) *Alcohol Interventions: Historical and Socio-cultural Approaches.* New York: Haworth.

Saunders, D.G. (1994). Posttraumatic stress symptom profiles of battered women: A comparison of survivor's in two settings. *Violence and Victims, 9,* 31–44.

Shepherd, J. (1990). Victims of personal violence: The relevance of Symonds' model of psychological response and loss theory. *British Journal of Social Work, 20,* 309–332.

Singer, M.I., Bussey, J., Song, L. & Lunghofer, L. (1995). The psychosocial issues of women serving time in jail. *Social Work, 40* (1), 103–113.

Stohr, M.K. & Mays, G.L. (1993). *Women's Jails: An Investigation of Offenders, Staff, Administration, and Programming.* Washington DC: National Institute of Corrections; U.S. Department of Justice.

Teplin, L.A., Abram, K.M. & McClelland, G.M. (1996). Prevalence of psychiatric disorders among incarcerated women. *Archives of General Psychiatry, 53,* 505–512.

Terr, L.C. (1991). Childhood traumas: An outline and an overview. *American Journal of Psychiatry, 148* (1), 10–20.

Van der Hart, Onno, Steele, K., Boon, S. & Brown, P. (1993). The treatment of traumatic memories: Synthesis, realization, and integration. *Dissociation, 6*(2/3), 162–180.

Veysey, B.M. (1998). Specific needs of women diagnosed with mental illnesses in U.S. jails in Levin, B., Blanch, & Jennings, A. (Eds.) *Women's Mental Health Services: A Public Health Perspective.* Thousand Oaks, CA: Sage.

Walker, L. (1984). *The Battered Woman Syndrome.* New York: Springer Publishing.

Weisheit, R.A. (1998). Trends in programs for female offenders: The use of private agencies as service providers. *International Journal of Offender Therapy and Comparative Criminology,* 35–42.

Wellisch, J., Anglin, M.D. & Prendergast, M.L. (1994). Drug-abusing women offenders: Results of a national survey. Washington, DC: National Institute of Justice: Research in Brief, 1–19.

Wolfe, V.V. & Gentile, C. (1992). Psychological assessment of sexually abused children. Chapter 5 in O'Donohue, W. & Geer, J.H. (Eds.) *The Sexual Abuse of Children.* Vol. 2. Hillsdale, NJ: Lawrence Erlbaum, Publishers.

Zetlin, P.A. (1989). A proposal for a new diagnostic category: Abuse disorder. *Journal of Feminist Family Therapy, 1* (4), 67–84.

Zupan, L. (1991). *Jails: Reform and the New Generation Philosophy.* Cincinnati, OH.: Anderson.

SECTION IV
Serving the Victims of Mentally Ill Offenders

16

Elder Abuse and Forensic Mentally Ill Abusers

Pat Brownell, Jacquelin Berman,

Aurora Salamone, and Adele Welty

Elder abuse and mistreatment has been identified as a significant social problem since the 1980s (Wolf, 1988; U.S. House of Representatives, 1990). Although available statistics on elder abuse and mistreatment are thought to significantly underrepresent this social problem, estimates have ranged from 3% to 12% of the older population affected by abuse, neglect or exploitation (Pillemer & Finkelhor, 1988; U.S. House of Representatives, 1990). As the population of older adults continues to grow, the incidence and prevalence of elder abuse and neglect is expected to increase as well.

While these estimates can be smaller or larger depending on how elder abuse is defined, there is a consensus that this is a serious social problem that threatens the safety and quality of life of many older adults. Media reports and early studies of elder abuse suggest that the term characterizes a family situation involving a frail, dependent older adult being abused or exploited by an uncaring or unscrupulous abusive family member (Wolf, 1998). Is this what elder abuse really looks like? Professionals in the field of aging and criminal justice reveal an alternative picture of elder abuse and maltreatment.

CASE EXAMPLE

Annie G., a 76-year-old widow, lives with Robert G., her 55-year-old son who suffers from schizophrenia, paranoid type. Annie cooks, cleans, and shops for both of them in spite of an arthritic condition that limits her mobility and causes her intermittent pain. When

Robert is compliant with his medication schedule and attends his adult day care program regularly, he is able to care for himself with limited assistance from Annie.

However, Robert is often non-compliant with taking his medication. When this happens, he stops attending his program and begins frequenting a bar in the neighborhood. The alcohol he consumes exacerbates his psychiatric condition and depletes his income from Supplemental Security Income (SSI) which is needed for household expenses in addition to Annie's small Social Security check. On these occasions, he begins to demand money from Annie and threaten her if she does not give it to him. His demands can escalate into verbal and physical abuse as well. In the neighborhood bar, Robert is viewed as a troublemaker. Bartenders and management have called the police on several occasions because of his behavior and, as a result, he has been hospitalized or incarcerated.

Upon discharge from the hospital or release from jail, Robert always returns home to his mother. While she has attempted to explain to hospital discharge planners and jail or prison officials that she is unable to manage him when he stops taking his medication, they have told her that his only other housing option is a men's shelter. Annie has heard that mentally ill homeless residents of the shelter have been threatened and even injured by other residents. As fearful as she is of her own safety when Robert stops taking his medication and begins to drink alcohol, she is even more concerned about his well-being. Robert is her only child and she has raised him alone since her husband died 32 years ago. Before he became ill, Robert studied to be an accountant, and was a loving and dutiful son. This is the memory of Robert to which Annie clings.

DISCUSSION OF CASE AS ILLUSTRATION OF ISSUES RELATED TO ELDER ABUSE AND CRIMINAL OFFENSES BY MENTALLY IMPAIRED ABUSERS

The situation described above is an example of elder abuse, defined as financial, emotional or physical mistreatment of an adult, age 60 years and above, by a family member or significant other (Wolf & Pillemer, 1984). For those whose only knowledge of elder abuse comes from the media or anecdotal information, this situation may not appear to be representative of this type of abuse. Unlike many of the stories about elder abuse in the popular press, Annie—although somewhat physically impaired with arthritis—is the caregiver of her abuser Robert, her middle-aged son.

Robert, far from being a cold and calculating abuser of a dependent elderly relative, is himself impaired and dependent on his victim, his mother. His abusive behavior is linked to fluctuations in his illness that limit his insight into the consequences of this behavior for himself and others. The behavior in question, which is not only confined to his home, has resulted in his arrest and incarceration or involuntary hospitalization on several occasions. Robert is an example of a forensic mentally ill abuser.

Experts recommend an interdisciplinary approach to elder abuse (Hwalek, 1988). Elder abuse and mistreatment may have service implications for providers of health and mental health services, as well as income security, housing, preventive, and protective service implications for victims. However, service providers may neglect to consider overlapping service needs of the abuser. This is due to the fact that, according to aging service providers, victims will often not act to protect themselves if they are unable to ensure the well-being of their batterer (Dundorf & Brownell, 1995).

To serve victims of forensic mentally ill abusers, service providers may need to move beyond the traditional aging service systems to engage mental health, substance abuse, and criminal justice systems as well (Brownell, Berman & Salamone, 1999). Professionals in these service systems should be aware of elderly parents' vulnerability to abuse and exploitation when considering whether they can be a resource for a mentally ill adult child.

In the case of Annie and Robert, unnecessary victimization occurred for two reasons. First, Annie was unable to advocate successfully for Robert because of her mistaken belief that she remained his only resource and buffer to incarceration, unwanted hospitalization, and homelessness. Second, Robert was not provided with service alternatives upon discharge or release from his frequent hospitalizations and incarcerations because professionals within these systems viewed Annie as a resource available to house and care for Robert, rendering arduous efforts to identify transitional or supported therapeutic housing alternatives unnecessary. As a result, Annie, Robert, and their community were all ill-served by the failure of mental health and criminal justice systems to effectively collaborate in identifying and creating, when necessary, appropriate community-based resources and policies to ensure safety for Annie and treatment for Robert.

DEFINITIONS OF ELDER ABUSE AND NEGLECT

The most common definitions of elder abuse and neglect include physical, psychological, financial, and active (intentional) and passive (unintentional) neglect (Wolf & Pillemer, 1984). Elder abuse and neglect definitions are categorized according to the behaviors of the abuser, intent of the abuser, and perceptions and, to some extent, the decisional capacity and health status of the victim. According to Wolf and Pillemer, these may include:

- Physical Abuse: the infliction of physical pain or injury or physical coercion (confinement against one's will).
- Psychological Abuse: the infliction of mental anguish.
- Financial Abuse: the illegal or improper exploitation and/or use of funds or other resources.
- Active Neglect: refusal or failure to fulfill a caregiving obligation, including a conscious and intentional attempt to inflict physical or emotional distress on the elderly victim.
- Passive Neglect: refusal or failure to fulfill a caregiving obligation by caregivers who lack the knowledge, skill or ability to provide adequate care, rather than a conscious and intentional attempt to inflict physical or emotional distress on the elder (Wolf & Pillemer, 1984).

Acts representing elder abuse and neglect, while distressing and even harmful to the elderly victim, are not necessarily defined as criminal in nature. To be regarded as criminal, the acts must meet criteria defined by state penal codes. In addition, characteristics of the abuser may be taken into account when a determination is made as to the degree of his or her culpability. In some states, neglecting to provide a frail older adult with needed medication or food may be considered a criminal act unless the alleged perpetrator were found to be incapable of fulfilling a caregiving obligation due to mental or physical incapacity. On the other hand, even a mentally impaired abuser may face criminal prosecution for abusive acts toward an older adult relative if defined as misdemeanor or felony level crimes by state penal codes.

In New York State, Section 260.25 of the Penal Code states: "A person is guilty of endangering the welfare of an incompetent person when he knowingly acts in a manner likely to be injurious to the physical, mental or moral welfare of a person who is unable to care for himself because of a mental desease or defect. Endangering the welfare of an incompetent adult is a Class A Misdemeanor."

The following are examples of abusive acts perpetrated by adult children against aged parents that rise to the level of a crime. They were identified in a study of elder abuse based on reports to the New York City Police Department in 1992 (Brownell, 1998). These include:

Physical abuse: Rape; Assault One, Two and Three; Attempted/actual robbery/physical; Menacing/physical; and Harassment/physical.

Financial abuse: Grand larceny, Robbery/financial; Attempted grand
   larceny; Larceny; Forgery; Menacing/financial; Criminal mis-
   chief/financial; Petit larceny; and Harassment/financial.
Psychological abuse: Menacing/psychological;   Criminal trespass/psy-
   chological; and Harassment/psychological.

The following are examples of narratives written by law enforcement
officers responding to 911 calls on elder abuse:

Robbery
   [84-year-old] Victim states [29-year-old] perp (son) came to his
   door and repeatedly banged on the door. The parents had an order
   of protection stating that he was not to come to his parents' residence and not to harass them. The father reluctantly let him in
   and then perp threatened father with bodily harm to give him $80
   for drugs.
Harassment, psychological
   [78-year-old] Victim states [34-year-old] perp (son) has been constantly harassing victim but perp flees when police respond. Victim
   informed by neighbor that perp told her he was going to kill his
   mother (victim). Victim is in fear of her life—son is an alcoholic,
   drug user, and was recently released from prison (on parole).

In both examples, the perpetrators were identified as impaired due to
substance abuse problems (Brownell, 1998).

THEORIES OF ELDER ABUSE AND MALTREATMENT

When elder abuse was first identified as a social issue of concern, practitioners, researchers, and policymakers focused on the characteristics of
the victim as primary risk factors. Frail and dependent elderly in the "old-
old" age category (85 years and above) were considered to be at greatest
risk of victimization, with overwhelmed caregivers or opportunistic relatives the most likely abusers.
   Some researchers, most notably Steinmetz (1988), sought an explanation of elder abuse that was interpersonal and interactive. In a study of
dependent elderly mothers and caregiving daughters, Steinmetz posited
that stress associated with caregiving could lead to abusive behavior by
daughters toward their elderly mothers. The burden of caregiving was
exacerbated by caregivers who limited the autonomy of frail elders in their
care, leading to learned helplessness on the part of the victim. Once the
victim learned to be more independent, the caregiver felt less pressure

and was less likely to behave in an abusive manner. Alternatively, formal in-home services that lessened the caregiving burden could lead to an increase in "quality time" for both informal caregiver and older family member, and decrease intrafamilial stress. This represents a type of elder abuse or maltreatment that rarely rises to the level of a criminal act.

While early studies of elder abuse based on small, agency-based convenience samples (Lau & Kosberg, 1979; Steinmetz, 1981) focused on victim characteristics, some abuser characteristics were also noted. Abuser impairments such as chronic substance abuse and mental illness were identified in some early studies as risk factors in elder abuse (Quinn & Tomita, 1997). However, as with the domestic violence movement, the characteristics and needs associated with abusers were considered to be of secondary concern compared with those of victims.

The intergenerational cycle of violence, adapted from theories of child and spouse abuse, hypothesizes that family members abuse older adult relatives because they have been exposed to abuse in the family or have learned that abusive behavior is acceptable. This has not been found to be as applicable to elder abuse as with other forms of domestic violence (Korbin, Anetzberger, Thomasson & Austin, 1991).

The abuser dependency theory has been cited as having greater validity in explaining elder abuse than abuse of younger partners or children. Adult children have been cited as perpetrators of elder abuse more frequently than spouses or partners, and are more likely to fit this profile of elder abuse (Wallace, 1999).

Explanatory theories of elder abuse that focused on the abuser, such as abuser dependency and abuser pathology, began to emerge out of later, more methodologically sophisticated research. Increasingly, the characteristics of abusers are seen to have stronger predictive power for elder abuse than characteristics of the victims (Wolf, 1999). While studies have increasingly identified characteristics of the abuser as a highly significant factor in elder abuse, few have focused on the abuser specifically. A qualitative study of elderly mothers and caregiving sons found that abuse and neglect were associated with personality disorders and substance abuse on the part of the sons (Anetzberger, 1987).

Other studies suggest that victims who provide support and care for impaired adult children are at risk of abuse, which appears counterintuitive. The theoretical explanation is that of social exchange theory (Pillemer & Finkelhor, 1989). The application of social exchange theory to elder abuse requires an adaptation from the theory as originally proposed (Dowd, 1975). As theorized in relation to elder abuse, the impaired abuser is ashamed of his/her dependency on the victim and seeks to diminish the victim through mistreatment or change the perceived balance of power and assume control over the relationship with the victim.

The explanatory theory of elder abuse that may best reflect the profile of elder abuse perpetrated by forensic mentally ill family members is that of abuser pathology (Wolf & McCarthy, 1991). According to this theory, abusers have mental disorders that cause their abusiveness independent of their victims' behavior or characteristics (Wallace, 1999). As noted, studies from the 1970s have included findings that significant numbers of abusers have been hospitalized for serious psychiatric disorders, such as schizophrenia (Wolf, 1994; Wolf, Strugnell & Godkin, 1984). Elder mistreatment has also been associated with abusers' addiction to alcohol or other drugs (Quinn & Tomita, 1997).

While researchers have begun to identify psychiatric impairments of the abuser as greater risk factors in elder abuse than victim care needs, little is known about the nature of abuser pathology or impairments as they relate to elder abuse. Some qualitative studies, most notably that of Anetzberger (1987), have examined the interrelationship between abuser pathology and victims with high-care needs among sons and their elderly mothers for whom they are providing care.

The New York City Department for the Aging (DFTA) undertook a survey of 401 older victims of reported domestic abuse requesting assistance from the DFTA Elderly Crime Victims Resource Center to examine the relationship between elder abuse, abuser pathology, and the criminal justice system (Brownell, Berman & Salamone, 1999; Salamone, Berman, Eidlisz & Lipton, 1998).

Data from the study highlight the significant connection between mental health issues and perpetrators of elder abuse. Almost three-fourths (74%) of the abusers in the study suffered from a mental health problem, including substance abuse. In addition, significant differences emerged among the different categories of abusers. Compared to the unimpaired abusers in the survey, the impaired abusers are more likely to be physically abusive and also more likely to be financially and psychologically abusive.

A forensic history also differentiated the impaired from the unimpaired abusers. Virtually all previously or currently incarcerated perpetrators were either mentally ill or substance abusers. Interestingly, the profile of elder abuse perpetrators is strikingly similar to prisoners described in a recent study conducted by the National GAINS Center (1997). The prisoners in this study are significantly more likely to be mentally ill or substance abusers than the general population.

The study findings reflect a significant connection between abuser impairment and elder abuse. About four-fifths of the abusers in the study suffered from an impairment, including mental illness and substance abuse, or both (Brownell, Berman & Salamone, 1999). Compared with unimpaired abusers, impaired abusers are more likely to be violent. In addition, drug abusers were found to be more likely than other categories of abusers to be financially abusive and mentally ill abusers more likely to be identified as psychologically abusive.

PREVENTION AND INTERVENTION STRATEGIES

It is interesting to note that victims of impaired abusers in the DFTA study were less likely than victims of unimpaired abusers to accept services for themselves alone. They appeared to be reaching out for assistance not only for themselves but also for their impaired abusers. In the case example of Annie and Robert, Annie still expressed considerable caring and concern for Robert in spite of his abusive behavior which she attributed to his illness and not to willful intent on his part.

The unwillingness on the part of the victim to accept services that do not address the needs of the abuser has been identified in several studies as a significant barrier to service delivery for elder abuse victims (Vinton, 1988; Brownell, Berman & Salamone, 1999; Barker, 2000). However, victims' refusals to accept services for themselves if their abusers cannot be served or refuse to accept services can have disastrous consequences. The case of Mary Bowe illustrates this point (Dugger, 1991, A1):

> The only relative who never gave up on Tracey Bowe was her grandmother, Mary Bowe. In return, Tracey stole her grandmother's good silver, a radio, a camera, a silver chain, a diamond ring, and a set of dishes. Tracey and her boyfriend lived rent-free in Mary's house, where they smoked crack".

When Mary, a recent retiree, finally refused to provide any more support to Tracey and her boyfriend and threatened to call the police, they killed her.

PREVENTIVE SERVICES FOR AT-RISK ELDERLY

There are ways that older adults can protect themselves from abuse, maltreatment, and exploitation. Refusing to provide housing or resources for substance abusing or dangerously mentally ill relatives is one protective strategy: failure to do so is illustrated by the tragedy of Mary Bowe. Ensuring that sufficient in-home assistance is available to support available caregivers or ensuring services for potentially abusive dependent relatives is also important.

Area aging agencies, under Title III of the Older American Act, are required to provide information and referrals for elderly crime victims, including those victimized by family members. Adult protective services programs, which are state- or county-operated case management agencies, may provide assistance for cognitively or physically impaired elders or their mentally impaired abusers. Local law enforcement and district attorneys offices are also resources for elder abuse victims abused by family members or significant others who may be impaired by mental illness and/or substance abuse. Recent policy changes in civil commitment procedures, such as "Kendra's Law" in New York State, provide easements to involuntary treatment for dangerous mentally ill family members decompensating in the community.

Assessing the cognitive capacity of an older adult at risk of abuse or exploitation is essential (Lachs & Pillemer, 1995). Like adults of any age, older adults have the right to make decisions about their lives that may seem to reflect poor judgement, unless they lack the capacity to understand the consequences of their decisions. Assessments by Adult Protective Services that reveal the need for involuntary intervention are important. However, the unimpaired older adult who refuses services may need ongoing support in the form of persistent telephone contact until that person is ready to make changes in his or her life to ensure protection from harm (Dundorf & Brownell, 1995).

Assessing the mental status of potential abusive family members is also important when making an assessment for elder abuse as a form of domestic violence. According to Decaire (2000), certain mental and personality disorders have been associated with violence and criminal behavior. These include Paranoid Personality Disorder, Antisocial Personality Disorder, Borderline Personality Disorder, and Narcissistic Personality Disorder. Substance abuse, particularly in combination with Borderline Personality Disorder or psychosis, has also been associated with violence and criminality (Porr, n.d.)

INTERVENTION STRATEGIES FOR ELDER ABUSE AND MISTREATMENT

Planning and implementing effective intervention strategies for elder abuse and neglect victims and family members require effective and multifaceted assessments and interventions. Three main categories of interventions include social services, health and mental health services, and use of the legal and criminal justice systems. While not mutually exclusive, decisions as to which option to utilize are dependent on a number of factors. These include the mental and physical characteristics of both victim and abuser, the preference of the victim and the intent of the abuser, and whether the abusive acts meet the standard of a crime as defined by state penal codes.

Examples of services that are available for victims of elder abuse include the following:

Social Service Interventions

1. adult protective services, which are government managed or funded case management services for victims (and/or perpetrators) who are cognitively or physically impaired and are unable to protect themselves from harm, lack capacity to understand the consequences of decisions that can put them at risk of harm, and are a danger to themselves or others;
2. community-based services for older people age 60 and above, funded through the Older Americans Act and supplementary funding, and provided by a not-for-profit or area agency on aging;
3. victim services that provide counseling for crime victims as well as concrete services like changing broken locks and providing emergency funds for food and rent; and
4. court-mandated program and services, including batterers' programs for perpetrators of abuse, and giving the victim a cell phone programmed to call 911.

Health and Mental Health Interventions

1. medical and mental health (including substance abuse) services for older victims of abuse who require treatment for medical or mental health conditions that precede or result from abuse;
2. medical and mental health (including substance abuse) services for impaired perpetrators of abuse; and
3. home health and nursing care for victims of abuse who choose to stay in their homes but remain at risk of abuse or exploitation.

Legal and Criminal Justice Interventions

1. guardianships for victims who are at risk of exploitation and lack capacity to manage their finances or protect themselves from harm (a person who lacks capacity for informed consent cannot execute a power of attorney, but can be a candidate for guardianship);

2. orders of protection to enable law enforcement officers to arrest abusers if they violate the orders and threaten victims;

3. police, district attorneys, and services of the State Attorney General for older people who fall victim to scams and other non-familial forms of exploitation. Types of crimes committed by family members, significant others, and strangers that can be prosecuted in New York State include assault, menacing, rape, murder, trespassing, burglary, larceny, robbery, and extortion; and

4. powers of attorney can be used for an impaired victim capable of informed consent to avoid exploitation, if in the hands of a trustworthy friend or family member. However, it may also be a means by which an untrustworthy person can exploit an elderly victim. Unlike a guardianship, which must be assigned by a court of law, a power of attorney does not have equivalent legal safeguards. As a result, great care must be exercised in its use.

In the following section, social service and criminal justice remedies will be discussed in greater detail.

SOCIAL SERVICE INTERVENTIONS

Service Remedies: Assisting the Victim

Counseling with victims of abusive adult children with mental illness or addiction problems must focus the victim's attention on how the habitual interactions between victim and abuser are evolving and how to go about changing them. One way to educate victims about changing their relationships to their abusers is the concept of tough love (Winter, 1986). This concept dictates that sometimes being a good parent or spouse means utilizing civil and criminal justice authorities and all the legal ammunition necessary—mental hygiene warrants, orders of protection, injunctions, eviction, and civil commitment—to get the abuser out of the house and away from the victim (Kaplan, 1997).

While aging service providers have proposed this philosophy to their clients, they have not focused sufficiently on what options are available for these mentally ill relatives and the emotional anguish incurred for the parents who love them if they do not get necessary treatment. A survey done through the National Alliance for the Mentally Ill (NAMI) reported that of 1,156 respondents, 89% were parents, usually mothers. They were asked to document the aggressive and violent behavior in the home by their mentally ill adult children, such as hitting or punching, and destructive acts such as breaking or throwing things.

Thirty eight percent of the sample perpetrators were judged to be violent, that is, assaultive and destructive. Another 5% were deemed threatening or potentially violent. The preferred living arrangement for 96% of respondents was sending the abusers out of the home. Some turned to the criminal justice system and the perpetrators were arrested and sent to a psychiatric facility.

Although the graying of America is a well-known phenomenon (Serow, Sly & Wrigley, 1990), the graying of the mentally ill and their caregivers is less well-known. Studies show that the primary caregivers for these individuals are elderly parents caring for their chronically mentally ill offspring (Leibowitz & Light, 1996). Primary caregivers for the mentally ill are parents, often in their late 50's and 60's, and many parenting caregivers are significantly older than this (Lefley, 1987; Greenberg, Seltzer & Greenley, 1993). While studies on parental caregiving of mentally ill relatives to date have not specifically examined elder abuse as an outcome, they have identified high levels of emotional stress, lower levels of life satisfaction, and depression among caregivers (Lebowitz & Light, 1996).

Service Remedies: Assisting the Batterer

Domestic violence advocates often resist the option of providing services to the batterer on the grounds that finite resources should be targeted to the victim. In cases of elder abuse and neglect, however, it is often necessary to assist the abuser to ensure that the victim will accept services. Particularly in the case of an impaired abuser, studies have demonstrated that an older victim is often very protective of an abuser if that person is an impaired adult child, grandchild or spouse/partner (Brownell, Berman & Salamone, 1999).

Focusing on the abuser's needs is not a popular concept in elder abuse cases or in other forms of domestic violence. Part of this issue is one of conflict of interest. Can a worker serve both the victim and the abuser? Another is that of available funding. In a world of limited resources, should workers advocate for services and treatment for populations they are not authorized to serve? There are no easy answers to these questions. The first step is education. Service providers in all public and private sectors must not only understand the interrelationship of their service mandates, but what services exist and how they can be coordinated in the most effective way to assist elder abuse victims and their impaired abusers.

The second step is to form working relationships with providers in other disciplines and in other areas of practice. Developing memoranda of understanding between providers who are not authorized to provide services for each other's clients is one way to ensure that referrals are made expeditiously. These steps are not costly and can be very effective. However, the services must be available when the referrals are made. This can be a challenging and costly undertaking. According to Tatara (1995), about 30% of abusers are adult children struggling with alcoholism, drugs, unemployment, and other mental and emotional problems. Tatara emphasizes that unless programs to address these problems become more accessible as well as effective elder abuse will not be curtailed.

EXAMPLES OF SOCIAL SERVICE AND AGING SERVICE PROGRAMS

The New York City Department for the Aging (DFTA) is the largest area agency on aging in the country. DFTA, directly and through a network of community-based agencies, sponsors crime prevention activities for older New Yorkers, and provides counseling and supportive services to elderly victims of crime and elder abuse in New York City. Through the Elderly Crime Victims Resource Center, DFTA staff provide direct services to clients 60 years of age and older who are victims of elder abuse. This program differs from Adult Protective Services in that it serves all older adults seeking services. Impaired older adults who appear to be at imminent risk of harm and unable to protect themselves from harm due to cognitive and/or physical limitations are referred to the New York City Adult Protective Services program (called Protective Services for Adults). New York State does not have mandatory reporting of non-institutional elder abuse. All referrals to both the DFTA Elderly Crime Victims Resource Center, as well as Adult Protective Services, are made on a voluntary basis.

The assistance provided by agencies like the New York City Department for the Aging Elderly Crime Victims Resource Center (ECVRC) can be critical, however, to the safety and well-being of elder abuse victims of impaired abusers. A case example follows:

> Mrs. Gonzolez is an 86-year-old woman living with her 46-year-old son, Geraldo, who suffers from a mental illness. Geraldo is on parole after serving time for the possession and sale of cocaine. He has a history of violence and is considered dangerous.
>
> Mrs. Gonzolez called the Elderly Crime Victims Resource Center of the New York City Department for the Aging because Geraldo was in a rage, punching holes in the walls of her apartment, throwing pots at her and threatening to kill the entire family. A caseworker took the call and contacted the police. Geraldo was arrested and brought to a psychiatric emergency room where he was evaluated and admitted to the hospital. The caseworker contacted Geraldo's

parole officer to report that he had been arrested and hospitalized and that he was in violation of his parole. The parole officer called the hospital, but the social worker refused to share information regarding her patient, citing confidentiality.

While he was in the hospital, Geraldo repeatedly called his mother and said he would come home and kill her. Upon the urging of the caseworker, Mrs. Gonzolez went to Family Court and obtained an Order of Protection which excluded Geraldo from the house and prohibited him from calling his mother and threatening or harassing her. He persistently violated the order while in the hospital.

The caseworker from ECVRC consulted with the legal department for the hospital and cited Mental Hygiene Law permitting the disclosure of information to a law enforcement agency. Under direction from the legal department, the hospital social worker then revealed to the Parole Officer Geraldo's date of discharge. Geraldo was arrested and awaits a parole hearing. The case worker also contacted Geraldo's lawyer to request that mental health treatment be mandated by the court under New York State's new Kendra's Law, as an alternative to incarceration.

As noted in the discussion on the New York City Department for the Aging study, elderly victims of abuse by impaired family members are less likely to accept services for themselves if services are not also made available for their abusive loved ones. Therefore, it is essential that services are developed or expanded for the mentally impaired (including substance abusers) living in the community as one strategy for ensuring the safety and well-being of their elderly family members.

THE CRIMINAL JUSTICE SYSTEM

Since the mid 1950s, America has adopted the policy of deinstitutionalization for the mentally ill (Barton, 1966). However, an unintended consequence of this policy shift has been a dearth of community-based mental health services in addition to greatly diminished institutional treatment options (Grob, 1994). Advocates for the mentally ill have decried the lack of housing for the mentally ill as well as the lack of supportive services in the community. Jails and prisons are now being used as hospitals for the mentally ill (Barr, 1999). According to a study by the Urban Justice Center and The Correctional Association of New York, on any given day there are close to 8,000 people with mental illness in New York State prisons and jails. A new awareness of this issue has emerged for aging services providers, that is, how to stop or prevent abuse of elderly clients in their homes by mentally ill adult children who have nowhere else to go.

As the DFTA study showed, these victims are the least likely to report the abuse or accept services. Many of these seniors have had their family members involuntarily committed many times, only to have the abusers returned to them by the hospital within weeks, on medication and temporarily stable. However, within a short period of time, usually a month, the abuser stops taking medication and the cycle begins again. According to service providers, elderly parents do not want their children arrested and they do not want their children to be homeless on the street or in a shelter where they will not receive treatment for their illness. However, most interventions to prevent or stop abuse are directed toward the victim, not the perpetrators.

Domestic violence in this population has a potentially devastating effect on family members who must live in tense and fearful home environments. Violent patients are more likely to be living at home with parents who have limited income, more likely to abuse alcohol, and less likely to comply with medication orders. The response of parents to violent behavior of their mentally ill relatives was indicative of tension, fear, and anger which restricts their lifestyles and reduces their quality of life. The tension and anger created in these circumstances may also exacerbate the anti-social behavior of people with mental illness.

This validates previous research on the role played by family members as it increases the probability of relapse by mentally ill patients in the home (Sullivan, 1994). Separating family members who are mentally ill from their parents seems to be advantageous to both the abuser and the victim. Finding appropriate residential treatment for mentally ill abusers is essential for the protection of older family members as well as the mentally ill family members who are potential or actual perpetrators of elder abuse.

However, it poses a striking challenge to providers of aging services, mental health providers, and the criminal justice system. Aging services providers are not funded to provide services to younger, possibly mentally ill or chemically addicted (MICA) impaired younger adults, yet it will be necessary for these providers to become acquainted with programs to help these abusers in order to help elder abuse victims. Elder abuse victims may not cooperate in a plan for their own safety or take action against their abusers if doing so means turning them over to the criminal justice system or putting them out on the street. Aging service providers must therefore learn new systems for intervention and form linkages and coalitions with providers of services for these populations.

According to the Urban Justice Center, people with mental illness in jails and prisons are victimized and segregated (Barr, 1999). They lose contact with their families and community mental health treatment providers and also lose housing income and insurance. While they may receive some basic mental health services in jail, they are eventually released without referrals to community treatment or any of the supports to prevent them from resorting to previous behaviors.

Unfortunately, the criminal justice system is often the only recourse for parents of mentally ill young adults who are violent. It is also a resource of last resort for aging services providers in order to keep their clients safe at home. It is not the best solution. It does, however, afford an opportunity to intervene in cases of treatment-resistant persons with mental illness, giving them an avenue for getting help (Barr, 1999). It is an opportunity that aging services providers must investigate in order to adequately serve their abused clients with mentally ill adult children.

It appears, then, that there is a significant risk of elder abuse among families of mentally ill young adults. Interventions in these cases may be hampered by a lack of information on the part of aging services providers regarding services available to the younger mentally ill population. But there is an equally meager knowledge of resources on the part of mental health providers regarding services for the elderly abused parents of their clients. Many of these parents are the younger (60 to 74 years of age) independent elderly, but some are aged, frail, and vulnerable and cannot care for themselves or their mentally ill son or daughter. As a last resort, service providers turn to the criminal justice system.

BENEFITS OF USING THE CRIMINAL JUSTICE SYSTEM

Elder abuse victims are subjected to a wide variety of criminal offenses by offspring (Brownell, 1998, 1999). These range from harassment (including stalking), menacing, assault, robbery, forgery, and even rape. The litany of criminal offenses by offspring read no differently than those committed by strangers against the elderly. However, while elders can take measures to protect themselves against stranger crime by refusing to admit strangers into their homes, avoiding leaving their homes in the evenings, seeking well-protected outdoor environments, and maintaining well-secured residences, these measures often offer limited protection against abusers who are offspring or other family members. When older adults report abuse to the police, complaint reports are filed that can be useful at a later date if they decide to apply for an order of protection against their abusers. A study of New York City Police Department (NYPD) police complaint reports filed by older victims of abuse by adult children in New York City (Brownell, 1998) found that a significant number of elder abuse victims are willing to report abuse to the police on their own or cooperate once the report is made by a third party witness.

Advocates of mandatory reporting for elder abuse suggest otherwise.

They claim that elderly victims of domestic violence by offspring will not report abuse to the police, much less state willingness to prosecute their abuser. While the findings of the study appear to challenge this, it is not possible—given the scope of the study—to determine if there were many more victims who did not report. However, the elderly victims in the NYPD study demonstrate that elder victims of abuse are not only capable of advocating on their own behalf but also view the police as a valuable resource and as allies in ensuring protection from abuse (Brownell, 1998). The candor with which some of the victims in the study shared intimate and potentially embarrassing details of the abuse to the responding police officer suggests a level of comfort on the part of the elderly victim in speaking to the officer. This, in turn, supports findings from the literature on the trust older people feel toward police (Yin, 1985). It also suggests that local law enforcement can play a valuable role within communities in identifying and responding to elder abuse.

RECOURSE TO THE CRIMINAL JUSTICE SYSTEM: CONTROVERSIES AND CONSEQUENCES

The use of the criminal justice system in addressing elder abuse has always been controversial (Wolf, 1999). Some recent studies have highlighted the prevalence of the mentally impaired in U.S. jails and prisons (Barr, 1999). Prison guards are not trained in working with mentally impaired inmates or in recognizing symptoms of mental illness. As a result, many inmates suffering from major mental illnesses are viewed as troublemakers and treated accordingly: i.e., beaten or placed in solitary confinement for extended periods of time.

Honberg (1996) states that one significant reason the mentally impaired are incarcerated is that family members are forced to call the police to intervene because of threatening or destructive actions of a mentally ill or substance abusing family member. He cautions families not to accept or risk personal injury at the hands of a mentally ill or substance abusing member. At the same time, family members should realize that the police have a vastly different agenda from theirs. Law enforcement agents may be required by law to initiate a process that can have lasting effects on the family. The case vignettes presented earlier in this chapter illustrate possible repercussions. The likely objective of the family, however, is to protect its members while trying to link the mentally impaired family member with appropriate services.

IMPLICATIONS FOR PRACTICE AND POLICY

Discharge Planning

Program initiatives that can serve to protect elderly family members while assisting mentally ill abusers include offender reintegration assistance through organizations such as the Fortune Society, forensic intensive case management (ICM) programs, and alternative sentencing projects managed by counties and district attorneys' offices.

Diversion

Outreach teams comprised of police and mental health professionals, including forensic social workers, have proven useful in assessing and diverting the severely and persistently mentally ill (SPMI) from arrest and incarceration (Lamb, Shaner, Elliot, DeCuit & Foltz, 1996). Other initiatives include assigning intensive case management (ICM) teams to SPMI offenders before release from jail/prison allowing social workers to certify SPMIs for emergency short-term hospitalizations, and making crisis services available 24 hours a day with an 800 number.

Alternative funding sources for psychiatric services and medication can remove barriers to community-based treatment for mentally ill abusers lacking third party health insurance or active Medicaid coverage. Training for judges and police to recognize the need for treatment and treatment options for mentally ill abusers can result in diversion to more appropriate service alternatives for those SPMIs and substance abusers who are required to make court appearances.

Treatment

Substance abuse treatment in prisons and in the community is inadequate to meet ongoing demands, in spite of research findings that substance abuse is a significant risk factor for violent behavior (Murdoch, Pihl & Ross, 1990). All treatment, including hospital beds in detoxification units and residential treatment programs and intensive case management, should be available on a priority basis for substance abusers who are also abusive to elderly relatives and friends. Training for substance abuse counselors and program staff could help sensitize those working with substance abusers to the issue of elder abuse and inform them of programs and services available to assist older family members.

CONCLUSION

Significant progress has been made in the last 10 years in understanding elder mistreatment, developing methods of intervention, and disseminating information. Many of the intervention strategies focus on the needs of the victim, however. Further research is needed on mental impairments of abusers and the relationship to elder abuse and mistreatment.

However, findings from this and other studies suggest that, in cases of domestic abuse of older people involving impaired abusers, the risk of elder abuse may be most effectively reduced in many cases by addressing the needs of the abusers. This may include improving service coordination and expanding services among mental health, substance abuse, criminal justice, and aging service systems. Forging new and stronger service provider partnerships is the challenge of the future.

Elder abuse is a complex phenomenon. It may include the learned interactions of a dysfunctional family, criminal activity, substance abuse, mental illness or organic incapacity. It requires extensive awareness on the part of interdisciplinary teams of professionals, public education, and a system-wide approach to address the problems. It also requires services that are adequately funded and available to serve the family as a target system rather than individual members of the family who are competing for resources.

It is not necessary or often not even practical to separate the needs of some family members to the disadvantage of others. Education for both professionals and older adults directed at prevention of abuse should be available in all communities. In this way, a community-wide awareness can be developed that abuse of the elderly is not acceptable and that there are professionals available who can intervene and provide both services and support to families in need.

REFERENCES

Abelman, I. (1992). *Report on incidence of adult abuse on the protective services for adults caseload in New York State.* New York: State Department of Social Services.

Anetzberger, G. (1987). *The etiology of elder abuse by adult offspring.* Springfield, IL: Charles C. Thomas.

Barker, N. (2000). *Unpublished Dissertation.* New York: Fordham University.

Barr, H. (1998). *Prisons and jails: hospitals as a last resort.* New York: Urban Justice Center.

Barton, W.E. (1966). Trends in Community Mental Health Programs. *Hospital & Community Psychiatry.* September, 1966.

Bernheim, K.F. & Lewine, R.R.J. (1979). *Schizophrenia: symptoms, causes, treatments.* New York: W. W. Norton.

Biggs. S., Phillipson, C. & P. Kingston (1995). *Elder abuse in perspective.* Buckingham, MK: Open University Press.

Brownell, P. (1998). *Family crimes against the elderly: elder abuse and the criminal justice system.* New York: Garland Publishing.

Brownell, P., Berman J. & A. Salamone (1999). Mental health and criminal justice issues among perpetrators of elder abuse. *Journal of Elder Abuse and Neglect, 11*(4), 81–94.

Butterfield, F. (1998). *Prisons replace hospitals for the nation's mentally ill. New York Times,* March 5, 1998, A1.

Decaire, M. (2000). *Mental disorders and crime: personality disorders.* www.suite101.com/article.cfm/forensic/psychology/32037

Dowd, J.J. (1975). Aging as exchange: A preface to theory. *Journal of Gerontology, 30,* 584–594.

Dugger, C. (1991). *When love doesn't conquer: crack and murder.* New York Times, October 13, 1991, A1.

Dundorf, K. & Brownell P. (1995). Elder abuse—what is it; what can be done about it?. *The Family Advocate,* American Bar Association, V. 17, No. 3, 81–3.

Greenberg, J., Seltzer, M.M. & Greenley, J.R. (1993). Aging parents of adults with disabilities: the gratifications and frustrations of later life caregiving. *Gerontologist, 33,* 542–550.

Grob, G.N. (1994). *The mad among us: a history of the care of America's mentally ill.* New York: Free Press.

Honberg, R. (1996). Mental illness and the criminal justice system. *AMI-FAM. Reporter,* May/June 1996, Vol. 17(3), 9–10.

Hwalek, M. (1989). *An Illinois plan for a statewide elder abuse program.* In Filinson, R. and Ingman, S. (Eds.) Elder Abuse: Practice and Policy. New York: Human Science Press, 196–207.

Kaplan, R. (1997). Interventions and support for relatives of the mentally ill. *NAMI Advocate,* July/August 1997, 8.

Korbin, J. E., Anetzberger, G. J., Thomasson, R. & Austin, C. (1991). Abused elders who seek legal recourse against their adult offspring: findings from an exploratory study. *Journal of Elder Abuse and Neglect, 3*(3), 1–18.

Lachs, M. S. & Pillemer, K. (1995). Abuse and neglect of elderly persons. *New England Journal of Medicine, 332,* 437–443.

Lamb, H.R., Shaner, R., Elliot, D.M., DeCuit, Jr., W. J. & Foltz, J.T. (1996). Outreach by police/mental health team prevents criminalization of individuals with mental illness. *AMI-FAMI Reporter,* 17 (2, 6).

Lau, E. & Kosberg, J. (1979). Abuse of the elderly by informal caregivers. *Aging,* 10–15 (September/October).

Lefley, H.P. (1987). Aging parents as caregivers of mentally ill adult children: an emerging social problem. *Hospital & Community Psychiatry, 38,* 1063–1070.

Lebowitz, B.D. & Light, E. (1996). The aging caregiver of psychiatric patients: healthcare perspectives. *Psychiatric Annals, 26*(1), 785–791 (December).

Murdoch, D., Pihl, R. O. & Ross, D. (1990). Alcohol and crimes of violence: current issues. *The International Journal of Addictions, 25,* 1065–1081.

National GAINS Center (1997). The prevalence of co-occurring mental and substance abuse disorders in the criminal justice system. *Just the Facts.* Spring 1997.

Pillemer, K. & Finkelhor, D. (1988). The prevalence of elder abuse: a random sample survey. *The Gerontologist, 281,* 51–57.

Pillemer, K. & Finkelhor, D. (1989). *Causes of elder abuse: caregiver versus problem relatives.* American Orthopsychiatric Association, 59, 179–187.

Porr, V. (n.d.). *Facts about substance abuse and borderline personality disorder.* New York: Treatment and Research Advancements Association for Personality Disorders.

Quinn, M. & Tomita, S. (1997). *Elder abuse and neglect: causes, diagnosis and intervention strategies.* Second Edition. New York: Springer Publishing.

Salamone, A., Berman, J., Eidlisz, S. & Lipton, S. (1998). *Mental health issues and service needs among perpetrators of elder abuse.* Poster presented at the 51st Annual Meeting of the Gerontological Society of America, November, 1998, Philadelphia, PA. New York City: Department for the Aging.

Serow, W. J., Sly, D.F. & Wrigley, J.M. (1990). *Population aging in the United States.* New York: Greenwood Press.

Steinmetz, S. (1981). Elder abuse. *Aging,* 6–10 (January/February).

Steinmetz, S. (1988). *Duty bound: elder abuse and family care.* Newbury Park, CA: Sage.

Sullivan, R. (1994). *Court allows holding of patients who may become dangerous after release. New York Times,* December 11, 1994, A7.

Tatara, T. (1995). *Elder abuse.* In Edwards, R.L. (Ed.) Encyclopedia of Social Work, 19th Edition. Washington, DC: NASW Press, 834–842.

Vinton, L. (1988). *Correlates of elder abuse.* Unpublished Doctoral Dissertation, University of Wisconsin, Madison, Wisconsin.

U. S. House of Representatives (1990). *Elder abuse: a decade of shame and inaction.* Washington, DC: Government Printing Office Publication No. 101–752.

Wallace, H. (1999). *Family violence: legal, medical, and social perspectives.* Second Edition. Boston: Allyn & Bacon.

Winter. A. (1986). Elder abuse. *Modern Maturity,* October–November Issue, 52–57.

Wolf, R.S. (1999). *The criminalization of elder abuse.* Presentation: Pan American Congress '99, San Antonio, Texas, February 23, 1999, Symposium on Social Policy II Elder Abuse.

Wolf, R.S. (1988). Elder abuse: ten years later. *The Journal of the American Geriatrics Society* 36, 758–762.

Wolf, R.S. (1994). Elder abuse: a family tragedy. *Aging International,* Vol. 21 (1), 60–64.

Wolf, R.S. (1998). Studies belie caregiver stress as key to elder mistreatment. *Aging Today,* November–December Issue, 9.

Wolf, R.S., Hodge, P. & Roberts, P. (1998). Elder abuse and neglect: Prosecution and prevention. *Critical Issues in Aging, 2,* 35–38.

Wolf, R.S. & McCarthy, E. R. (1991). Elder abuse. In Ammerman, R. T. and Hersen, M. (Eds.) *Case studies in Family Violence.* New York: Plenum Press.

Wolf, R.S. & Pillemer, K. (1984). *Definitions of elder abuse and neglect.* New York: Governor's Task Force on Elder Abuse.

Wolf, R.S., Strugnell, C. P., & Godkin, M. A. (1984). *Elder abuse and neglect: final report from three model projects.* Worcester, MA: University of Massachusetts Medical Center, University Center on Aging.

Yin, P. (1985). *Victimization and the aged.* Springfield, Illinois: Thomas C. Charles.

17

Identifying and Addressing the Needs of Victims of Mentally Ill Offenders

Gerald Landsberg and Marjorie Rock

PROJECT BACKGROUND

It is only since 1982 that the United States has formally addressed the needs of victims of crime. In that year, the President's Task Force on Victims of Crime recommended that a series of actions be taken to promote the involvement of victims in the justice system and promote financial restitution to crime victims. Currently, all states guarantee that crime victims can participate in the criminal justice process, yet there are important gaps in understanding the dilemma posed by certain victims who remain under-represented.

One significant group of victims who have not been considered in overall victim needs legislation has been victims of offenders with a mental illness. The Office for the Victims of Crime was eager to engage in an exploration of the problems encountered by this group of victims as well as to formulate some recommendations for enhancing services to this group. Therefore, the intention of this project—conducted by the Institute Against Violence of the Ehrenkranz School of Social Work of New York University—was to explore the needs of victims of mentally ill offenders and to make suggestions for better meeting their service needs. The intention of the project was, in no way, to cast blame on any one group of individuals or to excuse the actions of any one group of individuals but to explore the relationships between all those who work with the mentally ill and with victims.

Following an extensive process of exploring the issues, it became apparent that there was a serious need for different constituencies representing the mentally ill, their families, members of the criminal justice and law enforcement communities, and victims rights organizations to work together to understand the problems faced by the mentally ill and persons who were victimized by those with a mental illness. The training products that were developed as a result of this project, described later in this chapter, are meant to bring people together to engage in discussion about the issues as well as to initiate community-level programs and services for all parties.

RESEARCH AND DATA COLLECTION
PHASE OF THE PROJECT

The initial phase of the project presented the process of discovery and exploration of the problem of what happens to victims of mentally ill offenders. It reports on the scope and complexity of the problem and makes recommendations for improved service delivery mechanisms. The findings are the result of a year-long study conducted by New York University's Ehrenkranz School of Social Work and funded by the Office for the Victims of Crime (OVC). The purpose of the study was to define the problem of what happens to victims of mentally ill offenders, to understand the magnitude of the problem, and to offer recommendations of best practices for serving the victims.

Definitions:

For the purpose of this project, we defined mentally ill offenders as those who, before or after arrest, were diagnosed with a major psychiatric condition as defined on Axis I of the *Diagnostic and Statistical Manual* of the American Psychiatric Association (DSM-IV, 1994). These conditions included schizophrenia and other psychotic disorders, mood disorders including major depressive and bi-polar disorders, and schizo-affective disorders. We did not include in the definition sexual offenders or those with developmental disorders, learning disabilities, personality disorders or primary substance abuse disorder (without a psychiatric disorder). The offenders have committed a criminal act or engaged in violent behaviors that would be adjudicated as a criminal act. Therefore, we excluded verbal assaults or threats, misdemeanors, and similar behaviors which may cause the recipient to feel victimized but are not prosecuted as violent felonies. The definition of victim included both family and non-family members and "stranger" victims.

Project Activities and Findings

Project activities included: (1) an extensive review of the relevant literature in this area; (2) surveys of selected states with respect to the relevant
laws and regulations affecting this population; and (3) four focus groups
across the country. Three state or city groups were organized in Brooklyn,
New York, Kansas City, Missouri and Portland, Oregon. The regional groups
included representatives from crime victim compensation boards, victims
assistance programs, elder abuse prevention agencies, district attorney
offices, police departments, courts and local chapters of two national advocacy groups, the National Alliance for the Mentally Ill, and Parents of
Murdered Children.

The fourth focus group, held in Washington, D.C., brought together
representatives from national organizations in mental health, victim assis-
tance, and criminal justice including the Department of Justice, the
National Institute of Corrections, the American Bar Association, the
National Mental Health Association, the National Center for Victims of
Crime, the National Sheriffs Department, the United States Attorney
General's Office, the National Alliance for the Mentally Ill, and the VINE
Company, a computer program database that provides victims with offender
release status and notification information.

However, there has been strikingly little research specifically conducted
on victims of mentally ill offenders. Recently, Steadman H.J., Mulvey, E.P.,
Monahan, J., Robbins P., Appelbaum, P., Grisson, T. Roth L.H. & Silver,
E. (1998) reported that, when a mentally ill person engages in violence,
the victim is primarily a family member (51.1%) or a friend or acquaintance (35.1%). Strangers comprise 13.8% of victims of mentally ill offenders (Steadman et al., 1998).

Underscoring the findings of the Steadman study, each focus group
concluded that the overwhelming majority of victims of mentally ill offenders were family members or close acquaintances rather than strangers.
Although few statistics exist from agencies, participants anecdotally estimated that between 70% and 75% of victims fall into the family or close
acquaintance category. This finding is particularly important in light of
exaggerated fears in the general population confirmed by media hype
that often paints the mentally ill as threatening people, lurking in neighborhoods and ready to attack unsuspecting strangers, such as the media's
titillating focus on high-profile mentally ill offenders, such as President
Ronald Reagan's attempted assassin, John Hinkley, John. Lennon's killer,
Marc Chapman, or recent events on New York City subways or the
Washington Capitol case suggest that strangers to the mentally ill are at
high risk; in reality, those who suffer most as victims are family members.

"Once in a blue moon," according to a district attorney from Brooklyn, "you see a case where someone is on the subway and gets assaulted by someone who is mentally ill. But it's really not what you see habitually. And it's much more routinely cases involving family members."

Despite the overwhelming evidence that violence is directed at family members, it is still important to acknowledge that friends/acquaintances and strangers can be victims. Understanding these victim populations and their needs is crucial to effectively aid them.

Family Members as Victims

Given the significant proportion of family victims, we focus in substantial detail on the impact on this population as described by our focus group participants. The crucial concerns of these victims are the fear of stigma, feelings of guilt, and a desire to see the family member get help. In this light, it is not surprising that our focus group participants, especially family members, report that "family member victims vastly underreport their victimization." The family reaction to the mentally ill member is often cloaked in denial and integrated into a web of "family secrets."

These participants suggested that denial also takes other forms, such as contesting that offending behavior has taken place. Additionally, family members experience offending behaviors incrementally and may become so immune to the mentally ill person's escalating aggressiveness that they may be unaware that they are being victimized. They may not even recognize dangerous behavior.

Even in the cases where family members recognize dangerous behavior, report their victimization, and seek services for themselves and their families, they are often disillusioned by the response of the legal and mental health communities, according to focus group members. For the most part, family victims want to get treatment for the offender. They are searching, often pleading, for treatment rather than punishment. Yet when they call for help, more often than not, the offender is incarcerated. Time and time again, the victims of mentally ill offenders turn to the criminal justice system as a last resort, only to find that neither the mental illness in question nor their victimization is well understood.

Focus group members consistently reported that as a result of deinstitutionalization, shrinking psychiatric hospital services, and lack of community resources, jails have become the "de facto mental hospitals of the '90s." The criminal justice system is particularly ill-equipped to provide support for the family victim or services for the offender. It is neither the function nor the design of prisons to treat mental illness or provide services to victims. Scarce mental health facilities and inadequate community mental health services were common themes in all the focus groups.

When a victimized family member attempts to find help for the offender and in its place is faced with the offender's incarceration, there is guilt and reluctance to seek help in the future. This is particularly true for elder family members. The elderly may endure victimization by a mentally ill child or grandchild, the care of whom is often key to the victim's living at home rather than in a nursing facility. An advocate for the elderly in the Kansas City group explained that the elder abuse victim thinks "it's better for me to be able to stay in my home and put up with this than for me to let you do something and end up in a nursing home."

Additionally, elder family victims may have a strong sense of obligation toward caring for their mentally ill offspring. They may indeed feel responsible for their offspring's psychiatric condition. In the absence of appropriate services for the mentally ill offender and the aging family victim, both suffer needlessly and often silently. (The issue of the mentally ill as abusers of their elderly parent is a crucial one and demands further investigation. An ongoing study by the New York City Department of Aging suggests that three-fourth of these elderly abuse victims are abused by their mentally ill adult children.)

Non-Family Victims

Our group of participants suggested that, when a stranger is victim of a mentally ill person, the victim is more likely to report the crime to law enforcement officials. Unlike the family member, the stranger rarely has reason to protect the offender from incarceration and punishment.

When victims of mentally ill offenders become involved with the legal system, (like most victims) they perceive the criminal justice system as a daunting maze. Not only are they confused by the way the case is tried but they are also often excluded from the judicial process itself. When they are included, they are considered solely as a witness for the prosecution. Victims frequently feel used in the roles as mere evidence givers.

Although they share many concerns and problems of crime victims in general, the victims of mentally ill offenders have special needs, especially pertaining to the criminal justice system. The court system, as it deals with the mentally ill offender, engages in procedural complexities, such as plea bargains, insanity defenses, diversion programs, and (often inadequate) notification laws. Non-family members are shut out of the legal process. It's difficult for these victims to comprehend that an offender may be found not guilty by reason of insanity (NGR) or guilty but mentally ill (GBMI). Often the victim is not informed about the workings of the court system and the significance of its decisions.

"Victims want to be included," said a focus group participant who is a member of Parents of Murdered Children. "Victims are re-victimized by being excluded. Once you're a victim, you're a victim for the rest of your life. I got a life sentence when my daughter was murdered. The guy that murdered her did not get a life sentence."

Besides not understanding legal procedures, non-family victims of mentally ill offenders are often barred from obtaining information by confidentiality laws which go into effect when the perpetrator is diagnosed as mentally ill. The laws often pit victims' groups against advocates for the mentally ill.

One of the most difficult legal conditions for the victim to accept is the adjudication, Not Guilty by Reason of Insanity (NGRI). By virtue of the "not guilty" portion of the verdict, the victim is no longer legally recognized as a victim. The evidence is clear that they and their loved ones have been victimized, yet the perpetrator is declared "not guilty."

After an NGRI finding, the victims of mentally ill offenders are largely neglected by the legal system. They are not served by victims' advocates and are often removed from court activities after the verdict. Even the records of the offender may be removed from the courts and placed within the jurisdiction of the department of mental health.

Further, in many states, victims of mentally ill offenders are not only excluded from hearings pertaining to release but also are not even notified if offenders escape from custody (study by the National Center for Victims of Crime). Lack of notification is especially problematic when cases are diverted from the criminal justice system to the mental health system, and the "veil of confidentiality" (as one participant put it) falls over the entire proceeding.

Recommendations

The recommendations that follow emerge, primarily, from the suggestions of focus group participants and, secondarily, from the literature reviews and telephone interviews conducted by the NYU Project staff. Due to the emerging nature of these issues and, as noted by focus group participants, the lack of specific research defining the needs of victims of mentally ill offenders, the following recommendations should be considered as preliminary findings:

- Public education should take up the problem of mental illness and victimization, with an emphasis on identifying, educating, and serving both family and non-family victims of the mentally ill offender.
- Training and education need to be geared toward mental health, criminal justice victims assistance, and aging services professionals.
- Increased coordination of services for victims of mentally ill offenders on a local, state and federal level is critical.

- Outreach is a crucial task to aid family and non-family members. This is often crucial for victims in rural areas and victims unable to access needed services; mobile out-reach teams offer an important need expanded potential.
- Legal initiatives should seek to include victims in legal proceedings, refine victim notification laws and extend eligibility for victim compensation and assistance.
- There is great room for improvement in discharge planning and after-care for mentally ill offenders; such planning and care should include family member victims.
- Research on the incidence and impact of crimes committed by the mentally ill is needed especially related to the prevalence of crimes against families and non-families; exploring support systems for victims, evaluating effective intervention and service provision for victims of these crimes is necessary; also, further research on the impact of parental mental illness on violence against children is essential.

TRAINING PRODUCTS

As we have noted, the issue of victimization of family, friends and strangers by the mentally ill is becoming an increasingly important topic for discussion by families, advocates, mental health providers, law enforcement, and victims' assistance professionals and agency service providers in the community. This training initiative developed by the Institute Against Violence of the Ehrenkranz School of Social Work of New York University with funding from the Office for the Victims of Crime of the United States Department of Justice is designed to inform, educate, and most importantly, promote local community dialogues on the issues. It is our hope that through this training initiative, consumers, family members, advocates, mental health professionals, law enforcement and victims assistance personnel, agency service providers, and other interested parties can establish planning and discussion groups to *collectively develop local programs/services and ongoing educational/informational activities.* Further, the objective is not only to ensure attention to the needs of the victims but also to examine strategies to better serve the mentally ill victimizers. The issue of victimization of families and strangers is not without controversy and is seen through differing perspectives. It is important that these perspectives be shared at the community level so that collaborative strategies for action can be developed.

As part of the training initiatives, the following products have been created:
- Training Video (25 minutes in length)
- Video Discussion Guide (to assist in identifying topics/questions for discussion following the video)

- Informational Brochures for:
  - Family Members
  - Mental Health Professionals
  - Law Enforcement Professionals
  - Staff of Aging Service Agencies
  - Victims Assistance Staffs
  - Each of these brochures provides an overview of the problems of victimization, identifies key problems that each group needs to be aware of and indicates resources and books on the topic as well as additional resources to obtain further information.

STRATEGIES FOR PROMOTING COMMUNITY DISCUSSIONS AND ACTIONS

Effective strategies designed to promote community discussion and action require that a *single organization or group take a leadership role.* This initial leadership can come from a mental health advocacy group, a family group, a mental health agency, a criminal justice organization, or a victims assistance or an agency service organization. The leadership or organization needs to spearhead key initial tasks on the project. These tasks would include:

- Identifying key organizations/individuals concerned about the issue (even if only peripherally);
- Gathering data on the nature and scope of the problem in the local community;
- Meeting individually with key contacts in the community to inform them about this problem and your interests in addressing it;
- Convening at an initial forum/meeting at which the video is shown, followed by discussion from all participants, and arranging for additional meetings; and
- Developing a group plan for further actions and a timetable for action steps.

REFERENCES

Steadman, H.J., Mulvey, E.P., Morahan, J., Robbins, P., Appelbaum, P., Grisson, T., Roth, L.H. & Silver, E. (1998). Violence by people discharged from acute psychiatric inpatient facilities and by others in the same neighborhood. *Archives of General Psychiatry, 55,* 393–401.

SECTION V
Perspectives From the Legal System: Issues for Mental Health Professionals

18

A Judge's Perspective

Martin G. Karopkin

Recent studies demonstrate that mentally ill defendants make up a significant part of our jail and prison population (Ditton, 1999). What is most remarkable, in light of this, is how infrequently mental illness is an issue before the court in criminal cases.

The extent to which mental illness becomes an issue in criminal cases is dependent on many factors. The most significant are the seriousness of the crime and the manner in which the mental illness manifests itself. A case involving an unprovoked assault on a stranger will, by its very circumstances, almost certainly raise the question of the mental condition of the accused. Similarly, other crimes involving bizarre or irrational behavior will, ordinarily, prompt an inquiry into the defendant's mental condition. Even where the alleged criminal conduct is not, in and of itself, irrational, a defense attorney representing someone in a serious case may seek to raise the defendant's mental condition as an issue as a way of mitigating the circumstances in order to avoid a long jail sentence.

When mental illness becomes an issue two legal channels exist to address it. Severe mental illness may render someone "unfit to stand trial." In order to be found unfit a defendant's illness must be so severe that he is unable to understand the proceedings against him or to assist in his own defense.[1]

A mentally ill person who is found fit to stand trial may attempt to pursue what is commonly referred to as the "insanity defense." In New York State a person may be found *not guilty* if he can establish that "at the time of the conduct, as a result of a mental disease or defect, he lacked substantial capacity to know or appreciate either the nature and consequences of such conduct or that such conduct was wrong."[2]

While these are important issues, they involve only the most extremely troubled individuals and the number of cases that fall into these categories is very small, probably, amounting to less than 1% of all criminal matters[3] (Callahan et al., 1991).

The vast majority of cases where mental illness is a factor go largely unnoticed. It is this unidentified group of cases that accounts for the large number of mentally ill individuals in our penal facilities. These cases fall into no simple category. They cover the entire spectrum of criminal matters that come before the court. Usually there is very little about the crime or the defendant to make the case stand out. For example, a drug user who is mentally ill will appear before the court charged with drug possession in the same manner as does anyone else who uses drugs.

Identifying mental illness as a factor in the case is something that usually does not occur. For the judge, even one inclined to look for issues of mental illness, the job is difficult because a judge has very limited direct contact with a criminal defendant. Judges usually rely on the defense attorneys who have that contact to inform them if mental illness is an issue. This, however, does not always happen. Attorneys may not recognize the symptoms of mental illness or they may, out of concern that knowledge about a client's mental illness will hurt that client's chances for release, withhold that information from the court.

Indeed, knowledge about a defendant's mental illness may cause the prosecutor or judge to become concerned about public safety. A prosecutor or judge who has been made aware of a defendant's mental illness may reject a plea involving a sentence of community service or other non-jail option on the theory that a mentally ill defendant is not responsible enough to carry out that kind of sentence. It may also result in the setting of bail in a situation where, without knowledge of the defendant's mental illness, no bail would have been set.

Even when a judge is sympathetic to the needs of the mentally ill and wants to be helpful, few, if any, special services are available. It is difficult to adequately express the level of my frustration at confronting situations requiring immediate decisions that will result in a defendant's release or jail confinement, with no treatment alternative available. Worse still is the fact that often the only way to insure treatment is to send the person to jail.

One possible alternative would be to have a defendant sent for a psychiatric examination to determine if a civil commitment to a hospital or mental health facility is appropriate. Inpatient psychiatric care, however, can only be ordered when a defendant presents a danger to himself or others. This standard is simply not reached in most cases. Moreover, under New York law, a judge presiding over a criminal case cannot make a referral for such care unless the prosecutor is willing to dismiss the criminal case. [4] This is something prosecutors are, often for good reason, reluctant to do.

One of the ways in which this situation can be changed is by screening defendants for mental illness early in the criminal process and earmarking their cases for special treatment. For the past few years, I have had the privilege of presiding over night court arraignments in Brooklyn, New

York. I have come to the view that the arraignment process offers a unique opportunity to bring about change in how we handle cases involving the mentally ill.

Arraignment is the proceeding in which a criminal defendant makes his or her first appearance before a judge. It is the point of transfer from the police to the criminal justice process. It is the place where the formal criminal charges are first set forth. In most cases, it is the point at which a defense attorney becomes involved in the case and, in most situations, marks the first time the defense attorney and client meet. It is also the place where the first, and often most critical, decision is made about whether a defendant will be released or held in jail.

In New York City and other large urban districts the arraignment courts are busy calendar parts handling a high volume of cases ranging from minor infractions to the most serious crimes. Often these courts operate all day and evening. In New York City, each of the five boroughs has a day arraignment part seven days a week. Four of the boroughs, Manhattan, Brooklyn, the Bronx, and Queens, have night arraignments that run to 1:00 a.m. every day. In Manhattan, arraignments run all through the night three days each week. In 1999, approximately 370,000 cases passed though the arraignment process in the five boroughs of New York City. In 1998, that number was over 400,000.

Because many minor cases are disposed of at arraignment and decisions about release or jail are made at this proceeding, the difficult problems regarding mentally ill defendants present themselves more frequently and with greater urgency than at any other point in the criminal process. It is one of the reasons why the arraignment part offers an extraordinary opportunity to serve as a focal point for bringing about change. Another is the physical location of the defendants in the pre-arraignment process. Defendants awaiting arraignment are in custody close to the courtroom. They literally have nothing to do and no place to go while awaiting their court appearance. The situation presents a good opportunity to screen defendants by conducting interviews. The purpose of this screening would be to make a preliminary determination as to whether a defendant is mentally ill and if that person requires and is willing to receive treatment.

Of course, what is needed is not only screening but comprehensive follow-up. If treatment is to supplant jail as a means of dealing with the mentally ill, immediate availability of such treatment and, in many cases emergency housing, is essential. In some cases a defendant will need to be escorted directly from court to an appropriate inpatient or residential facility. Fortunately, just such a project is envisioned for the Brooklyn night arraignment part. Once it is in place, it should offer the judge an alternative between jail and unsupervised release.

Whether the case is resolved at arraignment or makes it way through the criminal process towards trial, early identification of the matter as one involving a mentally ill defendant will go a long way to achieving a fair and reasonable result. The key to success of this project will be the development of programs specifically for mentally ill criminal defendants. If the goal of treatment rather than jail is to become a reality, the programs to which defendants are referred must assure judges that public safety and other community concerns are adequately addressed. There must be feedback and communication with the court about the defendant's progress and assurance that the jail alternative is working for the individual defendant and for the community at large. As prosecutors and judges gain confidence in the ability of programs to provide reasonable alternatives to jail, the project can be expanded. This is our goal and this is our hope.

Notes

1 New York State, Criminal Procedure Law, article 730.

2 New York State, Penal Law, section 40.15.

3. Of approximately 100,000 criminal cases handled in Brooklyn, N.Y. in 1999, Dr. Thomas O'Rourke, Director of Forensic Psychiatry at Kings County Hospital, reports that there were approximately 300 requests for "fitness" examinations, less than half of which resulted in a finding that the defendant was unfit to proceed.

4 New York State, Mental Hygiene Law, section 9.43.

REFERENCES

Callahan, L.A., Steadman, H.J., McGreevy, M.A. & Robbins, P.C. (1991). The volume and characteristics of insanity defense pleas: An eight-state study. *Bulletin of the American Academy of Psychiatry and the Law,* *19*(4), 331–338.

Ditton, P.M. (July 1999). *Mental health and treatment of inmates and probationers.* Bureau of Justice Statistics Special Report, NCJ 174463. U.S. Department of Justice.

19

Social Workers as Advocates for Mentally Ill Criminal Defendants/Inmates*

Heather Barr

Is it a social worker's job to advocate for a client within the criminal justice system?

Imagine for a moment that you are a social worker in a shelter for homeless people. One of your clients is a woman who has been diagnosed with schizophrenia and has been living on the streets and using crack cocaine. Gradually through persistence and your skill at engaging people, you get her to stay in the shelter every night, to take antipsychotic medications regularly, and to stop abusing drugs. You spend many hours talking with her about moving on to supportive housing, do a great deal of work with her about what the experience of living in this housing will be like, and prepare her for the interviews she will have to go through to get into housing. Finally, the client feels she is ready and you begin the application process.

One morning you come to work and read in the logbook that she did not sleep in the shelter the previous night. You ask other clients if they have seen her, and several tell you that they heard she was arrested the previous night on the street outside the shelter, but they do not know what she was charged with.

What do you do? Do you know where people are taken after they arrested, or how to find out whether someone has been arrested? If she's in jail, do you know how to ensure that she gets the right medications while she is there? Does the work that you have been doing with her over the past year have any bearing on what sentence she should receive if she is guilty of a criminal offense?

---

* Sections of this chapter appear in other Urban Justice Publications.

Dedicated social workers don't just help people; they also *fight* for people. New social workers inherit a rich history of advocacy, and many of the best advocates I know are not lawyers, but social workers. People with mental illness, particularly those who are homeless, are today at great risk of finding themselves in the criminal justice system. This risk is so great that I believe social workers cannot do a competent job working with people with mental illness *unless* they understand the criminal justice system and develop skills in criminal justice advocacy. The first part of this chapter will explain why it is so important that social workers advocate to try to keep their clients out of the criminal justice system and, failing that, to minimize the damage that the criminal justice system will do to their clients. The second part of the chapter talks about some of the specific areas where advocacy for a mentally ill criminal defendant is most crucial and can be most effective.

WE HAVE A NEW COMMUNITY MENTAL
HEALTH SYSTEM—IT'S CALLED JAIL

Jails and prisons are the United States' new psychiatric institutions. People with mental illness in this country have been caught in a horrible collision between a collapsing mental health system and an ever-expanding criminal justice system. Across the country, attention is finally being paid to the problem researchers describe as "the criminalization of mental illness" and "transinstitutionalization"—the movement of people with serious mental illness from community psychiatric hospitals into jails and prisons.[1] While this problem has recently received considerable attention, solutions are a long way off.

Since the beginning of "deinstitutionalization" in the 1970s, psychiatric hospital systems across the country have down-sized drastically.[2] Nowhere in the country were community mental health services and supportive housing developed quickly enough to meet the needs of discharged patients. As a consequence, hundreds of thousands of people with serious mental illness, began living in communities that did not have enough of the supportive services necessary to give them a real shot at community living. Worse yet, when there was a crisis and a person required hospitalization, there often was no longer a treatment bed available. What there was, however, was tens of thousands of new jail and prison beds. The result? People with serious mental illness who needed care found themselves in the only institutions that did not turn them away—jails and prisons.

The incarceration of thousands of people with serious mental illness is having tragic consequences nationwide. A Department of Justice report, issued in July 1999, found that about 16% of jail and prison inmates nation-wide have mental illness—a total of over a quarter million incarcerated Americans with mental illness. In many jurisdictions, jails have become the primary treatment provider for poor people with mental illnesses. Rikers Island (New York City's jail complex) and the Los Angeles County jail have become our nation's largest psychiatric facilities.

"But my client is mentally ill. He doesn't belong in jail."

Often a social worker calls me and says something like, "My client was arrested on Thursday night. He's charged with robbery. He doesn't belong in jail—he's mentally ill. I need help." Unfortunately, the social worker is wrong; the fact that the client has a mental illness probably will not help him get out of jail.

Why? Because in the eyes of the criminal justice system, the fact that someone has a mental illness does not usually make them any less of a criminal. Most states have only two legal mechanisms for taking into account the psychiatric condition of a defendant, and neither of these mechanisms is of any help to most criminal defendants with mental illness. These two mechanisms existing in most states are competency evaluations and the not guilty by reason of insanity defense.

"Competency" refers to the defendant's competency to stand trial. The U.S. criminal justice system requires that in order to stand trial on criminal charges, an individual must be competent to assist in his/her own defense. When a judge has reason to believe that a criminal defendant may, because of mental illness or developmental disability, be unable to assist a defense attorney, state laws typically require the judge to order that the defendant undergo a psychiatric examination.

When a competency exam is ordered, the case is delayed while the defendant is evaluated. If the defendant is found competent, the case will proceed as usual. Where a defendant is found not competent, the consequences vary. In some cases, the charges may be dismissed and the defendant hospitalized; in others, the defendant will be hospitalized and medicated in an effort to restore competency so that the case may proceed in the future. Standards for competency are often very narrow and most people are found competent; a person may be floridly psychotic, yet still legally "competent."

The other legal mechanism available to mentally ill defendants is the not guilty by reason of insanity defense (often referred to as an NGRI defense). This defense asks a judge or jury to find that although the defendant did commit a criminal act, at the time of the offense, he/she, because of mental illness, could not appreciate the nature and consequences of the criminal conduct or could not appreciate that the conduct was wrong.[3] Some states have also adopted a Model Penal Code provision that provides that a defendant can also be found not guilty if he/she, although able to appreciate the wrongness of criminal conduct, nevertheless lacks "substantial capacity to conform his conduct to the requirements of the law."[4]

NGRI defenses are used fairly infrequently because they are expensive and generally require a defendant to take the substantial risk of going to trial with little chance of avoiding conviction. NGRI defenses often fail, even in cases where it is very clear that the defendant was psychotic at the time of the offense. For example, Andrew Goldstein, a schizophrenic man who pushed a woman off a New York City subway platform, was recently convicted and sentenced to 25 years to life in prison after unsuccessfully arguing that he was not guilty by reason of insanity. One explanation for why people like Mr. Goldstein are not successful in asserting NGRI defenses may be lack of understanding on the part of a jury about what the consequences of an NGRI verdict will be. Unless a judge specifically instructs a jury otherwise, jurors often believe that a defendant found not guilty by reason of insanity will either be released immediately, or will be released after a short hospitalization. The truth, in most states, is the absolute opposite; defendants found not guilty by reason of insanity are typically sent to forensic psychiatric hospitals for many years, sometimes for much longer than they would have spent in prison had they been found guilty.

In addition to the fact that the NGRI defenses often fail, there are a number of other reasons that they are used infrequently. A trial on an NGRI defense typically requires both the prosecution and the defense to have expert witnesses—at prohibitive cost. A defendant may prefer a finite prison sentence to a hospitalization that may last much longer. Or the defendant may simply prefer the experience of being in prison to that of being in a hospital. Finally, some defendants with serious mental illness refuse to permit their defense attorneys to use an NGRI defense because they do not believe they suffer from a mental illness.[5]

Neither the competency evaluation nor the NGRI defense comes close to addressing the needs of criminal defendants with mental illness. Both standards ("not competent" to proceed and "not responsible") are very narrow; the majority of criminal defendants with mental illness are found to be organized and coherent enough to understand the proceeding against them and are, under NGRI standards, legally responsible for their actions. Thousands of these "competent" and "responsible" defendants are seriously mentally ill, however, and should be dealt with differently in ways that address their mental health needs.

The Door Keeps Revolving

Police, courts, jails, and prisons are not adequately prepared to deal with a woman who stands in traffic yelling at voices she hears in her head, or a man who stalks a celebrity thinking she is his wife. Police are more likely to arrest people with mental illness than the non-mentally ill.[6] Once arrested, people with mental illness are incarcerated longer and have less access to alternative to incarceration programs than non-mentally ill offenders.[7] As a result, even people with mental illness charged with minor misdemeanors can end up spending significant time in jail. For example, I recently spoke to a schizophrenic homeless man who is facing a year in jail for jumping over a subway turnstile.

While incarcerated, people with mental illness receive limited psychiatric care or none at all. Psychiatric services in many U.S. jails and prisons are shockingly under-funded and poorly-run; even in "better" jails and prisons, they rarely approach the quality of good community care.[8]

During incarceration, any psychiatric treatment inmates receive in the community is disrupted. When inmates with mental illness are released from jail or prison, they often do not receive any discharge planning.[9] People with serious mental illness therefore leave correctional facilities without any supply of the medication they have been taking. They are also generally not referred to mental health services or assisted in obtaining benefits or housing. The result? They swiftly find themselves in trouble with the law and once again find themselves back in jail. This is the cycle that has criminalized many people with mental illness and made jails and prisons America's new psychiatric institutions.

What Happens to Mental Health Consumers in Jail and Prison?

The vast majority of people in the criminal justice system are not dangerous and are not incarcerated for long. With increasing punishment of "quality-of-life" crimes, more people with mental illness than ever, particularly the homeless mentally ill, are charged with misdemeanors.[10] They spend days, weeks or perhaps months in jail,[11] then return to the community where they will need help reintegrating into society, remaining psychiatrically stable and staying out of trouble. People with mental illness sentenced to prison terms (a year or more) are not gone forever either. The majority of people sent to state prisons have committed a nonviolent offense and will be released eventually; the longer they have been incarcerated the more difficulty they are likely to face reintegrating into the community.

Things do not go well for people with mental illness behind the walls of jails and prisons. By the time most people with mental illness leave the criminal justice system, the problems they came in with have only gotten worse.

Victimization

People with mental illnesses have difficulty protecting themselves while incarcerated. Jails and prisons are harsh, dangerous environments for inmates, and are especially so for inmates with mental illness Common symptoms of mental illness can include bizarre and disorganized behavior which make psychiatrically disabled prisoners vulnerable. Bizarre behavior often annoys correction staff and other inmates and leads to victimization. Disorganization makes prisoners with mental illness easy prey for aggressive fellow prisoners and makes it difficult for prisoners with mental illness to follow the many rules or a jail or prison. Finally, untreated mental illness may make inmates' behavior erratic, alarming others and provoking violent responses from guards and other inmates.

Institutionalization

Like all prisoners, inmates with mental illness learn institutional behaviors that help them cope with incarceration but complicate their successful transition back to the community. Some of these behaviors may include aggressiveness and intimidation of others or, conversely, extreme passivity, manipulative behavior and reluctance to discuss problems with (or "rat" to) authority figures.[12] These behaviors create barriers to engagement in mental health services and treatment. Former prisoners may also associate the structure of mental health treatment facilities, such as hospitals and supportive residences, with prison, and behave accordingly toward staff and fellow patients. Mental health professionals working with ex-prisoners need to understand the genesis of these behaviors and respond in a way that builds trust rather than being punitive.

Segregation

Inmates with mental illness may be punished for disruptive behavior in ways that exacerbate their illnesses. The standard punishment for disobeying prison or jail rules is "punitive segregation"—locking inmates in small single (or occasionally double) cells for 23 or 24 hours a day. Better known as solitary confinement, this punishment prevents contact with the general population, prohibits participation in programs or prison work, and often denies the inmate access to reading materials or hygiene products. A person with mental illness who has not violated rules, but whose presence in the general population is deemed by correction officials to be disruptive, may be placed in administrative segregation. Despite the kinder-sounding name, administrative segregation is just as isolating as punitive segregation and often as restrictive in terms of movement and privileges. It is not uncommon for prisoners to spend years at a time in punitive or administrative segregation.

People with mental illness are particularly likely to find themselves in punitive or administrative segregation due to behavior that is symptomatic of their illness.[13] For example, studies in Ohio in the early 1990s found that hundreds of inmates had been placed in disciplinary cells for no reason other than mental illness.[14] "Acting out" psychotic behavior and even suicide attempts by inmates with mental illness are sometimes treated as discipline problems; an inmate in a California prison received a disciplinary write-up for committing suicide—several days after his death![15]

The conditions in punitive and administrative segregation create great psychological stress and can cause symptoms of mental illness to appear even in inmates with no prior psychiatric problems. Segregated inmates are also at risk for suicide. A recent study examined 9 suicides that occurred within 24 months at a large metropolitan jail. The author found that of the nine suicides, eight were segregated from the general population of the jail at the time of their death.[16]

The dangers of segregation have been recognized by courts in many prisoners' rights cases. For example, in 1995 a federal court held that, "Social science and clinical literature have consistently reported that when human beings are subjected to social isolation and reduced environmental stimulation, they may deteriorate mentally and in some cases develop psychiatric disturbances."[17] Another federal court, presented with allegations regarding the misuse of administrative segregation in New York State prisons, held that, "A conclusion . . . that prolonged isolation from social and environmental stimulation increases the risk of developing mental illness does not strike this Court as rocket science."[18]

Psychiatric care in punitive and administrative segregated units is often especially bad. Even though mental health counselors may make rounds in segregation units, actual contact with individual prisoners, in the form of conversation or counseling, is infrequent. The cumulative effect of isolation, reduced supportive services and sensory deprivation will often leave the inmate with mental illness functioning at a lower level than before incarceration.

Stigma

People with mental illness who are or have been incarcerated are perhaps the most marginalized people in our country. They suffer the stigma and consequences of both mental illness and criminality; they are predominantly poor and of color, and they are often battling substance use and additional problems including homelessness and illnesses such as tuberculosis and AIDS. They are cut off from mental health services available to non-offenders, and their psychiatric problems isolate them from advocates for "normal" defendants and prisoners. Finally, when people with mental illness leave jail or prison, they often find that community mental health programs are reluctant to work with them because they have become "criminals."

How to Advocate for a Client in the Criminal Justice System

No one needs an advocate more than a mental health consumer involved in the criminal justice system, and the most powerful and effective advocates for these individuals are very often community mental health workers. You have the power to affect how the criminal justice system deals with your client, but you need to be prepared for it to be an experience that is frustrating, confusing, even Kafkaesque. You may encounter mental health workers who don't appear to care about helping people, defense attorneys who think treatment is worse than jail, judges who speak with great authority about things they know nothing about, prosecutors who will only consider treatment programs that don't exist (locked ones!), and a court system that regards your client as a docket number, not a person.

When a client of yours is arrested, chances are that you have an opinion about what should happen with the case. Don't let the fact that the court is intimidating and lawyers are not always friendly prevent you from being heard. Remember, chances are that no one making decisions about the case—neither the police, the judge, the prosecutor, nor even the defense attorney—is ever going to know the defendant as well as you probably do. The police make split-second decisions based on fragments of information. The judge and prosecutor will never speak to the defendant at all, and the defense attorney, unless he/she is being paid a great deal, will probably speak with the defendant for about 15 minutes every time there's a court date. If you are a social worker from a community treatment provider who knows the defendant well, then you have information that could be crucial in determining the outcome of the case.

There are three key challenges facing a social worker advocating for a client who has become involved in the criminal justice system. One, can you get the person out of the system entirely? Two, how will you make sure the person gets appropriate psychiatric treatment and is safe while incarcerated? And three, what can you do to try to affect the disposition of the case in a way that will get the client treatment rather than simply a jail or prison sentence?

Prior to Arrest—Trying to Stop the Arrest

First, don't assume that there's nothing you can do to prevent an arrest. Police in most jurisdictions have broad discretion in deciding who to arrest, who to hospitalize, and who to ignore. I have seen cases where people who have committed what could be viewed as very serious crimes (even attempted murder) have been hospitalized and never charged. If someone you care about is in a situation where he/she could be arrested, and you are fortunate enough to be there, ask the police not to arrest the person. Be assertive without making the police feel that you do not respect their authority. Say something like, "I know he shouldn't have done that, but he just needs to get his medication. I'll come with him—can you drive us to the hospital?"

Even after an arrest has occurred, you may be able to get the person in effect "un-arrested." Find out where the person is being held and go there. Talk to the police and ask if they can drop the charges or, if not, at least let the person out to come back to court later. Offer to take as much responsibility for the person as you feel comfortable doing.

After Arrest—Getting Someone Psychiatric Treatment in Jail

When a person you care about who has a mental illness has been taken into police or corrections custody, you have a real crisis on your hands. Your first priority will almost certainly be trying to make sure that the person is safe and gets appropriate treatment while in custody. Not only is it important that the person have continuity of care at this stressful time, but the person's very life may be in danger—most people who commit suicide in jail do it in the first couple of days in custody.

The good news is that most or at least many jails have mental health services. The bad news is that it may be difficult to get in touch with jail mental health staff, especially in big cities. Jail mental health staff may resist talking to you because of concerns about confidentiality. If this happens, be firm. Say something like, "Look, I'm not asking you for any information right now. I'm calling to give you some information. My client was arrested last night and he is in your jail. He has a mental illness. His diagnosis is schizophrenia and he should be getting 10 milligrams of Zyprexa and one milligram of Cogentin twice a day. He has a history of suicide attempts and you need to put him on suicide watch right away. When you speak to him, please ask him to sign a release so that you can speak to me about his condition. I will call you back tomorrow morning."

Take the name and number of the person you spoke with and call back when you said you would. Follow up regularly. Find a way to balance respecting the fact that the people who work in jail mental health services have too much to do and too few resources with letting them know that you're involved and you're not going away.

After Arrest—Influencing What Happens with the Criminal Charges

There is a cliché that is heard many times in law school—it says there are two things you don't want to watch being made, one is sausage and the other is law. The courts where criminal cases are heard can seem very much like an assembly line where defendants go by on a conveyor belt. The highest priority is speed, not the rights and needs of the individual, and no one really gets their "day in court." As an advocate for someone in this position, your job is to stop the conveyor belt, to say to the court, "Hold everything, this is not an object on an assembly line. This is a human being with special needs and you'd better pay attention."

But how do you do this? Clearly you can't just march into court and scream "Stop!" (though you will earn my eternal admiration if you do!). And even if you have a good understanding of how the system works and when and where the appropriate points of intervention exist, courts, lawyers, and particularly judges can be intimidating. You're not imagining it. I often think that the main thing I learned in law school was how to use big words that no one else can understand, so that I and all the other lawyers can preserve our mystique, prevent nonlawyers from understanding legal issues, and protect the financial well-being of our profession.

Social Workers and Lawyers

In advocating for a client of yours who is in the criminal justice system, you will encounter lawyers. It is therefore worth spending a moment talking about the relationship between lawyers and social workers. Lawyers often have little respect for anyone who is not a lawyer (except for doctors, their natural enemy), and in many lawyers' view, social workers are pretty low on the food chain. Law school teaches arrogance and reinforces a sense of privilege that many people brought with them to law school. At my school, the law school graduation was at Carnegie Hall and the social work graduation was in the university gymnasium. Even some lawyers who work in organizations that also have social workers on staff, for example many public defender and prosecutor's offices, may not understand what social workers do and may choose not to collaborate with social workers. There is no excuse for this behavior, but if you want to be an effective advocate for your client, you need to be prepared for it and cool-headed about dealing with it.

Why Do You Need to Talk With Your Client's Defense Attorney?

There are two reasons that you need to talk to the defense attorney. The first reason does not necessarily have to do with advocacy—it is simply that the defense attorney has information you may want. The defense attorney is the only person in the criminal justice system who has direct contact with your client. The defense attorney will know the client's version of the "crime" and will have a sense, as soon as he/she meets the client for the first time, of what is likely to happen with the case. The defense attorney gets information from the prosecutor about what the police and/or the complainant in the case say happened, as well as any statement the client may have made to the police. The defense attorney will also know what the client wants to do, such as planning to plead guilty or go to trial, and whether the client is interested in trying to get a disposition that includes mental health and/or drug treatment. If you need information about what is going on with your client's case, the defense attorney is your best source of information.

The second reason to talk to the defense attorney is that you may have information the attorney needs, and you may be able to work with the attorney to help your client. The defense attorney probably does not know very much about the client's psychiatric problems and history. Most defense attorneys have no specialized training in mental health; they may neglect to ask the client about mental health issues and may miss even obvious clues that the client has a mental illness. Even if the client tells the lawyer that s/he has a mental illness and takes medications and is in a program, it may not occur to the lawyer to talk to the program about these issues. By contacting the lawyer, you educate him/her about the client's mental health problems and what supports are available to the client in the community to help her/him stay out of trouble in the future.

You generally cannot talk to the judge on your own initiative. S/he will never return your phone calls, and while you may have the opportunity to address the judge in person on a court date, you should do so only with the defense attorney's approval and assurance that what you plan to say will be helpful to your client.

Similarly, do not talk to the prosecutor without the defense attorney's blessing. Information that you think will help your client may actually be harmful in the hands of a prosecutor. Even the simple disclosure that an individual has a mental illness may lead the prosecutor to fight harder to keep the person in jail. If you disclose harmful information about your client to a defense attorney, that attorney is bound by professional ethics to never disclose that information. A prosecutor, on the other hand, is charged with protecting public safety and if you give a prosecutor any information that can be used to harm your client, it probably will be used to do so. Even if you find the defense attorney challenging to deal with, you must remember that the defense attorney is the only person in the criminal justice system whose job it is to look out for the needs and rights of the defendant.

If the Defense Attorney and I Have the Same Client, Why Isn't S/he More Helpful?

Where do you start when you advocate for someone who is charged with a crime? You must start with the person's defense attorney. Sadly, nearly every time I speak to social workers about advocating for mentally ill criminal defendants, I hear bitter complaints about defense attorneys, particularly public defenders—stories of unreturned phone calls, abrupt conversations, or just plain refusals by attorneys to speak with their clients' social workers. Why is this? The answer is that while some attorneys may just be rude, the problem is usually one of resources, money, and caseloads—and, often, different views of the client's "best interest."

"You have a right to an attorney. If you cannot afford one, one will be appointed for you . . ."

The U.S. Constitution provides that every person charged with a crime has a right to an attorney, whether or not the defendant has money to hire one. Unfortunately, the right to an attorney does not seem to include the right to an attorney who actually has the time to do a thorough job on every case or the breathing room to return phone calls. Public defenders may be representing 60 or 70 or 150 clients at one time. These caseloads are not their choice, but rather are a function of how much money states and localities are willing (or not willing) to pay to provide lawyers for people accused of being criminals. With that many cases, a defense attorney likely has a hard time remembering many clients' faces and names—your job is to convince the defense attorney that this is a special case.

Many public defenders chose their jobs for some of the same reasons that inspired you to go to social work school—the desire to help people in trouble, concern about the rights of disenfranchised people. Other lawyers representing poor criminal defendants may have a struggling tax law practice and have decided to supplement it by picking up a few criminal cases. In some jurisdictions, attorneys are even assigned against their will to represent indigent criminal defendants according to a rotating schedule. Understanding which type of defense attorney your client has, for example a public defender versus an attorney who only does criminal defense occasionally or part of the time, can help you assess whether your client is getting competent representation. One thing virtually all defense attorneys representing poor criminal defendants share, however, is that they have far too many cases and too few resources to devote a great deal of time to ta single case.

A free lawyer is better than a cheap one

Knowing all of this, you might assume that anyone who can possibly come up with the money to hire a lawyer should do so. This is not necessarily the case, however. People who are wealthy enough to spend a substantial amount of money on a defense attorney should do so—and will probably be required by the court to hire their own lawyer. But people who have limited funds and who can meet the criteria to get a court-appointed lawyer should be extremely cautious about selling the car or mortgaging the house to hire a lawyer instead.

Why? Because, in general, a free lawyer is better than a cheap one. A lawyer who takes a case for a low fee has to take a lot of cases to earn a living—and thus can't devote much time to any one case. A cheap lawyer may also be cheap because s/he is not a very good lawyer. Or he/she may practice tax or real estate law most of the time and just pick up a criminal case once in awhile. Someone who is a great real estate lawyer is, almost by definition, not likely to be a great criminal defense attorney. Inexpensive lawyers often have no support staff—not even a secretary or paralegal, let alone a social worker. In fact, I've encountered lawyers in private practice doing criminal defense who do not have fax machines or answering machines, and offices where when you call, you can hear a television in the background and you know the lawyer is working out of his/her living room.

Finally, there is virtually no oversight of lawyers in private practice. If you are dealing with a lawyer working in a public defender agency and you are very dissatisfied with the lawyer's work or cannot ever get in touch with the lawyer, you can speak to the lawyer's supervisor. Lawyers in private practice have no supervisor.

What is the client's best interest? (Or, lawyers are from Mars,
social workers are from Venus)

Sometimes social workers and lawyers seem to speak languages so different that they cannot communicate at all. I have seen this arise most often when discussing the best interests of a client who has a social worker, has mental health and/or substance abuse treatment needs, but is also facing criminal charges.

Imagine that you have been working as an outreach worker and have been trying for several months to engage a particularly hard-to-reach client. The client is a man with paranoid schizophrenia who is living on the streets, refusing psychiatric treatment and shelter, and using crack cocaine and alcohol every day. Your efforts to engage the client seem to be going nowhere and you are concerned that his lifestyle places him at great risk. One day you receive a phone call from the court because the client has been arrested and has shown your card as a contact person. You rush down to the courthouse and find the defense attorney who has been assigned to represent your client.

The defense attorney tells you that the client has been arrested for possession of crack cocaine. Because the client had only four bags of crack, the offense is a misdemeanor, punishable by up to a year in jail.[19] You feel suddenly inspired; while of course you don't view it as a good thing that you client has been arrested, you wonder whether this might not provide the opportunity you've been looking for to break through the client's resistance and help him get off the street and into treatment. You start outlining for the attorney the treatment plan you would propose for the client—an 18-month residential MICA program, assistance obtaining benefits, day treatment, medical care—in the hope that, with your assistance, the defense attorney can suggest to the prosecutor and judge that rather than being sentenced to a year in jail, the client should be mandated to comply with this treatment plan.

The lawyer interrupts you. "This is a bullshit case," he says. "And the guy's only got a couple misdemeanor and no felony priors. I know this A.D.A.; she'll give me two weeks jail time on this case and I'm gonna have the guy take it." With that, the lawyer walks away to deal with some other cases. A few minutes later, your client's case is called, the client pleads guilty to criminal possession of a controlled substance, and he is sentenced to two weeks in jail. Two weeks later, when you go out to do outreach, you see him back on his usual corner with a bottle of malt liquor.

What just happened? Well, what just happened was that you and the defense attorney had different views of what was in the client's best interest—and the defense attorney's view trumped yours. Defense attorneys have an obligation to look out for the legal best interest of their clients, while social workers are concerned about a more holistic view of what is in a client's best long-term interest. Defense attorneys are also less likely than social workers to substitute their own judgement for the client's—in fact, they are ethically prohibited from doing so. Often these two perspectives are irreconcilable, particularly when a defense attorney has an opportunity to get a client out of the system quickly and a social worker would rather use the opportunity to get the person into treatment. A few defense attorneys do not see getting a client into treatment as being part of their job under any circumstances; most are happy to consider their clients' treatment needs, but only when the treatment intervention is proportionate to the sentence that would otherwise be imposed. For example, if a month later the same client is arrested for selling crack cocaine, and is facing a minimum of two years in prison, the same defense attorney may be begging you to come to court and advocate for the client to go to an 18-month MICA program instead—because this time the client is in a lot more trouble, so 18 months of treatment seems proportionate.

This system can be maddening to a social worker because of course there is often no relationship between how much trouble the client is in and how badly he/she needs treatment. Social workers may be frustrated by a sense that the client will have to commit a serious offense before the criminal justice system will ever do anything to help the individual. A social worker may also feel that it is only through criminal justice intervention that a particularly resistant client will ever become engaged in treatment— and wish the system was more intrusive about mandating treatment.

While these perspectives are certainly valid, it's worth stepping back for a moment and remembering what a toxic place the criminal justice system is and how destructive being in that system is to people's physical and emotional well-being. It is because that system is so destructive that defense attorneys fight so hard to minimize the contact their clients have with the system. While it's clearly a mark of progress that courts have become more amenable to sending offenders to treatment as a disposition in a criminal case, the cost of obtaining treatment through the courts can be very high.

For example, the client described above may have a choice of taking a sentence of two weeks in jail, or being mandated to an 18-month MICA program. But if, three weeks into the program, the client leaves the program and goes back to the streets, he will very likely be sentenced to more than two weeks in jail—perhaps the full year—as punishment for having been "given a chance" and failed. Faced with those options, any competent defense attorney would advise the client to take the two-week sentence. Even if the client desperately wanted treatment, the defense attorney would have to advise the client to do the two weeks in jail and then seek treatment voluntarily after release—when the consequence of failure in treatment will not be so high.

Can We Stop the Criminalization of Mental Illness?

People with mental illness do not belong in jail and prison. Sending them there wastes money, wastes lives, lets the government off the hook for its broken promise of deinstitutionalization, and perpetuates the ridiculous notion that the best response to every social problem is to incarcerate people. Many of the "crimes" that mental health consumers end up in jail for today would be viewed as symptoms if we had enough residential and hospital treatment beds.

In the last year or two, the issue of people with mental illness in the criminal justice system has become a hot topic—witness the Geraldo Rivera show and lots of other tabloid television on the issue, several excellent *New York Times* articles, a multitude of conferences, and the recent Department of Justice report. But those of us who care about mental health issues—consumers, families, friends, treatment providers and advocates—should not assume that being in the spotlight will fix the problem.

The criminalization of mental illness is just one symptom of much broader problems with crumbling mental health systems across the country, but it may be the most tragic symptom. We must make federal, state and local officials realize what they have done by incarcerating hundreds of thousands of mental health consumers. Everyone who cares about mental health must work together to stop criminalization and demand a real community mental health system, regardless of whether someone you care about has been arrested—yet.

Notes

1. See generally Torrey, E.F., Steiber, J.E., Zekiel, J., Wolfe, S.M., Sharfstein, J., Noble, J.H., & Flynn, L.M. (1992). *Criminalizing the Seriously Mentally Ill: The Abuse of Jails as Mental Hospitals.* Washington, DC: Public Citizen's Health Research..

2. For example, in New York State, prior to deinstitutionalization, our state psychiatric hospitals housed over 90,000 on any given day. Today the census is 6,000 state-wide. Within a few years, this number will sink to 4,500.

3. For an example of this type of law, see New York State Penal Law §40.15.

4. ALI, Model Penal Code and Commentaries (Official Draft and Revised Comments), §4.01, Comment, p. 168 (1985).

5. For example, many people will recall the case of Colin Ferguson, the man who killed a number of people in a shootout on the Long Island Rail Road. Mr. Ferguson fired his defense attorneys because they wished to pursue a not guilty by reason of insanity defense. He then went to trial representing himself and was convicted of murder.

6. Teplin, L.A. (1984). Criminalizing Mental Disorder: The Comparative Arrest Rate of the Mentally Ill. *American Psychologist, 39*(7), 794–803.

7. Rock, M.A. & Landsberg, G. (1996). County Mental Health Directors'

Perspectives on Forensic Mental Health Developments in New York State. *Admin. and Pol'y in Mental Health,* 25(2), 327–332.

According to the New York City Health and Hospitals Corporation, the average length of stay in the New York City jail system for mentally ill inmates is 215 days, compared with a 42 day average stay for all inmates. Butterfield, supra note 8.

8. For more on the problems with U.S. correctional mental health services, see Amnesty International's excellent 1999 report on the U.S., "Rights for all." Available at www.amnesty.org.

9. Failure to provide discharge planning to jail inmates with mental illness is the subject of a major class action lawsuit currently pending against New York City. The lawsuit, Brad H. v City of NY, challenges New York's practice of dropping seriously mentally ill jail inmates off in the middle of the night in a high crime neighborhood with $1.50 and two subway fares and no medicationor assistance obtaining treatment benefits or housing. In July 2000, the judge ordered the city to begin providing discharge planning. The plaintiff class is represented by my agency, the Urban Justice Center, as well as the law firm of Debecoise and plimpton abd New York Lawyers for the Public Interest.

10. For example, a 1996 study in Austin, Texas, found that 63% of public order offenses involved alcohol or substance abuse, a third of public order arrests were of repeat offenders, and two thirds of repeat offenders were homeless. "Clearly, those who have no permanent residence and those suffering from addiction are particularly prone to commit these crimes, and to circulate in and out of the municipal justice system," the report concluded. Patricia G. Barnes, *Safer Streets at What Cost?* 84 A.B.A.J. 25 (1998) *quoting* BROKEN WINDOWS & BROKEN LIVES: ADDRESSING PUBLIC ORDER OFFENDING IN AUSTIN (Center for Criminology and Criminal Justice Research at the University of Texas at Austin).

11. For example, the average length of stay in New York City jails is 46 days for detainees and 37 days for sentenced inmates. City of New York, Mayor's Management Report: Preliminary Fiscal 1998 (Vol. II) 15.

12 SPECTRM Training, Bronx Psychiatric Center (March 5, 1998). SPECTRM is a treatment and risk management program designed for work with mentally ill ex-offenders.

13. Rold, W.J. (1992). Consideration of Mental Health Factors in Inmate Discipline. J. of Prison & Jail Health 11(41), 43-44.

14. Bill Sloat, Mentally Ill Inmates Sealed Off from *Care, Plain Dealer,* Sept. 9, 1994, at 1A.

15. Bill Wallace, Suicidal Inmates Often Ignored— Until Too Late, *San Francisco Chronicle,* Oct. 4, 1994, at A1.

16. Hayes, L.M. (1997). From Chaos to Calm: One Jail System's Struggle with Suicide Prevention. *Behavioral Sciences and the Law* 15(4), 399–414.

17. *Madrid v. Gomez,* 889 F. Supp. 1146, 1230 (N.D. Cal. 1995).

18. *McClary v. Kelly,* No. 90-CV-0501A, slip op. at 14 (W.D.N.Y. Apr. 30, 1998).

19. This is just an example. Laws governing what is a criminal offense and how serious the consequences are for different offenses vary widely from state to state and even from one part of a city to another. For example, the case described above might turn out very differently in Queens than in Brooklyn.

20

Observations of A Criminal Defense Attorney

Mary Elizabeth Anderson

Mentally ill clients present particular challenges for attorneys, and especial ones for criminal defense attorneys. The role of any attorney is, of course, to advocate for her client, zealously, within the bounds of the law.[1] The lawyer must assist the client to understand the charges and the court proceedings; to advise the client as to whether it is advisable to go to trial or to work out a plea and, if a plea is to be entered, to ensure the best possible terms with respect to the sentence. Above all, criminal defense attorneys understand their role to be one of attempting to gain dismissal of the charges or, if this is not feasible, seeing that their clients serve as little time as possible incarcerated.

Persons with mental illness are unlike other criminal defendants in many ways. Many of them are unable to assist their attorneys or to make the decisions that other clients make with ease: They are unable, or unwilling, to tell you where and/or with whom they live; they often want to follow courses of action that are not in their best interests. Such clients may be unaware of where they are or why they have been arrested. They may want to go to trial for reasons that do not comport with reality. For instance, a client charged with stalking may insist on taking a losing case to trial in order to see the complaining witness one more time so as to give the witness another opportunity to see how the accused loves her. Or a client may insist that he needs to go to trial to prove the existence of a conspiracy against him wherein the complainant originally gained power over the accused by placing germs inside of the accused's shoes which bored their way through the soles of the accused's feet, thus enslaving him and making him part of the masses controlled by the government-sponsored cabal.

Mentally ill clients may insist that the judge grant them relief that makes no sense whatsoever—a client who asserts that he will plead guilty to breaking a window at the hospital emergency room only if the judge will order the hospital to remove the computer chip the hospital previously implanted in the client's brain. (The prosecutor's recommendation had been for the client to receive a sentence of "time served.") Mentally ill offenders often see themselves as victims and insist that the complainants be brought to trial or ask the court to call as witnesses persons who have no connection to the case.

For these above illuminated and diverse other reasons, many defense lawyers find representing the mentally ill an uncomfortable obligation. Some attorneys prefer to avoid such representations altogether. Other attorneys enjoy working with the mentally ill, but find aspects of the representation quite frustrating.

Most of the seriously mentally ill persons who are arrested for crimes are indigent. Many of them live on the street; others live in shelters or in rooming houses; a smaller number live in mental health residences or with relatives; a very few have their own apartments or houses. Most of them have no incomes or are supported by Supplemental Security Income, Social Security Disability, or other government assistance. Thus, due to their poverty, most mentally ill offenders are represented by public defenders or other court-appointed counsel.

Public defenders are, by and large, extremely competent practitioners who are zealously committed to advocating for poor people charged with crimes. For the better part of my years as a lawyer, I have worked alongside some of the most talented criminal defense attorneys in a public defender's office in New York City. My colleagues at the Legal Aid Society are creative, dedicated, and, as are public defenders in most jurisdictions, overburdened with cases and institutional assignments.

Many public defenders find representing the mentally ill particularly challenging, as such clients generally require a larger time commitment than other clients (and can try an attorney's patience as well). Often, it takes longer to communicate with a mentally ill person, and sometimes communication can be impossible altogether. If a client has relatives or other persons concerned with his welfare, the attorney can spend hours talking to these people. Also, mentally ill clients rarely tend to have triable cases, being "caught in the act" more often than other clients. Working out pleas for mentally ill people can take much longer than for a client who does not suffer from such illness, particularly if the prosecutor knows about the client's psychiatric condition.

To resolve the mentally ill client's legal situation, the attorney must act as she would with any other client. She must "advise [the] client fully on whether a particular plea to a charge appears to be desirable" (EC 7–7);[2] she must provide her client with sufficient information to make this decision. *See, e.g.,* MR 1.4; EC 7–7. If the client chooses to go to trial, the attorney must inform the client about the trial process and whether it is advisable to waive a jury, if the client is otherwise entitled to a jury trial. The attorney must also advise the client whether or not the client should testify in his own behalf. *See* ABA Standards Relating to the Administration of Criminal Justice, the Defense Function, Standard 4–5; MR 1.2; EC 7–7 and 7–8.

Naturally, for a mentally ill client to make these decisions, the client must be competent, or fit. Competence can vary, depending upon the charges and the complexity of the proceedings. At a bare minimum, a criminal defendant must have "sufficient present ability to consult with his lawyer with a reasonable degree of rational understanding . . . and . . . a rational as well as factual understanding of the proceedings against him" (*Dusky v. United States*, 362 U.S. 402 [1960]).

All states have procedures whereby the competence of a defendant can be ascertained. The question of competence is nonadversarial; the primary concern is the accused's mental state. The issue can be raised by the judge, the prosecutor, the defense attorney, or the accused himself.[3] Once the question is raised, some states make a competency evaluation by qualified psychiatric examiners mandatory. *See, e.g.*, N.Y. Crim. Proc. Law, Sec. 730.30(1). The fitness issue is one which cannot be waived; thus it can be raised on appeal, even if it was not raised at any earlier stage of the proceedings. The principle is simple: All accused persons have the right to understand the crimes with which they have been charged and the nature of the attendant proceedings; they must be able to assist their assigned attorneys in determining the course of action to take. No accused person can give up this essential right (*Pate v. Robinson*, 383 U.S. 375 [1966]).

If a client is found unfit to proceed, the client will be hospitalized. In most, if not all, jurisdictions, minor charges will be dismissed after a finding of unfitness. Serious charges will generally be held in abeyance until the accused is restored to fitness. *See, e.g.*, N.Y. Crim. Proc. Law, Secs. 730.40, 730.50.

Most persons with psychiatric disorders can be restored to competence through the administration of appropriate psychotropic medication coupled with psychotherapy and education about the court process. While the accused is hospitalized, the state's criminal procedure law and/or mental health law will tend to govern the conditions of his hospital confinement. *See, e.g.*, N.Y. Crim. Proc. Law, Section 730.60; N.Y. Mental Hygiene Law, Article 9. If the client cannot be restored to fitness, the client's fate should be governed by the standards set forth in *Jackson v. Indiana*, 406 U.S. 715 (1972). *See also* ABA Criminal Justice Mental Health Standard 7–4.13. While the client is committed for competency evaluations or hospitalized for restoration to fitness, he should earn credit for the time committed or hospitalized, and such time should be applied against any sentence ultimately imposed. *Id.*, Standard 7–4.15.

Often criminal defense attorneys can ignore their clients' psychiatric problems. Ignoring a client's mental illness is not callous; rather, the client's legal problems generally can be resolved without an attorney's dwelling on the client's psychiatric difficulties. And the defense attorney's job is, after all, to resolve the client's *legal* problems.

Moreover, attorneys are not trained to recognize psychiatric conditions. For this reason, unless an attorney knows from other experience how to recognize mental illness, she will usually fail to recognize mental illness in all but the most obviously depressed or psychotic clients. Even with the most extremely ill clients, if a defense lawyer can assist the client to resolve the client's case without focusing on the client's mental state, the defense lawyer should follow this course of action.

Since beginning my career as a public defender in 1990, I have been drawn to clients with mental illness. One of my first difficult assignments was to handle a case for a schizophrenic client who had been charged with trespassing in an area enclosed to exclude the public. The crime with which this client was charged carried a maximum sentence of ninety days. At the client's arraignment, the judge had ordered a competency examination; the client, after being examined by doctors, had been found unfit to deal with his case, due to his mental illness. And yet, as is often the case, the doctors who had conducted the examination had also directed the corrections health service to offer the client antipsychotic medication. When I met the client for the first time, handling the calendar call in the court part dealing with the fitness issue, the client had been incarcerated for over thirty days and had been receiving medication for almost two-thirds of that time. The client now wanted to plead guilty; I knew that the sitting judge would give a sentence of "time served" for the offense with which the client was charged. Yet the doctors' examination and concomitant findings mandated that the client be transferred from jail to a state psychiatric center. Such transfer takes, in New York City, an average of ten working days. How could I let this client, who appeared to me to be mentally ill but able enough to enter a guilty plea, remain incarcerated any longer?

I was a lawyer with less than three months' experience. To keep such a client in jail, for even a day longer, was anathema to me. I contacted our mental health specialist and asked him if it was permissible for me to argue to the judge that I had spent a half hour or so talking with the client and that, in my opinion, he appeared to be mentally sound and able to plead guilty to the minor charge he faced. My argument was based on this principle: In court, most opinions are inadmissible, unless they are opinions of qualified experts. One of the few subjects upon which ordinary witnesses can render an opinion is sanity. I reasoned that perhaps I could both advocate and "witness" for this client. My specialist agreed, and that's what I did. And the judge agreed with my argument and allowed the client to plead guilty. And I walked the client out of the court room, wished him well, and gave him a subway token and a couple of bucks.

Many mental health providers cringe when they hear lawyers tell about how they have walked such clients out of jail, back to the streets. Medical and social service providers know that the upshot of my having gotten the client out of jail was, more than likely, his return to the streets for another month or so, until his mental condition deteriorated and he committed another crime, only to end up back in the jail system again. But, as a young lawyer, I proudly walked this man out of jail, and I've done similar things for other mentally ill clients time and time again.

I don't lose sleep over this aspect of my job. Mentally ill prisoners are not treated well, and thus I believe the streets to be preferable to jail for a mentally ill client and, usually, preferable to hospitalization in a state psychiatric hospital. Clients who are transferred from jails or prisons to state psychiatric centers have more difficulty gaining release to community-based mental health services than those who are admitted to the centers from civil hospitals. (At least, this is the situation in New York.)

Public defenders prize freedom. For us, there is no thrill or professional accomplishment that can equal gaining liberty for another human being. As Toni Morrison has said: "The function of freedom is to free somebody else." It is especially precious to help free an impoverished person: a person who is already marginalized as a human being due to his very inability to purchase his justice. In this American society, where everything is bought and sold, it is a marvelous thing to obtain for a fellow human being a very valuable commodity—freedom—without paying a cent for it. Indeed, many of our clients think that we public defenders are not good, or even real, lawyers, because they don't believe that anything that is free can be of good quality. We often hear clients tell us that, if they thought their case were serious, they would hire a "real lawyer"—translate that, "paid lawyer," or "private attorney."

Not so amazingly, mentally ill clients generally do not worry about whether their attorney is good or bad, a public defender or a private practitioner. This dynamic is not important to them. They do tend to want to get out of jail, but not always. And rarely do they *want* to accept mental health services, but most of them will, if offered. Mentally ill clients tend to want to just keep on with where and how they were living, whether it be in a co-operative apartment bought for them by a generous relative (or purchased by the client himself, although this is more rare), or in a hospital or mental health residence, or in a shelter or on the streets. Usually, mentally ill clients have little insight into what brought them into the criminal system in the first place.

As a public defender, I find the legal predicaments of mentally ill defendants troubling, tragic, frustrating, and, yet, sometimes, very life-enlightening—there's nothing quite like observing a psychotic client tell a psychiatrist that the client knows the psychiatrist is an atheist (and, of course, the particular psychiatrist was), or like hearing another client explain how her actions were undertaken to create a "medicine the color of water" to assist in "the unassassination of President Kennedy." (She was charged with shoplifting shampoo, placing the shampoo in a clear plastic bag which also contained various assorted coins.)

Over the years, with assistance from a mentor attorney who specializes in competency and responsibility issues, I have made it my business to seek out clients with mental illness, helping them resolve their legal problems and, sometimes, their life problems.

Often, I can tell that a client has mental illness because of notations in his criminal history sheet, for example, a dismissal on competency grounds or a discharge from state prison to the office of mental health. I can suspect mental illness with particular crimes—menacing, assault on a stranger, harassing phone calls, arson, certain sex crimes. Other attorneys ask me to assist them with the representation of clients with psychiatric problems; attorneys leaving the office ask me to assume representation of their mentally ill clients. Sometimes, a mentally ill client is returned to court from a period of hospital commitment; I will pick up the restored case. Sometimes judges, prosecutors, civil advocates, health professionals, even court clerks, have asked me to accept assignment of mentally impaired people's cases.

Currently, nearly 70% of my caseload consists of clients with some type of psychiatric malady. I work quite closely with social workers and/or doctors in trying to resolve many of these cases. My role differs from the roles of doctors and social workers for obvious reasons. The primary reason, as I have mentioned, is that my duty as a defense attorney, to each and every client, whether mentally ill or mentally sound, is to ensure that I advise the client in a way that takes into account what is in his *legal* interest. Certainly what is in a client's legal interest is often intertwined with what is in the client's medical, social, and/or emotional interest, but not always. Usually, when I take into account all of the client's interests, if I can get a client out of jail, it is in the client's legal interest.

Obviously, there are times that getting a client out of jail may not be in his medical or social interest. The client may be leaving jail for the street, where he will not receive any medication or therapy. The client may return to a use of street drugs. The client may be suicidal or assaultive. None of these things can enter into the resolution of the client's legal problems if the client's legal problems can be resolved without a consideration of the client's psychiatric problems.

Naturally, when I discern that a client suffers from mental illness, I attempt to refer the client to appropriate services. However, due to my constant caseload pressures, I am usually unable to follow clients with closed cases. When a past client takes the initiative to contact me, looking for a referral to social services, I will assist the client by procuring such a referral, but I cannot provide monitoring of the referral. To attempt to do so would cause me to neglect the representation of current clients, which would be unprofessional and potentially unethical. *See* EC 6–1, 6–3, 6–4; DR 6–101(3); MR 1.1, 1.3, 1.4. Try as I would like to be a "multiservice" provider with the ability to follow up my clients' legal, medical, and social needs, I tend to be able to do this only for clients with open cases. And this aspect of my job—not having enough time or administrative support to assist my clients in the long term, to help keep them from becoming "repeat customers" of public defense services—is one of the things about my work that keeps me awake nights.

It is especially difficult to attempt to assist a mentally ill client who ends up serving a state prison sentence. The attorney loses complete contact with such a client—the client's case ends after the attorney has made her sentencing recommendations; another client quickly takes the previous client's place; an attorney's commitments to her current clients, and her personal life, overwhelm her ability to ascertain whether court-ordered or court-recommended treatment has been provided to the state-sentenced former client.

Who ensures that a mentally ill prisoner receives psychiatric treatment? How can an inmate earn his release to parole if he is not receiving treatment? Who ensures that the inmate receives that treatment? Who encourages mentally ill prisoners who are sometimes reluctant to admit mental illness to take the psychotherapeutic medications that can help them cope with the stress of incarceration? Who assesses whether the client is noncompliant with prison regulations, and thus requires punishment or isolation from other prisoners, or whether the client is actually having a psychotic episode and thus requires hospitalization or other medical treatment? Who provides discharge planning for mentally ill prisoners? To my knowledge, no one in the New York State prison system does this terribly well.[4] I have conferred with many forensic psychiatrists and psychologists and other professionals who have experience in other states, and it seems to be a nearly universal opinion that no state prison system in this country handles mentally ill prisoners in a way that comports with minimum mental health standards of treatment.

Once a client's case is closed, it is very difficult for any lawyer to maintain consistent contact with that client. If a client's legal problems have been solved, the defense lawyer, particularly a public defender, generally has little ability to solve that client's life problems, such as drug addiction or homelessness. Unfortunately, the client often becomes a "repeat customer," going in and out of jail until he is "lucky" enough to place himself in such a precarious position that he is able to qualify for program placement.

Defense lawyers try to ensure that their clients have as few conditions placed upon them as possible. We endeavor to keep a client from being subjected to conditions of sentence or release unless the client receives some significant benefit in return, for example, a non-criminal disposition, a misdemeanor conviction instead of a felony, or a sentence of no jail in a matter where the client would ordinarily serve time. For this reason, if a drug-addicted client is charged with a minor drug possession offense, a defense lawyer sees "time served," or even a short jail sentence, as infinitely more desirable than a drug program. If the same client is charged with a felony drug crime, a sentence of several months' time can be a better deal than five years of probation with drug treatment. And if the client is mentally ill, there are even more reasons for the defense lawyer to want the client to avoid having to comply with conditions of release or sentence. It's not that defense lawyers are naturally pessimistic people; we are realists. We have seen so many failures that we are inclined to believe that nearly all clients will fail (even though the actual percentage of successes may be acceptable in the opinion of others unconnected to the system).

This bleak attitude possessed by most defenders can frustrate the social workers who intercede on behalf of our clients. However, such pessimism is the least of the conflicts we attorneys have with our social workers. More often, the conflicts between lawyers and social workers center around one of these two issues: the length of time a client spends in jail and whether a particular setting is appropriate for the client.

Social workers who are employees of a public defender enjoy an advantage of sorts that many other social workers do not. In that they are employed directly by a public defense office, they do not have the same statutory reporting obligations that most other social workers have. In other words, whereas a social worker who hears about possible child abuse or neglect ordinarily may have an obligation to report the matter, a social worker employed as a regular employee of a public defender's office almost always has no such obligation. In fact, it would be a violation of the attorney-client privilege for the public defender's social worker to make such a report.

The attorney-client privilege extension to the public defender's social worker is not always perceived as an advantage by our social workers. If a social worker feels that a mentally ill client may pose a danger to the client's children, spouse, or elderly parents, the social worker cannot report the potential peril to the court or to any reporting agency. A social worker who is employed by an independent agency would have the ability, indeed may have a mandatory duty, to report or comment upon a dangerousness issue. *See Tarasoff v. Regents of the University of California*, 17 Cal. 3d 425

(1976). On the other hand, on most occasions when a hazard presents itself, the court is well aware of the danger—usually due to the nature of the crime (often wherein the potentially identifiable victim is the complaining witness in the case). Thus, the social worker who is bound by the attorney-client privilege generally need not worry about the social worker's inability to render an opinion in such a scenario.

More complicated is the situation wherein the attorney insists on the social worker's removing certain material from a report the social worker is preparing for court. Sometimes, a social worker's overall assessment can include matters that, while relevant for the social worker's purposes, may harm the client's position with respect to the criminal charges. In such a case, the attorney is bound by codes of ethics and disciplinary rules which provide, *inter alia,* that the attorney take no action to damage or prejudice a client in the course of the professional relationship. *See, e.g.,* DR 7–101(A)(3). *Compare* MR 1.6. The attorney's obligation to protect the client may override the social worker's professional opinion that certain information be included in the report to court. In other words, when the social worker is an employee of the attorney's office, the social worker's opinion takes a backseat to the attorney's. The attorney must not, of course, take any action that would constitute a fraud upon the court (i.e., counsel or her social worker could not state to the court that a schizophrenic client does not suffer from mental illness). *See* DR 7–102; MR 3.3.

Social workers and lawyers also have conflicts centering around the length of time that clients remain incarcerated or hospitalized. Social workers do not seem to feel the same urgency to "free" a client; rather, they seem to be more concerned that the program and the client are a good fit. Locating the most appropriate program for a client increases the client's chances of successful completion. However, attorneys can grow frustrated when a social worker is more concerned about "program fit" than "program placement" and, thus, prolongs a client's incarceration.

Finding a program for an incarcerated mentally ill client can take two to three times as long as placement for a client who does not suffer from mental illness. In part, this is because many of the programs which provide services for persons with psychiatric illness are run by smaller organizations that do not have the ability to conduct interviews of people who are in jail. Also, the very fact that the client is mentally ill can cause the judge and/or the prosecutor to veto the client's placement in certain programs.

The bottom line is that the court's proposed sentence of jail will often return the client to the streets more quickly than if the attorney were to find a program or mental health residence for the client. When a client is given the choice of (1) taking a plea and going free or (2) taking a plea and remaining incarcerated pending placement in a program or other residence, the client chooses going free nearly one hundred percent of the time.

This can frustrate a social worker who has spent countless hours attempting to gain program placement for a client. An example of the problem is illustrated by this case recently handled in our office: The client was 18 years old and had no criminal record. He was charged with a misdemeanor assault; the incident occurred while the client was high on drugs and also experiencing a first or second psychotic break. The maximum sentence for the offense, due to the client's age and lack of a criminal history, was four months in jail. The first-year attorney who picked up the case made a referral to our social work department immediately after the client's arraignment. A social worker, also in her first year with our office, was assigned to the matter quickly, and she promptly began the process of residential program placement. Due to the shortage of funding for mentally ill substance abusers, and due to the dearth of programs for juveniles with major psychotic disorders, a placement could not be completed before the client had served four months in jail. At the client's next court date, some four plus months after his arraignment, the assigned attorney was unable to appear on the case; she left instructions for a colleague who would cover the case for her that day. The colleague, who was senior to the assigned attorney, listened to the client's complaints about being detained such a long period on a first arrest, reviewed the court paperwork and the corrections' commitment records, and promptly pleaded the client guilty so he could get out of jail.

The junior attorney and social worker were up in arms: How could the senior attorney have returned this mentally ill client to the street with no supportive services?

While it may seem inhumane for a person to take the actions he did, the senior attorney acted appropriately in pleading this client guilty. There was no legal advantage that could have been gained by further incarceration of the client. He had served more than his maximum sentence; he was entitled to be released from jail. The assigned attorney and social worker had no right to substitute their judgment, *parens patriae*, for the client. The client, who was competent to proceed with his case, had an absolute right to choose his course of action.

Defense attorneys need constantly be mindful that there are certain decisions that the client, and only the client, can make. We are only the client's advisor; the client—even the client who suffers from mental illness—is free to reject our advice. Some defense lawyers are tempted to substitute their judgment for that which should be exercised by a mentally ill client. Obviously, the lawyer has no right to decide, for instance, that a client with mental illness cannot testify on his behalf because it is unwise for him to testify. If the client is competent to proceed, the client with psychiatric problems is entitled to make decisions in his case in the same way as is a client who does not suffer from such problems. The attorney must resist attempts to make choices for her clients who are mentally impaired.

Deciding whether or not to reveal a client's mental illness to the court, or the prosecutor, is difficult. Sometimes there is no hiding the matter; other times the only way a client's psychiatric problems would be revealed to the court is through disclosure by the defense lawyer. (If the client is competent to proceed in the case, his attorney must secure his permission before revealing the information; if the client appears to have competency problems, the attorney often must call the issue to the court's attention, but should not reveal attorney-client privileged matters.) Sometimes a client's psychiatric problems can garner sympathy for the client's situation and secure his release, and help him to avoid a criminal conviction. Other times the information can engender fear, causing a judge to set higher bail or mete out a more onerous punishment than is otherwise warranted in such a case or causing a prosecutor to refuse to make an offer that would be made to a client without psychiatric problems.

As of my writing this, in early 2000, the climate toward persons with mental illness in New York City, and across the country I would surmise, is one of fear. There have been a number of prominent incidents in my city in the recent past—schizophrenic Andrew Goldstein's pushing Kendra Webdale in front of a subway train, causing her death; an apparently psychotic individual crushing Nicole Barrett's skull with a brick—which have created a panic. Prosecutors are afraid to give mentally ill people access to alternative-to-incarceration programs; countless prosecutors have warned me that they do not want to be responsible for another "brick man" type of incident. Judges have similar fears.

It is a difficult time to be a defense lawyer who represents clients with mental illness. It is more difficult to be a mentally ill person accused of a crime.

Notes

1. American Bar Association (ABA) Model Code of Professional Responsibility, Ethical Consideration 7–1. *See also* ABA Model Rules of Professional Conduct, preamble ("As advocate, a lawyer zealously asserts the client's position under the rules of the adversary system.") and Rule 1.1; National Legal Aid and Defender Association Performance Guidelines for Criminal Defense Representation, Guideline 1.1.

2. "EC" pertains to an ABA Code of Professional Responsibility Ethical Consideration; "DR" refers to an ABA Code of Professional Responsibility Disciplinary Rule; "MR," to the ABA Model Rules of Professional Conduct. Approximately two-thirds of the states are "Model Rules" states; most of the remain-

ing states follow the ABA Code; a few states follow neither of these two sets of professional conduct rules, but have other professional conduct rules.

3. *See* R. Roca, *Determining Decisional Capacity: A Medical Perspective*, 62 Ford. L. Rev. 1177–96 (1993)(Discussion of the various forms of incompetency). Attorneys seeking guidance on whether to bring to the court's attention a client's potential incompetence can compare EC 7–11 and 7–12 with MR 1.14. An excellent discussion of this difficult issue can be found in *Ethical Problems Facing the Criminal Defense Lawyer: Practical Answers to Tough Questions*, Uphoff, Rodney J., editor, ABA Criminal Justice Section (1995)(Chapter 3: "The Decision To Challenge the Competency of a Marginally Competent Client: Defense Counsel's Unavoidably Difficult Position"). *See also* ABA Criminal Justice Mental Health Standards 7–4.1 and 7–4.2.

4. *See* H. Barr, *Prisons and Jails: Hospitals of Law Resort*, A Joint Report of the Correctional Association of New York and the Urban Justice Center (1999).

21

Someone Had to Stop the Spinning: The Prosecutor's Role in an Unlikely Alliance Called "Mental Health Court"

Lee Cohen and Lourdes Roberts

THE *INSANE* SYSTEM—A SUPERVISOR'S PERSPECTIVE

"Lee, we've got another one of those cases." I had only been the Assistant State Attorney in Charge of the County (Misdemeanor) Division for a few weeks, supervising 30 rookie prosecutors, and that announcement from my secretary was already all too familiar. No, it did not mean that a brand new attorney had passed out during his first jury trial or that another drunk celebrity had wrecked his Porsche on A1A. No, the call had to be coming from the Public Defender's Office. And it was about an inmate. So why were they calling me, the prosecutor, the guy who should be happy that their client was apprehended for violating the law? Simple, they just wanted me to drop charges. Why? Was it because we had the wrong guy, that a grave injustice had occurred, and that their client was innocent? No. They would admit that he probably did exactly what the police said he did. Was it because he was not a threat to society, would not hurt a fly, and had never been in trouble before and would never do it again? No, it was to the contrary on all counts.

When one of *those* calls came, it was usually concerning a defendant who was in custody on a minor charge, something like trespass for refusing to leave a convenience store where he was singing or shouting obscenities at the magazine rack. The defendant, who was obviously mentally ill, would have been arrested by an officer who would much rather do a quick dropoff at the county jail rather than waiting several hours for the defendant to be admitted at the nearest receiving facility for the mentally ill in crisis. The defendant would have a $25 bond that he could not afford and was usually on his way out of the jail en route to the "Crisis and Stabilization Unit" due to his smearing his feces all over his jail cell. Well, why were they calling a supervising assistant state attorney instead of a supervisor at the Department of Children and Families (D.C.F.) (formally know as the Department of Health and Rehabilitative Services)? I'm a prosecutor, not a social worker. The reason was that the Assistant Public Defender was calling this office was to advocate that charges be quickly "dropped" so that the client, after "stabilization," would not be returned to the jail where he would only decompensate in a matter of days, necessitating the calls all over again. It all made perfect sense except for one important factor— what about my duty to protect the public from the criminals who plague society, even those who stand on runways insisting that they are in a relationship with the President's daughter? And every decision evokes images from every prosecutor's biggest nightmare—reading that headline the next morning that the mentally ill trespasser whose charges the well-intentioned prosecutor had dropped today had become the cop killer of tomorrow.

Unfortunately, those calls kept coming during those first few weeks on the job, causing me more and more concern for the position this office was being put in. Therefore, a little personal investigation was conducted. First, the infamous "Unit 12," where the critically mentally ill are housed in the county's jail, was toured. I had already been at the state hospital covering Baker Act (involuntary civil commitment) hearings which had left an indelible impression in my mind, and it was doubtful that things had actually improved. Informal interviews were conducted with doctors at the facilities, a jail superintendent, public defenders, other prosecutors, and judges. Also reviewed were some, often humorous, police reports, rushed (and expensive) competency evaluations, and rap sheets long enough to wallpaper a large office. Very quickly one conclusion became painfully obvious, one that, other than the mentally ill defendants themselves, only a few people were cognizant of and even less were willing to admit: Despite the best efforts of those involved, the manner in which the criminal justice system was dealing with the mentally ill defendants, particularly those charged with minor offenses, was, pardon the pun—*insane!*

Imagine a courtyard shaped like a triangle with one revolving door at each point. At one point was the door to what was, at the time, the biggest provider of mental health services in the county, the Broward County Jail— a jail that four years ago was 600 inmates over capacity, and, under a federal mandate had third degree felons being released on their own recognizance. At another point was the second revolving door leading to a very short hallway known as the mental health community. The state government agency responsible for administrating the revolving door of mental health services in this community was the Department of Children and Families that had recently been described in a grand jury report as "a rudderless ship." In this hallway were three very small doors. The first small door was to the crisis units where the main goal was to stabilize (pump up with drugs) their patients in the throngs of psychosis as quickly as possible so that they could return to society (or the jail if that was where they came from). The second small door was to the civil state hospitals, which were at the time completing their reorganization, initiated decades before, called "deinstitutionalization." Finally, the third small door in this hallway was to the outpatient "providers" who attempted to provide mental health treatment for their "consumers" (a term that I used to associate with a fair exchange of goods and services). The last revolving door was the front door to the courthouse. In the misdemeanor courts, the response to this crisis was quick pleas of guilty and a sentence equal to whatever time they had already spent in jail, or dropped charges based on unfulfilled hopes and promises of meaningful psychiatric treatment. To make matters worse, in April, 1997, the Supreme Court of Florida, in a case called *Onwu v. State of Florida*, the Office of the Public Defender, with the assistance of the Department of Children and Families (surprise) persuaded the court to hold that county court judges did not have the legal authority to forensically commit to the custody of the Department, incompetent, potentially dangerous criminal defendants charged with misdemeanors. The judges, prosecutors, and defense attorneys involved in this system were well-intentioned, but without resources, most without experience or knowledge, and more than anything—with their overwhelming caseloads where "moving the case" was a priority, not breaking a spiraling cycle—without time. With 16 different judges in four different courthouses throughout the county, any of the scarce resources available remained hidden under a mountain of bureaucracy. These three doors were spinning furiously, flinging defendants/patients/consumers from one to the other. The real tragedy in this model is that our humane society of peace, security, and wellness was not in the middle of this courtyard—it was on the outside.

That was the situation in this county, a sight, more likely than not, that is mirrored by most major metropolitan areas. From the perspective of the State Attorney's Office, this revolving meant continuing criminal activity of what some classify as "petty offenses" (although you might not think it so petty if you owned that convenience store). It also meant felons getting out of jail to make room for the trespassers coming in. And it meant pressure to make quick decisions regarding how to dispose of cases involving possibly dangerous mentally ill defendants where everyone agreed jail was not the proper place for them but where there were no legal, safe or effective alternatives.

THE AD HOC COMMITTEE—
BIRTHPLACE OF A NATIONAL MODEL

A few years earlier, there was a group that, albeit from different perspectives, saw the same triangle-shaped courtyard that I did. The group known roughly as "The Ad Hoc Mental Health Task Force " was not elected, appointed, incorporated or chartered. It was organized and led by a well-respected (former prosecutor) circuit judge who at the time was the Administrative Criminal Judge for the Circuit Court, The Honorable Mark Speiser. He was assisted by Chief Assistant Public Defender Howard Finklestein, a media-connected "activist" for the downtrodden, particularly the mentally ill. The members of this task force included representatives from the bench, the Office of State Attorney Michael J. Satz (my boss), the Office of Public Defender Alan Schreiber, the Criminal Defense Bar, the Broward County Sheriff's Office (as well as its jail), the Department of Children and Families, and mental health services providers and advocates. Through the prestige and reputation that Judge Speiser lent to the effort and Howard Finklestein's ability to generate public opinion, this group's goal was to put its proverbial foot in the revolving doors and to add some semblance of sanity to the criminal justice system in its dealings with the mentally ill.

From this group of unlikely compatriots came the genesis of the Mental Health Court. It was dreamed of as a humane court where non-violent misdemeanants suffering from mental illness could be moved from the detrimental effects of their jail cells to meaningful treatment facilities and programs, without compromising public safety. Relentlessly, this group persevered, knowing that "if you build it, they will come" (despite the knowledge that "if they come, where will they go?"). Finally, pen was put to paper and an administrative order was drafted. While the defense and advocates were happy to include all of their "treatment in an environment conducive to wellness and not punishment" type flowery language, my duty was to ensure that the rules of criminal procedure were addressed such as speedy trial and discovery, in conjunction with reviewing the logistics of how cases entered and exited the court. Additionally, the State Attorney insisted that great care was taken to ensure that these humanistic goals never compromised the safety of the public. After the various factions had reviewed and revised the order, at a short yet memorable meeting, the matter was presented to the Chief Judge, The Honorable Dale Ross. Both Judge Ross and State Attorney Satz are what most would consider traditional, no-nonsense, law-and-order type guys, and most people who know them think it is highly ironic that these two would be such major participants in such an unconventional endeavor. Moreover, Judge Ross actually seemed bewildered that we were all able to so easily form a consensus on the matter, and after a surprisingly brief discussion, Judge Ross agreed that the creation of this court would not only promote judicial economy, better protect the public and the rights of defendants themselves, but more importantly, that it was the right thing to do. In May of 1997, Judge Ross signed the original administrative order creating a Mental Health Subdivision operational within the County Court Criminal Division and this nation's first Mental Health Court was born. (This order was recently amended as Administrative Order No. VI-00-I-1.)

The next step was to staff the court. The selection of judge was obvious. The newest County Court Judge at the time, The Honorable Ginger Lerner-Wren, was still in the process of acclimating herself with the intricacies of the law surrounding "driving under the influence" cases when Judge Speiser, on behalf of the Task Force, approached her about the position. Judge Wren, prior to taking the bench, had an extensive background in the area of mental health including working as an advocate for the mentally ill, the monitor in a class action suit on behalf of the residents of the State Hospital, and acting as the Public Guardian for this county. She eagerly accepted the challenge and has presided over the court ever since. Next, Howard Finklestein basically shamed D.C.F. and the largest community mental health provider into supplying a "system's liaison," someone who would act as a "boundary spanner," mustering whatever scant resources were available in the community. Because the court would have the capability of referring these individuals for emergency psychiatric evaluation, this individual would need to be a licensed clinical social worker. Assistant Public Defenders and Assistant State Attorneys were also assigned to the court. By the end of the first year, it became evident that for the sake of consistency, and in order to effectively note the progress (or lack thereof) of the defendants who participated in the court, this court could not be treated like other courtrooms in the county court where prosecutors are rotated in and out every four or five months. Therefore, Mr. Satz selected an experienced prosecutor, Assistant State Attorney Lourdes Roberts, as the court's first prosecutor. She will be describing in more detail the actual day-to-day workings of the court as well as some of her less conventional responsibilities later in this chapter.

DOES THIS THING REALLY WORK?

At least one Thursday per month, representatives from this office involved with the Mental Health Court are interviewed by a contingent from another county or state interested in the court. These groups are usually made up of assistant public defenders, judges, social workers, providers, and representatives from their jails. Usually the prosecutor is notably absent and, when inquiry is made as to his or her whereabouts, the response is often off-the-cuff comments concerning lack of interest or even opposition to the idea. Most prosecutors' offices, understandably so, often consider this concept, similar to other specialty courts like drug court, to be a liberal-minded diversionary court where guilty people are again cut a break in a system that is supposed to be striving for accountability. Other concerns are logistical such as how to decide and organize which cases go into the court, the application of the rules of criminal procedure, and their concerns about the defense using this more often lenient judge to inappropriately "judge shop." Finally mentioned is the usual lack of resources and manpower within their offices and how they are having difficulty keeping their felony divisions staffed, let alone creating another position to handle some new misdemeanor court.

In response to these concerns, it is asserted that Mental Health Court is not for everyone and is probably not needed in most jurisdictions. Unquestionably, if the social service agencies here were doing their job, and had the proper resources, we probably would not need the court here in Broward County. Inquiring prosecutors are advised how the court basically grew out of necessity and how this office's involvement was not motivated solely by altruistic goals but by a desire to better protect the public and increase the accountability of both the defendants and those responsible for their supervision. It is emphasized how their logistical concerns were carefully addressed in the drafting of the administrative order. The abuses, such as forum shopping, are deterred by the unique non-adversarial relationship that this office has with the Office of the Public Defender (in this matter), mainly due to the fact that, particularly in light of their "victory" in the *Onwu* decision, they need the court in order to keep their clients out of jail, to get them treatment, and, because they know that if our concerns are not addressed or if some catastrophe occurs within the court, the court will be instantly disbanded by all concerned. As Judge Wren always says, "Public safety is number one" and the prosecutors are the ones charged with preserving that in the creation, administration, and operation of the court. All of the other factions involved in this process, despite our differences, have eventually come to learn to accept and respect that fact, and to the extent appropriate, facilitate our fulfilling that responsibility. Even the advocates such as the members of the local chapter of the National Alliance of the Mentally Ill (NAMI) no longer consider this office as "The Evil Empire."

Usually, still not totally convinced, an interested prosecutor would ask, "Well, does this thing really work?" The answer is always the same, "Of course it works. Anything is better than what we had before." In that regard, using the previous situation as a baseline, the court was inevitably going to succeed. Pushed for specifics, discussed is the prosecutor's favorite catchphrase used when evaluating the effectiveness of any diversion-type program—recidivism. The problem is that there are no real statistics to give them (that is in the works) and they are directed to Assistant State Attorney Roberts who is in there day in and day out, seeing the same people as well as the new ones, their progress and their failures, who responds to questions about the recidivism rate with "very little." That is significant though. When you consider that before the creation of this court, the average now Mental Health Court defendant was getting arrested several times a month, if not a week, and now *may* re-offend once each year, that is considered great success. When you consider that the same defendant who, before the court's creation, would keep pleading out his cases or having them dismissed as he was on his way from the jail to the crisis unit was now being linked with the scant services available, being given a caseworker, and being assisted in securing benefits from the government, being required to return to the court about once a month for up to one year for a "status" (a term that in traditional courtrooms was used to describe the status of the case, not the defendant) where adjustments and re-evaluations of his treatment and placement can be made, that is considered success. For prosecutors trying to work an insane system full of risk, inequities, and apathy into one with consistency, responsibility, and accountability, success is measured by the court's ability to provide for better protection of the public as well as the defendants themselves.

WHAT'S NEXT?

There is still a long way to go. The Ad Hoc Committee continues to meet monthly. Judge Ross just signed the amended order which emphasizes the voluntariness of the court as well as codifying the procedures where this office occasionally reduces appropriate felonies to misdemeanors so that the defendants can participate in the court (only to have their case re-filed back to a felony if they fail to participate or benefit from the court). As the caseload increases and the staff gets more adept at determining the needs of the defendants, the lack of resources in the mental health community becomes even more evident. The committee did successfully lobby some very brave and enlightened heroes in the Florida Legislature and the Broward County Commission for some funding to create "Cottages in the Pines," a residential treatment facility with its 35 beds specifically earmarked for defendants in the Mental Health Court who do not need the strict confinement of jail but are not yet appropriate to be released into the community. Although that facility which is such an integral part of the success of this nation's first Mental Health Court is just a drop in the proverbial bucket, the latest news out of Tallahassee is that the Cottages are on the legislative chopping block. Regardless, all in all, the Mental Health Court might not be the panacea for all the deficiencies in how the Broward County criminal justice system deals with the mentally ill, having for its resources a fragmented community mental health system, the crisis units, and the jail, but it's a start. We might not have stopped the spinning of those three revolving doors, but at least maybe we have slowed them down.

COURT IS NOW IN SESSION—
THE PERSPECTIVE FROM THE IN-COURT PROSECUTOR

The prosecutor in the Mental Health Division is constantly faced with the dilemma of punishment, public safety, deterrence, or rehabilitation and treatment. Whereas a standard case may merit a jail sentence, a mental health defendant may need to be in a treatment facility. The balancing act gets even more complicated where there are issues of dual diagnosis: psychiatric needs and substance abuse. Many times there are more questions than answers. Is the substance abuse merely self-medication? Is the substance abuse the driving force of the defendant's problem? Are the defendant's intentions genuine or is he merely paying lip service to the court in order to avoid a jail sentence? At what point does the state recommend punishment rather than treatment for relapses involving substances? Although legally the court cannot order medication compliance, at what point does medication compliance become the "ticket" for remaining in Mental Health Court? How closely should the defendant be monitored? Does the defendant need to be remanded back into custody or just reprimanded for non-compliance with the conditions imposed? And the questions could go on and on. It is a constant balancing act. When all is said and done, prosecutors still have to be able to justify their actions concerning the handling of a particular case, if need be, to the community.

By its design, the Broward County Mental Health Court seeks to identify and intervene in cases involving mentally ill defendants as early as possible in the criminal process. Unlike other mental health courts around the country, Broward County's court serves principally as a pre-adjudicatory diversion program for misdemeanants. While there are certain situations where a defendant may be placed on probation with a specialized probation officer that reports to the court on the defendant's progress, most defendants have their cases "put on hold" while they deal with their mental health issues. The rationale of addressing these cases on a pre-adjudicatory scheme focuses on "decriminalizing" the mental health defendant, thus empowering him to take control of his condition. Jail and formal adjudication does very little in addressing the reasons for the individual's contact with the criminal justice system. In fact, such contact often triggers a rapid recycling through the criminal courts.

WHO GETS IN?

The Broward County Mental Health Court currently accepts and screens mentally ill defendants charged with a wide range of misdemeanor offenses. These offenses carry a maximum penalty of up to one year in the county jail. Because the court is primarily restricted to individuals who commit minor offenses, the court will accept individuals with prior convictions. On the rare occasions where a felony is reduced for the purposes of making the services of the Mental Health Court available to the defendant, his criminal history is often the determining factor. Before an individual is accepted into mental health court, a detailed criminal history is run through national criminal registries. Defendants with criminal histories that include violent offenses are closely scrutinized by the prosecutor to avoid involving defendants who pose a clear threat to the public safety. This is one of the instances where the prosecutor may request that the defendant be placed on probation and incorporate the mental health treatment into the conditions of probation. Another prerequisite for eligibility is that the person have an Axis I diagnosis of mental illness, a developmental disability, or organic brain injury or head trauma. Axis I is a primary mental health diagnosis which is a part of an assessment on several axes, each of which refers to a different domain of information to help clinicians plan treatment and predict outcomes. Axis I can include such diagnoses as schizophrenia, anxiety disorders, impulse-control disorders, and major depression. This criteria ensures that the court is focusing on the seriously mentally ill or the disabled population.

Many of the participants of the Mental Health Court are identified at their first appearance (bond hearing/probable cause hearing) before a magistrate within 24 hours of their arrest. There, clinical students assigned to the Public Defender's Office screen these in-custody defendants for any history of mental illness. Individuals who present with visible signs of mental illness or self-report a history of past mental illness are immediately referred to the Mental Health Court for further screening. Some of the referrals also come from judges in regular criminal divisions, criminal defense attorneys and even the jail personnel will make observations of inmates and ask that the Mental Health Court screen the individual. Defendants' families often contact the court to ask that their family member's case be accepted into the Mental Health Court due to a history of mental illness. If the defendant is an "active" client of a local mental health center the referral may even come from his or her caseworker.

WELCOME TO THE MENTAL HEALTH COURT. NOW WHAT?

It is estimated that as 30% of the individuals making a first appearance in the Mental Health Court are acutely ill and in need of referral to a receiving facility for an independent evaluation to determine whether an involuntary civil commitment is necessary under the Florida Mental Health Act. The Florida Mental Health Act, better known as the Baker Act (Chapter 394, Part I, Florida Statutes) promulgates the procedures for both voluntary and involuntary admission to a mental health facility and treatment therein. If the defendant is stabilized within a short period of time, he is then returned to the court for further action. At that time a status hearing is held and the issue of competency is raised for the first time. Competency to proceed is governed by the Florida Rules of Criminal Procedure and sets out the criteria for determining whether the defendant has the sufficient present ability to consult with counsel and whether he has the rational as well as the factual understanding of the pending proceedings. The issue of competency may be raised by any party or on the court's own motion. If competency is raised, the defendant is then ordered to undergo an evaluation to determine his mental condition. If the evaluation confirms incompetency, the criminal case cannot proceed and the defendant is under the jurisdiction of the court until such time as competency has been restored or jurisdiction has lapsed. The court maintains jurisdiction over a criminal misdemeanant for up to one year. While the defendant is in the community under a "Conditional Release Plan" due to his incompetence, the prosecutor will generally ask that reasonable conditions be set in order to ensure the safety of the community and also ask that the defendant participate in a competency restoration program. During this time, the court will set frequent and periodic status hearings in order to monitor the defendant's progress. If the defendant's competency can be restored, he is then able to resolve his case. If, at the end of a year, competency has not been restored, the court shall dismiss the case.

Another issue that is discussed at the defendant's initial appearance is the fact that his participation is totally voluntary. The defendant needs to understand that participation in Mental Health Court constitutes a commitment on his part to engage in treatment and effectively manage his condition. Several factors are evaluated at this time. Issues involving housing, ties to the community, the defendant's prior criminal history, and the defendant's feelings towards treatment are considered. Not all cases remain within this court for an extended period of time. If, for example, the defendant has strong community links and is an active client of a local mental health provider, the case may be disposed of immediately. This may be the case in a situation where the defendant has gone off medication for a period of time and had police contact. On the other hand, an individual who needs the oversight of the court to become engaged in treatment or has a significant criminal history will have to "prove" himself/herself to the court and to the prosecutor in order to obtain a lenient sentence. Following the defendant's agreement to participate in the court, the criminal charges are held in abeyance. No depositions are taken and no discovery is done. The entire focus of the case becomes the defendant's progress with his treatment. The defendant can be monitored for up to a year. The actual length of supervision will vary with each individual case, depending on the particular needs and the progress of each defendant. During the treatment process, participants regularly report to Mental Health Court so that the judge can review their progress. Status hearings are held on an as-needed basis, usually every two, three and eventually every four weeks as participants demonstrate satisfactory progress. At the end of that time the case may be dismissed by the state or the defendant will receive a more lenient sentence as a result of his positive participation.

MISSION CONTROL, WE'VE GOT A PROBLEM

Difficulties do sometimes arise that necessitate legal intervention. If the court or the state determine that the defendant is no longer sufficiently participating or benefiting from the program there are several options. First, the defendant's case may be transferred out of the Mental Health Court and the defendant is held to answer to the charges in a "regular" criminal court. Second, the defendant's conditions of release may be changed to a more structured program with closer supervision. Finally, the defendant may be remanded into custody if there has been a new offense or a substantial breach of the conditions of release while participating in Mental Health Court. At this point, the state must decide whether the violations and the level of the defendant's participation warrant expulsion from the program. These determinations must be done on a case-by-case basis. Obviously, in the case of a new offense, the state will take the position that the defendant is not effectively participating in treatment as evidenced by the commission of a new law violation. Many factors come into play in deciding what the next step should be. The defendant's level of participation, medication compliance, prior criminal history, circumstances surrounding the new offense, and willingness to continue with the program with additional and more stringent conditions are all considered at this point. It should be noted that, due to its voluntary nature, a defendant may ask to be transferred out of the Mental Health Court at any time, including at the time of a violation.

Generally, the court will complete its relationship with a participant when he has made the transition into the required treatment and supportive services. These may include housing, counseling, medication, training, and employment. When the criminal court is no longer needed to facilitate those connections, the participant is considered to have been "successful" and the case is resolved.

SUCCESS?

In conclusion, the experience as a Mental Health Court prosecutor is unique. The role is often times a blend of prosecutor, social worker, case manager, and probation officer. While there have been disappointments along the way in seeing some of our "success stories" return after a long absence from the criminal justice system, the Mental Health prosecutor eventually comes to the stark realization that the success of the court is not measured solely by looking at recidivism rates. The court and all its players operate with the knowledge that compliance problems will be common among its participants. If the pattern of arrest for petty offenders is even slowed because of intervention of the court, it has been a success. Success lies in the knowledge that mentally ill individuals have been expeditiously removed from a jail setting and diverted into a mental health forum while still ensuring the public is protected.

22

A Personal Experience

The Honorable Sol Wachtler

I can remember the day when "Beetlejuice" cut his throat. Don't ask me the origin of his name. I couldn't tell you that any more than I can tell you where the razor blade he used came from.

He was one of those seemingly lifeless patients who would walk stiff-legged through the unit, his joints and psyche affected by the powerful anti-psychotic "Haldol."

Beetlejuice is here on a study. Some federal judge in Tennessee is waiting to learn from the prison doctors if Beetlejuice is competent to stand trial. That is, can he understand the nature of the charges against him and is he able to assist in his own defense? The judge has been waiting, the doctors have been studying, and Beetlejuice has been doing the "Haldol strut" for six years. His trial will not be held until he is declared competent.

His case illustrates the difficulty the justice system has had for centuries in dealing with mental illness. When and if he is found competent to stand trial, and if he pleads insanity as a defense, the finder of fact—be it judge or jury—will have to determine not his current mental state but whether he was insane at the time the crime was committed—many years ago.

There is an incompatibility between the law and psychiatry. The law says that a person should be punished for his unlawful acts. Psychiatry assumes that behavior is caused by forces within the person or by the environment acting on the person and, after all, if a person is unable to control his or her conduct, it would be uncivilized to punish that person. In other words, the law simply asks the question: "Did he do the wrongful act?" and the behavioral sciences ask the question, "Why did he do the wrongful act?"

A psychiatrist or psychologist will not use the term insanity. Both the word and the definition belong in the lexicon of lawyers—and lawyers have been trying for centuries to establish standards and criteria which can be used to determine if a person can be held legally responsible for his crime.

The touchstone of all definitions for insanity came from an English case decided in 1843. It involved a man named David McNaughton, who suffered from what a psychiatrist in this century would describe as paranoia. He believed that the Prime Minister of England, Robert Peel, was part of a plot to destroy him. After dodging shadows and imaginary assassins all over Europe, he decided that the only way to rid himself of his tormentor was to kill him. He shot the person whom he believed to be the Prime Minister, in front of No.10 Downing Street. Unfortunately for the private secretary of Mr. Peel, and Mr. McNaughton, he shot the wrong man.

The McNaughton trial captured the public's imagination. For two days, medical experts convinced a jury that McNaughton was, indeed, delusional and therefore not responsible for his crime. He was committed to an "insane asylum" where he eventually died.

Despite the fact that he was never allowed to go free, the public and Queen Victoria thought it a travesty that someone so guilty should be allowed to escape the gallows. The high court judges were instructed to devise a definition of insanity which would assure that a civilized perspective be maintained without impeding justice. Thus, long before psychiatry was considered a science, the so-called McNaughton rule was formulated. It held that before a person can be successful in proving an insanity defense it must be shown that "at the time of committing the act, the accused was laboring under such a defect of reason, from a disease of the mind, as not to know the nature and quality of the act he was doing, or, if he did know it, that he did not know that what he was doing was wrong."

The McNaughton rule, after 150 years, is still the law in almost half the states. The remainder of the states have adopted variations of the Model Penal Code developed by the American Law Institute, a standard which softened the McNaughton rule insofar as it requires a defendant, not to "not know the nature...of the act he was doing"—as required by McNaughton—but only to lack "substantial capacity" to "appreciate" the nature of the act.

This liberalized test was the standard for the federal courts when John W. Hinkley, Jr. gunned down President Reagan on March 30, 1981. At his trial, 15 months later, Hinkley's lawyers managed to persuade a jury that Hinkley was responding to the forces of a diseased mind and that he did not "appreciate" what he was doing. Hinkley enjoyed the additional advantage of having the trial judge place the burden on the prosecution to prove Hinkley's sanity rather than placing the burden on Hinkley to prove his insanity.

Hinkley was found *not guilty by reason of insanity*, and was initially incarcerated in the same prison to which I was sent in Butner, North Carolina. A prison which has a "mental health" unit. He is now committed to St. Elizabeth's Hospital in Washington, D.C.

In 1984, partially as a result of the Hinkley verdict, Congress passed, and President Reagan signed into law, the Comprehensive Crime Control Act which revived the "right versus wrong" criteria of the McNaughton rule back into the insanity defense and placed the burden of proving an insanity defense on the defendant.

With this constricted definition of insanity, it is little wonder that so many defendants who are mentally ill are now incarcerated. Their mental illness is not recognized by the law as an adequate defense. It is for that reason that there are more people with diagnosed mental illness in our prisons than in state mental hospitals.

A recent U.S. Department of Justice report indicated that close to 300,000 inmates have mental illness—or 16% of the population in state jails and prisons. There are another 548,000 people with mental illness in probation—also 16% of that population.

The recent trial of Andrew Goldstein demonstrates the need to reappraise the law's flawed insanity defense. Mr. Goldstein is the schizophrenic who pushed a total stranger to her death in front of a subway train. His conviction of murder was a commentary, not only on the deficiency of our mental health systems, but also on the failure of the criminal justice system to adequately deal with or understand the nature of mental illness. The fact that Andrew Goldstein is a schizophrenic who had a history of violence is not disputed. The fact that he sought help for hospital treatment and community care is also a matter of public record. Here was a man who was severely mentally ill. This unpremeditated and irrational violence by a schizophrenic against a stranger would seem to be the very definition of an "insane act" and yet the jury found him guilty. Why? Because under the law of New York he was guilty.

After the trial, jurors indicated that they focused on Mr. Goldstein's state of mind the moment before he pushed Kendra Webdale onto the tracks. He had told the police that he "knew his act was wrong." Because he knew what he was doing and knew it to be wrong, he was not legally insane. The fact that he acted by psychotic compulsion or as a schizophrenic who is untreated for his disease might be expected to act would perhaps be persuasive to a psychiatrist, but it would not be a legal defense.

Perhaps it is time we considered modifying the insanity plea by taking it out of the mid-Nineteenth Century. A recognition of contemporary psychiatric treatment and means of alternative sentencing which would allow for the mentally ill defendant to be treated instead of warehoused would be a step toward civilizing our criminal justice system. Considering a plea of "guilty but mentally ill" instead of "not guilty by reason of insanity" would be another mark of progress.

That is not to say that a person who has exhibited a tendency to violence should be excused by virtue of mental illness. But he should be treated. Had Mr. Goldstein been found not guilty by reason of insanity, or had been allowed an appropriate plea, he most likely would have spent the rest of his life in a psychiatric hospital being compelled to take the medication which would have curbed his violence.

But this is not to be. Andrew Goldstein has been condemned to join the likes of Beetlejuice and thousands of other mentally ill prisoners. I can attest to the fact that prison is the worst possible place for these individuals—not only because of the prison environment, but because treatment is minimal. And we should remember, many of these untreated mentally ill prisoners will one day be released and jettisoned on our streets.

23

Implementing Kendra's Law

Neal L. Cohen, Stacy S. Lamon, and Norman Katz

In November, 1999, New York State entered what many believed would be a new era in community-based mental health care with the enactment of Kendra's Law. The statute, also know as the Assisted Outpatient Treatment Law, allows civil courts to order services in the community for non-compliant mentally ill patients. To be eligible, patients must be 18 or older and have been hospitalized twice over a three-year period because of treatment non-compliance. In addition, individuals can be eligible if they have made acts, threats or attempts of serious, violent behavior toward themselves or others as a result of non-compliance. When actual or potential violence is an issue, only one hospitalization within a four-year period is required. Several other variables are used to determine eligibility for assisted outpatient treatment (AOT). Individuals must be determined to be in need of treatment by clinicians, unlikely to voluntarily accept it, and unlikely to survive independently in the community without extensive supports.

In one sense Kendra's law is truly unique. It marks the first time that New York State has acted to mandate treatment outside a hospital setting. In another sense, however, the law represents a logical step in the evolution of the state's community-based care system. Historically, care for mentally ill people has been premised on a passive treatment model. The serious and persistently mentally ill (SPMI) population in the community was expected to take medications and appear at clinic appointments without assistance. While the failure of this approach was apparent almost from deinstitionalization's onset, a wider recognition of its shortcomings did not become evident until the homelessness crisis of the mid-1980s. Media coverage indicated that large numbers of very sick, fragile people were receiving little or no treatment in community settings. In response, government, mental health providers, consumers and their families recognized the need to make services in the community more client-focused and more assertive.

The changes have been substantial and varied. Widespread homelessness among the SPMI population helped establish the idea that supportive housing was an essential element in a community-based system of care. Hospital diversion programs and assistive community treatment teams helped address the chronic instability of SPMIs and reduce their need for repeated hospitalizations. There also has been rapid growth in day treatment and a variety of community support programs that address the day-to-day needs of SPMIs. With funding provided for community-based care, New York City's Department of Mental Health has started or enhanced 144 programs for SPMIs. In addition, a wide variety of existing programs now offer a more aggressive approach to medication management and a growing number of clients are being assisted through case management programs.

Underlying this transformation in services is a recognition that traditional clinical assumptions about patient autonomy and independence in the treatment setting may not be as applicable for those with serious and persistent mental illnesses. A growing number of social workers, psychiatrists, psychologists, consumers and their families, including those with a firm commitment to the civil liberties of people with mental illnesses, now believe that some SPMIs may require ongoing external supports to enter or stay engaged in treatment. The programmatic changes resulting from this evolving clinical paradigm created the crisis management, supportive housing, day treatment, case management and medication management programs, and clinical services that provide the infrastructure for service delivery under Kendra's Law.

Enactment of Kendra's Law

In the late 1990s, New York's mental health community was in the midst of an extended debate about court-mandated, community-based treatment. Several civil commitment bills had been introduced in the State Legislature which ordered a study of court-mandated treatment. Conducted at Bellevue Mental Center, the study (Policy Research Associates, Inc., 1998) offered inconclusive answers on the impact of court orders upon treatment outcomes. It did, however, validate the efficacy of intensive community-based services, especially the use of case managers. Despite the study, the debate over civil commitment might have remained unresolved, but on January 3, 1999 an event took place that brought discussion to an abrupt end. On that date, Andrew Goldstein pushed a young woman, Kendra Webdale, to her death in front of an oncoming subway train.

Goldstein was seriously mentally ill with a long history of sporadic and unsuccessful treatment. His story, detailed in a widely read *New York Times* article (Winerip, 1999) prompted the enactment of Kendra's Law and of the New York State Office of Mental Health's plan to infuse substantial new dollars for community-based mental health care. More than $125 million was allocated for an infrastructure to implement assisted outpatient treatment (AOT), including the hiring of more case managers, expanded day treatment programs, and strengthened hospital discharge planning.

The speedy enactment of a civil commitment statute required New York's counties to create AOT programs without any immediate new funding in only 90 days. This proved difficult. However, the absence of a rigid implementation plan prior to the law's effective date had an unexpected result. It allowed localities to experiment with procedures to implement Kendra's Law. The result is considerable variation. AOT teams are exercising discretion on whether or not to seek court orders. Some are putting effort into getting patients with a history of non-compliance into treatment without a court petition. Other teams are making greater use of the courts. Researchers and practitioners will undoubtedly attempt to compare and evaluate program models and treatment outcomes under Kendra's Law.

Kendra's Law: Initial Results

In New York City, AOT teams now operate at four public hospitals: Bellevue Medical Center, Woodhull Hospital, Elmhurst Hospital Center, and North Central Bronx Hospital. New York State has an AOT team for patients released from its psychiatric hospitals. A sixth AOT team for Rikers Island Correctional Facility, which annually releases thousands of seriously mentally ill individuals, has been formed. The teams evaluate patients recommended for mandated outpatient services and petitions the court when they determine that civil commitment is warranted.

In the nine months since the law became effective (November 8, 1999 through August 11, 2000), over 1,000 potential candidates were referred to AOT teams (New York City Department of Mental Health, Mental Retardation and Alcoholism Services [DMHMR&AS], 2000). Investigations were initiated in 1,023 cases by AOT teams and other petitioners (hospitals and other services providers); 837 of these were completed. Almost a third (31%) resulted in petitions being filed with the court. Of the 255 petitions filed, court proceedings were concluded for 229 people. The court granted mandatory treatment orders in response to 88% of filed petitions (201). In 8% of the cases (18), petitions were withdrawn by the original petitioner. Only 4 percent of filed petitions (10) were denied by the court. However, it is important to note that these results may reflect the fact that AOT teams were careful in selecting only those individuals who would benefit from a court order (see Table 1).

Table 23.1 Assisted Outpatient Treatment Activities in New York City— First Nine Months*

Activities	Number	Percentages
Investigations initiated	1023	100% of investigations initiated during the first nine months of operation, 11/8/99 through 8/11/00
Investigations in process	186	18% of investigations in process as of 8/11/00
Investigations completed	837	82% of investigations completed by 8/11/00
Investigations concluded without petition or alternative	487	58% of investigations did not produce petitions
Investigations resulting in alternative voluntary services	95	11% of investigations resulted in alternative services
Investigations producing petitions	255	31% of investigations resulted in petitions filed in court
Petitions awaiting adjudication	26	10% of petitions in process in court as of 8/11/00
Petitions concluded	229	90% of petition proceedings concluded by 8/11/00
Petitions granted: court orders	201	88% of petitions resulted in court orders
Petitions denied	10	4% of petitions denied by the court
Petitions withdrawn	18	8% of petitions withdrawn by the petitioner

Source: DMHMR&AS, 2000

* November 8, 1999 through August 11, 2000

For this reason, two-thirds of all cases investigated by an AOT team never proceeded to court. Yet, this does not mean that these individuals went without treatment. Since the effective date of Kendra's Law, an alternative mechanism for providing services to non-compliant patients has evolved. Teams regularly identify individuals who, though eligible for AOT, will voluntarily accept case management and other treatment services. With their consent, services are provided without a court petition. From November 8, 1999 through August 11, 2000, 95 individuals volunteered to receive AOT services in New York City. This number represents 11% of the cases for which investigations were concluded.

A voluntary approach to implementing Kendra's Law has obvious benefits. It avoids the time, effort, and expense of a court hearing and it provides the individual with access to all needed services. There is also good reason to believe that this voluntary approach will succeed. Individuals who accept intensive services are, in many respects, analogous to the control group of the Bellevue study. That group remained in treatment at an almost identical rate to those who received services with a court order. The voluntary alternative developed by the AOT team has another critical advantage. AOT patients who accept services and then stop treatment still can be taken to court. Their failure to remain in treatment gives the court additional evidence that a more coercive approach is required.

While it is impossible to provide a comprehensive assessment of Kendra's Law at this early date, figures tabulated by the Department of Mental Health suggest that the statute is having a positive effect. The law appears to be providing better, more comprehensive services to a growing number of patients. The number of petitions granted by New York City courts is steadily increasing. From November, 1999 through March, 2000, only 24 petitions were granted, an average of five a month. In April, 2000, the numbers began to increase with 29 petitions granted in the city. The increase became more pronounced in May when 55 petitions were granted. From June through August an average of 37 petitions per month were granted (see figure 1).

The number of patients accepting voluntary treatment without a court proceeding has also increased over the same period. The willingness of patients to avoid civil commitment hearings suggests several things. First, AOT teams are growing increasingly sophisticated in their ability to influence patient treatment decisions. Second, the statute's threat of commitment may be an effective motivating factor in getting patients to accept and stay in treatment. Additionally, faced with the opportunity to receive an enhanced services package, many will accept it with or without a court order.

On more than one occasion, a patient's desire for assisted treatment has been demonstrated during court proceedings. During one proceed-

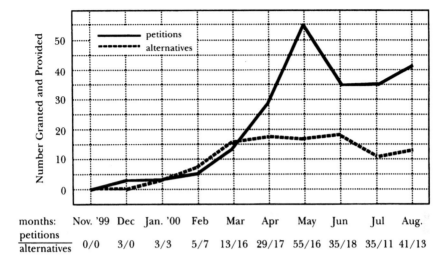

months:	Nov. '99	Dec	Jan. '00	Feb	Mar	Apr	May	Jun	Jul	Aug.
petitions / alternatives	0/0	3/0	3/3	5/7	13/16	29/17	55/16	35/18	35/11	41/13

FIGURE 23.1 AOT Petitions Granted and Alternative Voluntary Services Provided in New York City.

ing, when a judge questioned the inclusion of a specific medication in a treatment plan because of previous noncompliance, the AOT candidate spoke up, saying that he was willing to "try the medication again." The patient felt he could stay on the medication with the help of a case manager. In another case, a patient provided the AOT team with the names of mental health care professionals who could testify to make the petition stronger.

Some may argue that these examples may simply indicate the confusion exhibited by many AOT candidates or illustrate that these particular candidates might have accepted services voluntarily. But they may also underscore that AOT clients have an interest in treatment and perceive the petition process as an insurance policy in which the mental health care system guarantees them appropriate services. The individuals described above had long histories of non-compliance but both wanted help. For AOT candidates like them, a court proceeding may be perceived as part of a process requiring accountability from clients, as well as social service and mental health care systems.

There is another potentially significant trend to emerge from early data collected on Kendra's Law. AOT teams outside of New York City are far more likely to recommend that non-compliant patients voluntarily accept treatment alternatives that do not involve the issuance of court orders. Alternatively, their New York City counterparts make more extensive use of the courts. During the first nine months of AOT ending August 11, 2000 in New York City, voluntary alternative treatment had been offered in 95 cases and 201 petitions were granted by the court (DMHMR&AS, 2000). This represents an approximate 1:2 ratio of alternative treatments to petitions. The proportions are very different outside of New York City. During approximately the same time period, the New York State Office of Mental Health indicates (New York State Office of Mental Health, 2000) that for counties outside of New York City some form of voluntary alternative treatment was offered in 442 cases and the courts granted petitions in only 40 cases. This represents an approximate 11:1 ratio of alternatives to petitions.

The disparity between New York State and the city may be explained by the choice of many counties to offer voluntary alternatives services to patients who may not strictly meet the statutory requirements of Kendra's Law. In addition, the specific type of alternative treatment varies significantly from county to county. For both reasons, a clear comparison of New York City's use of voluntary alternative treatment service to that of other counties cannot be exact. There remains a strong indication that significantly fewer voluntary alternatives to treatment are offered in New York City than elsewhere in the state.

Several factors may explain the disparity. The difference in petition rates may indicate that New York City-based AOT teams see more non-compliant patients. It may also reflect the historical difficulty of insuring patient cooperation in a complex, urban environment. However, the disparity may also indicate philosophical and clinical differences in implementing Kendra's Law. City AOT teams may be more predisposed to the use of coercive measures because of a long-term inability to actually secure sufficient resources for more assertive treatment programs and because of the ongoing frustrations involved in addressing the needs of a subgroup of highly complex patients with extended histories of repeated hospitalizations. Whatever the reasons, the geographic disparity in implementing Kendra's Law needs to be thoroughly investigated. Research is also required to determine the impact of assertive treatment with or without a court order. It will be interesting to see if future research duplicates the findings of the Bellevue study which suggest that the provision of intensive services was as important as a court order in maintaining patients in treatment.

Another area for future investigation is the impact of Kendra's Law on the legal system. For the first time, New York has a statute that regularly exposes judges to mentally ill people, case records, and treatment options. Hopefully, this first-hand knowledge will make the legal system more sensitive to the burdens imposed by severe mental illness. While petitions under Kendra's Law are reviewed by civil court judges in State Supreme Court, the statute may soon have an impact on both the civil and criminal courts. The reason is that in New York there is considerable overlap between the civil and criminal courts. Civil court judges are frequently assigned to the criminal court for specific periods of time and many criminal court judges move to the civil courts. With greater judicial awareness, the courts may become more concerned about the "criminalization" of mental illness and this may insure a more realistic response to a fragile, disorganized population that is too frequently jailed for minor offenses.

A Model for Implementing Kendra's Law:
The Directly Observed Therapy Program

Kendra's Law is not without precedent in New York State. It resembles the state's Directly Observed Therapy (DOT) Program. This highly successful initiative introduced in 1992 insures that patients with active infectious tuberculosis comply with medication regimes. DOT, like Kendra's Law, was not designed for all TB patients. It was targeted to those who would not take medications. Trained health care workers were assigned the task of ensuring that TB medications were taken. Compliance was assured through a variety of direct observation techniques. Kendra's Law and the statute creating DOT have much in common. Both laws require compliance and both can mandate hospitalization. What is striking about the city's experience with DOT is the degree to which it succeeded without using involuntary hospitalization. From 1992 to 1998 less than 2% of DOT patients were hospitalized by an order of the Health Commissioner.

DOT may be a good predictor of the future impact of Kendra's Law because of the overlap between the populations targeted by both initiatives. No systematic studies of DOT patients exist, but anecdotal evidence suggests that a disproportionate percentage of those in the program had a concurrent diagnosis of TB and a mental and/or substance abuse illness. The threat of involuntary commitment combined with the offer of less coercive forms of help had a positive effect on this subgroup of TB patients. Hopefully, it will have a similar effect on those subject to Kendra's Law.

DOT also illustrates the importance of effective case management in assisting noncompliant patients. From its beginning, DOT was more than a medication management program. Health care workers came to understand that insuring compliance with medication regimes was often contingent on stabilizing the lives of many DOT patients. To achieve that, DOT staff often became informal case managers helping patients to get social services, income supports, housing and mental health, substance abuse, and other health-related services. Illustrative of this is a DOT case chronicled in an article in *The Nursing Connection*, a publication of New York City's Department of Health (Barton, 1998).

The case involved an Asian-American female with TB and a long his-

tory of severe mental illness. Treatment for her TB had been unsuccessfully attempted on three occasions. Each time the patient stopped taking
her medications before the end of the treatment cycle. Success came when
DOT staff combined medication management with mental health care
and linkages to organizations in the Asian-American community that could
address the patient's comprehensive needs. Similarly, Kendra's Law patients
frequently have multiple, interdisciplinary needs that must be addressed
concurrently if they are to remain stable in the community. DOT offers a
model of how case managers can address a complex set of support needs.

Recommendations for Implementing Kendra's Law.

In the first year of implementing Kendra's Law, New York City appears to
be succeeding at bringing comprehensive assistance to people at highest
risk for repeated hospitalizations. AOT teams have described multiple
instances where results were achieved after years of failed treatment
attempts. There are, however, several measures that should be taken to
insure that the law's initial positive impact will grow in the future.

   *A. Hospitals need incentives to provide assisted outpatient treatment to addi-
tional eligible patients.* New York City Department of Mental Health data
indicate that hospitals refer the vast majority of patients to AOT teams.
Current efforts to shorten the length of stay for psychiatric illnesses decrease
the likelihood that cost-conscious hospitals will want to expend the
resources needed to secure civil commitment. This is particularly true
when hospitals confront patients with complex and multiple needs. Because
these difficult cases require the expenditure of considerable time, resources,
and staff, third party payors need to encourage hospitals to refer cases
requiring extensive discharge planning. Financial incentives to hospitals
are especially important because New York State has not yet acted to create special needs managed care plans for SPMIs.

   B. Case managers need enhanced authority. One of the major issues confronting the community mental health system, as it has moved toward
more assertive treatment models, is insuring the authority of case managers. The importance of case managers and the effectiveness of case management was underscored in a variety of studies (Bond, Miller, Kurmweid
& Ward, 1988; Borland, McRae & Lycan, 1989; Bush, Langford, Rosen &
Gott, 1990; Rife, 1991; Rubin, 1992). In the past, however, determinations
made by case workers have been frequently ignored or altered by insur-
ers, providers and clinicians. Because of this, case managers frequently
felt powerless. If Kendra's Law is to succeed, case managers must be granted
expanded managerial authority.

C. Standards are needed for evaluating the success of commitment orders and non-court-ordered treatment programs. The most significant finding of the Bellevue civil commitment study (Policy Research Associates, Inc., 1998) was that the community-based mental health system had the skills and expertise to keep patients in treatment. The success of the Bellevue effort may, however, have been premised, in part, on the fact that staff members knew their efforts were being evaluated. It can be argued that the study itself acted as an incentive, making providers more committed to achieving successful treatment outcomes. Mental health workers are offered few incentives or penalties for good or bad performance. Both are required if Kendra's Law's is to be a success. Performance outcome standards are also needed for AOT teams, hospitals and community-based providers. New York State and the City also need to be effective regulators, and judges must insure that their orders are properly implemented. Patients must also be held accountable and need to know that penalties for noncompliance will be enforced.

However, performance standards must be based on realistic expectations of treatment outcomes. The Bellevue study of civil commitment gives a realistic indication of what can be expected. While staff involved in the Bellevue study kept a higher than average percentage of patients in treatment for longer periods of time, a substantial number of subjects in the study stopped accepting services. These individuals dropped out of treatment regardless of whether they were getting services under court order or through a voluntary agreement to accept them.

D. Additional advocacy is needed to ensure the ongoing success of Kendra's Law. Improvements in community-based mental health care tend to come when the public believes the system to be in crisis. Kendra's Law fits into this pattern. It derives from the perception that violent mentally ill people are a danger to public safety. Over the long run, however, the success of Kendra's Law may have little to do with enhanced public safety. Mental health advocates (e.g., Barr, 1999) have repeatedly emphasized that the overwhelming majority of SPMIs are neither violent nor dangerous to themselves or to others. Recently, the MacArthur Violent Risk Assessment Study (Steadman et al., 1998) which looked at 1,000 mentally ill people found that individuals not abusing drugs or alcohol and in treatment are no more likely to be violent than are people without mental health problems.

Consequently, the real promise of Kendra's Law may lie in its potential to provide enhanced services to a segment of the SPMI population that has not accessed the types of programs available to them under this statute. Resources for intensive services must be incorporated into future state budgets and advocates will need to insure that government meets its obligations annually.

CONCLUSION

Less than a year after its passage, Kendra's Law shows progress in addressing the seemingly intractable problem of keeping non-compliant severely mentally ill people in treatment. The creation of AOT teams and their increasing effectiveness coupled with what appears to be an improving partnership between the mental health care and legal systems point toward more effective supervision of non-compliant patients. Equally, the growing ability of the mental health care system to provide patients with intensive services and the willingness of patients to accept them, with and without a court order, presage the emergence of a more effective system of community-based care. Kendra's Law is by no means a panacea for the New York's mental health care system but it appears to be a significant step along a continuum of improved services.

REFERENCES

Barr, H. (1999). *Prisons and Jails: Hospitals of Last Resort.* New York, NY: Correctional Association of New York and Urban Justice Center.

Barton, V. (1998). When a psychiatric disorder interferes with tuberculosis treatment. *The Nursing Connection, 6*(1), 4–5, New York, NY: Department of Health.

Bond, G., Miller, L., Kurmweid, R. & Ward, R. (1988). Assertive case management in three CMHCs: A controlled study. *Hospital & Community Psychiatry, 39,* 411–418.

Borland, A., McRae, J. & Lycan, C. (1989). Outcomes of five years of continuous case management. *Hospital & Community Psychiatry, 40,* 369–376.

Bush, C.T., Langford, M.W., Rosen, P. & Gott, W. (1990). Operation outreach: Intensive case management for severely psychiatrically disturbed adults. *Hospital & Community Psychiatry, 41,* 647–649.

New York City Department of Mental Health, Mental Retardation and Alcoholism Services. (2000, August 16), *Assisted outpatient treatment: Summary report* (Departmental Report). New York, NY: Author.

New York State Office of Mental Health. (2000). *Statewide AOT Report as of August 9, 2000* (State Office Report). Albany, NY: Author.

Policy Research Associates. (1998). *Research study of the New York City involuntary outpatient commitment pilot program* [report submitted to the New York City Department of Mental Health, Mental Retardation and Alcoholism Services]. New York, NY: Author.

Rife, J.C., First, R.J., Greenlee, R.W., Miller, L.D. & Feichter, M.A. (1991). Case management with homeless mentally ill people. *Health and Social Work, 16,* 58–67.

Rubin, A. (1992). Is case management effective for people with serious mental illness? A research review. *Health and Social Work, 17*(2), 138–150.

Steadman, H.J., Mulvey, E.P., Monahan, J., Robbins P.C., Appelbaum, P.S., Grisso T., Roth, L.H. & Silver, E. (1998). Violence by people discharged from acute psychiatric inpatient facilities and by others in the same neighborhoods. *Archives of General Psychiatry, 55*, 339–401.

Winerip, M. (1999, May 23). Bedlam on the Streets. *New York Times Magazine, The New York Times.*

SECTION VI
Screening Instruments

24

A Review of Screening Instruments for Co-occurring Mental Illness and Substance Use in Criminal Justice Programs

Nahama Broner, Randy Borum,

Laura Whitmire, and Kristen Gawley

This chapter provides a review of screening instruments for mental illness and substance abuse for use by court-based diversion programs, specialty courts or alternative to incarceration programs.[1] A crucial task for mental health professionals and programs working with this particular criminal justice population is to be able to appropriately identify a client with these problems and to match him or her with individualized services. An overview of diversion and programmatic trends in New York City is presented in Chapter 7.

We begin with a brief description of the scope of the problem of mental illness and co-occurring mental illness and substance abuse in the criminal justice system, and highlight the need for systematic screening. The

Preparation of this chapter was supported in part by Grant No. 1-UD8-TI 11213-03 from the U.S. Department of Health and Human Services, Substance Abuse and Mental Health Services Administration, Center for Substance Abuse Treatment and Grant No. MH16242-20 from the National Institute of Mental Health. The opinions expressed in this manuscript are strictly those of the authors and no endorsement by the funding agencies is to be inferred.

The authors wish to thank Roger Peters, Ph.D., Hunter L. McQuisten, M.D., Jayme Delano, C.S.W. and Stacy S. Lamon, Ph.D. for their review of drafts of this chapter and Valerie Raine, J.D., Jayme Delano, C.S.W. and their Brooklyn Treatment Court staff for their input and participation in this project.

review examines instruments for the screening of mental health problems, alcohol and drug abuse, and for personality disorders. The instruments reviewed were selected on the following bases: (1) they were cross-validated or demonstrated significant promise; (2) they could be administered by case management staff; (3) they were sufficiently brief to not overburden staff; and (4) they were non-proprietary and could be used without a fee. This chapter concludes with recommendations addressing the instruments reviewed and staff training for administration.

THE SCOPE OF THE PROBLEM

Research describing the scope of the problem of criminal justice contact for those with mental illness is extensive and focuses on police and those they arrest, emergency room populations, involuntary hospitalization, family members' perception of their mentally ill relatives, and jails and prisons as well as courts (Borum, 1999a). For example, 7% of police contacts involve mentally ill people in crisis as reported by major police departments (Deane, Steadman, Borum, Veysey & Morrissey, 1998); and a survey of 450 police officers in three U.S. cities noted that within the month prior to the survey police each responded to an average of six calls regarding mentally ill people in crisis (Borum, Deane, Steadman & Morrisey, 1998). In a survey of family members, the average number of arrests reported for their mentally ill relative was more than three (McFarland, Faulkner, Bloom & Hallaux, 1989). For those who had been involuntarily committed to a hospital and diagnosed with a serious psychiatric disorder, approximately 20% of the 350 surveyed reported that they had either been picked up by police or arrested for a crime within four months of their admission (Borum, Swanson, Swartz & Hiday, 1997).

In terms of jails and prisons, national surveys report that between 6% and 15% of all jail inmates and 10% to 15% of prison inmates have a severe mental illness (Lamb & Weinberger, 1998). Since mentally ill individuals are admitted to jails at approximately eight times the rate at which they are admitted to public psychiatric hospitals, there are now more people with severe mental illness in U.S. jails than in state hospitals (Torrey et al., 1993). Nearly three out of four, or approximately 70%, of mentally ill detainees also have a co-occurring alcohol and/or drug abuse problem (Abram & Teplin, 1991; Teplin, 1994). Although people with mental illness are at greater risk for arrest than the general population (Teplin, 1994; Rock & Landsberg, 1998), those with co-occurring substance use disorders are among the highest risk group, not only for arrest, but also for homelessness, HIV, violent behavior, poor treatment adherence, and a host of other negative, costly outcomes (Borum et al., 1997; Drake,

Bartels, Teague, Noordsy & Clark, 1993; Monahan, 1995; RachBeisel, Scott & Dixon, 1999; Steadman et al., 1998; Swartz, Swanson, Hiday, Borum & Wagner, 1998). Further, those who use alcohol or drugs and do not take their prescribed medication are three times more likely to be arrested than others with mental disorders (Borum et al., 1997), and their risk for violent behavior significantly increases (Swartz et al., 1999).

Finally, of particular relevance to the ultimate purpose of screening and assessment for individualized treatment planning and appropriate treatment matching, is the co-morbidity of other psychiatric disorders. Whether the population is defined as "co-occurring," whereby major mental illness and substance use disorders are equally present, or dually diagnosed where one or another diagnostic class predominates, other "less severe" disorders, which may have equally deleterious effects on functioning and treatment outcomes if untreated, are commonly present in both the primarily substance using populations or the primarily mentally ill criminal justice populations (Peters & Hills, 1997). These include posttraumatic stress, anxiety and phobia disorders along with chronic less severe depression, attention deficit and personality disorders (e.g., Haywood, Kravitz, Goldman & Freeman, 2000; Henderson, 1997; Peters & Hills, 1999; Teplin, Abram & McClelland, 1996; Wexler & Graham, 1993).

SCREENING FOR MENTAL ILLNESS AND SUBSTANCE ABUSE

The first step to effective management for this high-risk population is the development of systematic processes to screen for these disorders. However, there are currently few jurisdictions that systematically screen for mental health problems upon arrest, prior to or following the arraignment process, or upon entrance into the jails. Despite the remarkable prevalence of co-occurring disorders, their existence is not always evident from the defendant's arrest charge or mental status during booking. Unless the screening process is systematic, the target population may not be identified. As a result, they cannot be diverted into alternative programs or provided effective discharge planning—both of which may reduce recidivism.

In establishing a screening protocol, one preliminary question is: For what and how do we screen? With regard to mental health problems, most of the professional literature on the existence of co-occurring disorders in the criminal justice system has focused on the most severe mental disorders—schizophrenia, bipolar disorder, and major depression. However, as described above, other "less severe" disorders, such as anxiety disorders, are common among criminal justice samples and affect treatment outcomes (Peters & Hills, 1997), which may in turn affect recidivism. Specific recommendations for appropriate screening instruments may shift, depending on the type of client being referred to a specific court or court-based program, and thus the adoption of best practices must be flexible and based on the particular program parameters, including type of staff and client goals and needs. A drug using population being screened for co-occurring mental illness will have lower rates of co-occurring psychiatric disorders than those revealed within a mentally ill population being screened for co-occurring substance use disorders (Mueser, Drake & Miles, 1997; Peters & Bartoi, 1997). And the female population in these groups will likely be over-represented in terms of both serious substance use and trauma disorders, along with a host of other risk factors such as poverty, abuse histories, unstable social systems, and medical problems (El-Bassel, Gilbert, Schilling, Ivanoff & Borne, 1996; Fullilove et al., 1993; Haywood et al., 2000; Henderson, 1997; Holden, Rann & Van Drasek, 1993; Jacobson & Herald, 1990; Jordan, Schlenger, Fairbank & Caddell, 1996; Richie & Johnsen, 1996; Teplin et al., 1996). Further, the ethnic and racial composition of a program's target population will impact the choice of instruments for screening and assessment; to that end, the availability of instruments in languages other than English and the population(s) on which the instruments were developed and studied are described, as available, for each instrument reviewed below.

Finally, it is important to note that the purpose of screening is not diagnosis; it is, rather, the "flagging" of clients who need further assessment. The primary goal of an effective screening instrument is to identify the largest possible proportion of people who are likely to have a disorder. As a result, the number of people flagged will be somewhat over-inclusive. That is, although most of the people with a disorder will be flagged by the instrument, some of those flagged will be found not to have a disorder during a subsequent comprehensive assessment. This "false positive" effect has important implications for staff training, court dispositions and treatment matching: without understanding the purpose and characteristics of screening, individuals may be inappropriately labeled resulting in potential ramifications for treatment options and legal dispositions. Further, this chapter focuses solely on instruments developed to assess mental health and substance use problems in order for the collected information to be as reliable and valid as possible; this information must be placed in the context of a thorough history. Others have detailed a comprehensive list of screening and assessment components and methods for collection of that information (e.g., Peters & Hills, 1999). The screening phase, which can be conducted by non-licensed or "lay" staff, should lay the foundation for the assessment.

Assessment, on the other hand, does encompass diagnosis through structured assessment methods and collateral and self-report information, in part gathered by the program's case management or "screening" staff and integrated by the assessor, and should be conducted by a licensed trained mental health professional (Peters & Hills, 1999; Spitzer, 1983; Steadman, Morris & Dennis, 1995). Further, assessment is not static; it is a dynamic process which includes periodic reassessment over time and makes use of change measures for symptom severity (psychiatric and substance use) as well as other important domains (e.g., functionality, health, employment, risk for violence and criminal justice recidivism, etc.) (Broner, Borum, Whitmire & Gawley, 2000). The assessor should be aware of the impact of culture and ethnicity upon diagnosis (Substance Abuse Mental Health Services Administration [SAMHSA], 2000). Examples of misdiagnosis for ethnic minority populations are well documented; for instance under diagnosis of depression and over diagnosis of psychosis are common for African-Americans (Drake, Alterman & Rosenberg, 1993; Fabrega, Mezzich & Ullrich, 1988; Fiander & Bartlett, 1997; Paradis, Horn, Yang & O'Rourke, 1999; Rayburn & Stonecypher, 1996).

METHODS

A series of comprehensive literature searches were conducted to identify appropriate screening and assessment instruments to include in this review. This began with a search for all relevant journal articles and books within the PsychInfo database from 1986 to April, 2000. In addition to the database search, we also reviewed information and documents from a number of governmental agencies, including: the Center for Substance Abuse Treatment (CSAT); National Institute on Alcohol Abuse and Alcoholism (NIAAA); National Institute on Drug Abuse (NIDA); National Institute of Justice (NIJ); and Substance Abuse and Mental Health Service Administration (SAMHSA).

Recommendations were also taken from the GAINS Report (Peters & Bartoi, 1997), one of the most comprehensive and thorough evaluations of instruments for use in this population. Finally, authors of the major instruments reviewed were contacted directly to answer further questions, provide feedback, and determine whether their current, not yet published research might have relevance to our review.

Eight meetings were held with the clinical, research, MIS, and administrative personnel from Center for Court Innovation's (CCI) Brooklyn Treatment Court (BTC) in New York City (Broner, Borum & Gawley, 2001). During these meetings, BTC was briefed on the status of this review and provided input about the instrument selection process. Two focus groups were held with the program's case managers both to obtain a thorough understanding of the needs and working process of their current screening, assessment, treatment matching and placement procedures and to involve front-line staff in the instrument selection process. Each focus group lasted two hours and included three observers and a focus group leader. The researchers/observers' notes were summarized independently; themes were extracted by a group of four researchers, reviewed with administrative personnel, and incorporated into our recommendations. Additionally, answers to a survey administered to New York City policy makers, criminal justice representatives, community treatment program executives, consumers, family members, and advocates (N= 65) about the nature of the populations served in their diversion, alternative to incarceration and court programs, staff education levels, and the need for screening and assessment were summarized and further informed the direction and scope of this review.

GUIDING PRINCIPLES IN INSTRUMENT SELECTION

Validity. We sought to identify the instruments with the strongest base of research support and validity. Very few screening instruments, however, have been validated within this specific population (a drug and alcohol using mentally ill population involved in the criminal justice system), and not all studies included ethnic, racial, gender, and socioeconomic breakdowns in their descriptions of instrument development, validity, and reliability studies. In validation and reliability studies where this information was included, it will be noted in the instrument review.

Brief administration time. We attempted to locate an instrument or combination of instruments that could be used to screen for mental illness and alcohol and drug use (including route of administration, frequency and quantity), and that could be administered in approximately 20 minutes.

Administration by non-clinical interviewers. Because many individuals in this client population have difficulty with language and/or literacy, it was determined that screening instruments should be interview-based instead of self-administered. As many criminal justice programs use non-clinical staff, we determined that the recommended instruments should be able to be reliably administered, with minimal training, by lay interviewers—those with little or no formal mental health training.

Minimal cost. Screening needed to be non-proprietary and available for use without associated fees. Unless otherwise stated, the instruments reviewed below are in the public domain.

Adequate scope of coverage. After assessing the needs of a number of programs in New York City, we identified screening instruments for the following problems: Anxiety Disorders (Generalized Anxiety Disorder, Obsessive Compulsive Disorder, phobias, Post Traumatic Stress Disorder); psychotic disorders (including all of the Schizophrenias, with rule-outs for substance induced psychotic disorders); mood disorders (Bipolar Disorder and Major Depressive Disorder); substance use disorders (alcohol and illegal drugs); Personality Disorders (screening only); and suicidality.

INSTRUMENT REVIEW: SCREENING FOR CO-OCCURRING MENTAL ILLNESS AND SUBSTANCE USE

Screening for Psychiatric Syndromes (see Table 24.1)

While there is a myriad of instruments that screen for the major psychiatric syndromes targeted in this review, and even more measures of psychiatric symptom severity, the universe of instruments meeting the requirements for this project is limited. There are definite advantages, mainly for research and validity reasons, to choose a single, comprehensive instrument over a combination of disorder-specific instruments; however, given the population involved, two of the instruments (the Referral Decision Scale, Teplin & Swartz, 1989, and the Addiction Severity Index, McLellan et al., 1992) have the advantage of having been validated in forensic settings. None, however, have been validated in both forensic and known co-occurring populations.

Structured Clinical Interview for DSM-IV Screen (SCID Screen)

The Structured Clinical interview for DSM-IV (SCID-I; First, Gibbon, Spitzer & Williams, 1996a) is a comprehensive structured interview published by the American Psychiatric Association to provide clinical and research diagnoses based on the diagnostic criteria in the most recent version of the Diagnostic and Statistical Manual of Mental Disorders (DSM-IV; American Psychiatric Association [APA], 1994). The SCID Screen (First, Spitzer, Gibbon & Williams, 1998) was not designed as an independent screening measure; rather, it was intended as an aid for administration of the full SCID-I by identifying modules that could be skipped and by preventing response biases that can develop as an interviewee realizes that denying symptoms can allow him/her to exit the interview more quickly (First et al., 1996a; First, Gibbon, Spitzer & Williams, 1996b).

The advantage of the SCID Screen is that it is based on the American Psychiatric Association's SCID-I and is directly linked to DSM-IV criteria. Additionally, most of the SCID is available in Spanish and is being translated into ten or more other languages. However, in its current form, it does not include items for mood disorders or for Post Traumatic Stress Disorder. Although screening items for these disorders could be added

Table 24.1 Summary of Psychiatric Screening Instruments

Screening Instrument	Training Level	Admin Time	Language Availability	Disorders Screened	Validity and Reliability
Structured Clinical Interview for DSM-IV Screen (SCID Screen), (First et al., 1998)	Unknown; Full SCID: Clinician administered w/ extensive training	Approx. 10 min.	Full SCID in 12 languages, including Spanish	Mood and PTSD disorders not in screen; can adapt SCID skip out questions	Reliability and validity studies of the screening version have not been done
Composite International Diagnostic Interview-Short Form (CIDI-SF), (Kessler et al., in press)	Lay interviewer w/ training	Approx. 10 min.	Full CIDI in 25 languages, including Spanish	Substance Use Disorders are DSM-IIIR-based other disorders are DSM-IV-based disorders. No Psychotic and PTSD disorders are not measured	No reliability or validation studies of the Short Form currently published; complicated scoring

Table 24.1 (continued)

Screening Instrument	Training Level	Admin Time	Language Availability	Disorders Screened	Validity and Reliability
Addiction Severity Index, Psychiatric Subscale (McLellan et al., 1992	Lay interviewer w/ training	Approx. 10 min., psych. subscale only	Spanish and eight other languages	Index of psychiatric symptoms; does not screen for specific disorders	Initially validated among men in chemical dependency programs; subsequently used with women and in forensic settings; inter-rater reliability poor with inpatients
Mini-International Neuropsychiatric Interview (M.I.N.I.), (Sheehan, Lecrubier, Janavs, et al., 2000a)	Lay interviewer w/ training	Approx. 15 min.	37 languages	All major Axis I DSM-IV disorders; modular format allows choice	M.I.N.I. validated against full versions of SCID and CIDI with good results in psychiatric and control subjects; validation studies not conducted among co-occurring or forensic populations. Inter-rater reliability high, with test-retest lower
Referral Decision Scale (RDS), (Teplin & Schwartz, 1989)	Lay interviewer	Less than 10 min.	No translations cited in current literature	Psychotic, bipolar, major depressive disorders	Extensive validation in forensic populations with ethnically diverse subjects; good validity and reliability, but with high false positive rates in several studies and question if disorders can be discriminated from each other

by including the first, skip-out questions from the respective modules, our primary concern about its use in court-based diversion screening is that the instrument was not designed for use as a stand-alone measure, and there are no data available regarding its sensitivity (ability to accurately identify people who have the disorder) and/or specificity (ability to accurately identify those who do not have the disorder) when used in this capacity. Since a trained clinician must administer the SCID-I, the SCID Screen may also require a higher level of professional training than is typically available in court-based programs. The utility of the SCID-I as a full assessment instrument has been extensively reviewed (e.g., for a summary see Broner et al., 2000; Segal, Hersen, & Van Hasselt, 1994).

Composite International Diagnostic Interview—Short Form (CIDI-SF)

The CIDI-SF (Kessler, Andrews, Mroczek, Ustun & Wittchen, in press) was designed as a screener or short form of the World Health Organization's Composite International Diagnostic Interview (CIDI), version 1.0 (World Health Organization [WHO], 1990). The advantages of the CIDI-SF are the brevity of administration time (less than ten minutes), its connection to the CIDI, an instrument used in large-scale epidemiologic studies, and its ability to be administered by lay interviewers. Despite these features, the CIDI-SF is not completely based on the most current version of the DSM (substance disorders are based on DSM-III-R), and it does not screen at all for two critical disorders of interest: psychotic disorders and Post Traumatic Stress Disorder (PTSD). In addition, the instrument has not been validated in a sample other than the one on which it was first developed; therefore, it has not been validated in a forensic setting or with a sample of people with co-occurring mental health and substance use disorders. The format of the CIDI Short Form is also more difficult to follow than that of comparable instruments and could require a greater investment in staff training time to achieve proficiency.

Addiction Severity Index, Psychiatric Subscale (ASI-Psychiatric Subscale)

The Addiction Severity Index (ASI; McLellan et al., 1992) has been used extensively in clinical settings and research studies to assess substance use disorders. The ASI subscale that assesses psychiatric problems takes about 10 minutes to administer and consists of questions about psychiatric history, and the presence of psychiatric symptoms in the past 30 days as well as observer ratings based on the client's current presentation. Although scores on the ASI-Psychiatric Subscale are significantly correlated with having any DSM-IV Axis I psychiatric diagnosis (Dixon, Myers, Johnson & Corty, 1996), it does not offer any specific guidance regarding the type of disorder that is likely to exist. This would notably limit its utility for treatment matching. Moreover, the need for observer ratings may increase training time and introduce potential problems in obtaining consistent scores from different interviewers, thus, decreasing inter-rater reliability as demonstrated in a study of inpatients by Appleby, Dyson, Altman and Luchins (1997). The instrument was developed and validated on male clients entering chemical dependency programs (ethnic and socioeconomic sample characteristics were not reported) (Cosden, 1994), although it has since been used extensively in forensic samples and among women. The authors note that the ASI has been translated into nine languages; however, validation studies using these versions have not been published.

Referral Decision Scale (RDS)

The Referral Decision Scale (RDS) (Teplin & Swartz, 1989) is composed of 14 items from the Diagnostic Interview Schedule (DIS; Robins, Cottler, Bucholz & Compton, 1998; Robins, Helzer, Croughan & Ratcliff, 1981; Robins, Marcus, Reich, Cunningham & Gallagher, 1998)) selected for their statistical ability to identify people with lifetime diagnoses of major depression, bipolar disorder or schizophrenia. Using DIS diagnosis as a criterion, the RDS produced a sensitivity of .79 and specificity of .99 in a validation sample of jail admissions and sentenced inmates (Teplin & Swartz, 1989). The authors did not present data on the internal consistency, test-retest, or inter-rater reliability of the instrument.

In contrast to the scope of other screening instruments, the RDS only screens for three major psychiatric disorders: depression, schizophrenia, and bipolar disorder. Nevertheless, it is quite brief (14 items, one of which is used in two of the scales), easy to administer and score, and its development, as well as the establishment of population norms, occurred within criminal justice settings. The validation sample was predominantly young (mean age 26 years), male, mainly black (more than 80%), and had an average of 11 years of education; more than half were unemployed at the time of arrest (Teplin & Swartz, 1989).

Since the initial validation of the RDS in 1989, it has been evaluated with mixed results by other investigators in criminal justice settings. Although it has not yet been systematically validated in a forensic sample of individuals previously known to have co-occurring disorders, both chemical dependency and major mental illness affected many of the persons in the validation samples. In a sample of 790 men in an urban jail, the RDS was found to have excellent reliability (interrater reliabilities ranged from .89 to .93) and adequate validity, but the authors also found that it generated a large number of false positives (Hart, Roesch, Corrado & Cox, 1993); when these researchers adjusted the cut-off level for the depression scale (increasing the number of symptoms required for a positive finding from two to three), specificity levels improved. Even with these changes, however, the RDS made a large number of false positive errors relative to concurrent and subsequent full psychiatric assessments. This latter finding has generated much of the criticism of the RDS in the literature. In spite of replicating these findings, others have found that the RDS has good sensitivity and perhaps adequate specificity for this type of brief screener, making it a useful tool (DiCataldo, Greer, & Profit 1995; Veysey, Steadman, Morrissey, Johnsen & Beckstead, 1998). For example, in a multisite study of mentally ill jail detainees (90% were men; 43% were white, 53% black, and 4% Hispanic; the average age was 34), Veysey et al. (1998) note sensitivity rates ranging from .73 to .85 with specificity rates varying only from .16 to .31 when the RDS was compared to psychiatric diagnosis.

Rogers, Sewell, Ustad, Reinhardt, and Edwards (1995) tested the convergent and discriminant validity of the RDS in a sample of male inmates from the mental health unit in a jail, most of whom were of low normal or borderline intelligence with 11 years of schooling; 31% were black, 6% were Hispanic, and 54% were white. They found that the total RDS scale score had adequate internal consistency (alpha = .78), but that exceedingly high intercorrelations between the subscales for the three disorders limited the tool's convergent validity. Although the RDS may not distinguish which inmates have which disorders, these authors note that it may provide an adequate screening for general psychological impairment.

An additional problem with the RDS, based on the nature of the dual disorders population, is that substance induced mental disorders are not adequately ruled out. A possible solution to this problem and to the problem of the high false positive rates of the RDS might be to add a question to this instrument to rule out substance induced disorders. Because this rule-out was not built in to the instrument, however, its addition could affect the instrument's validity and reliability in unknown ways. Although the RDS is a relatively brief instrument and could be easily translated into other languages, there is no evidence in the literature that any translation has been attempted.

Mini-International Neuropsychiatric Interview (M.I.N.I.)

The only single instrument that both screens for all major DSM-IV Axis I disorders including the schizophrenias, mood disorders, anxiety disorders, substance dependence, and eating disorders, has a brief suicidality screen, and has an administration time of approximately 15 minutes is the Mini-International Neuropsychiatric Interview (M.I.N.I.; Sheehan et al., 2000a). The instrument was specifically designed to be used by both clinicians and lay staff, after limited training. The instrument is composed of a series of independent modules for each disorder, with the number of questions in each module ranging from a low of 2 to a high of about 20. In each module, the first two to three items determine whether the entire module needs to be administered. By having a skip-out exit strategy overall administration time can be reduced. The modular structure also allows the user to choose which disorders are to be screened and to eliminate modules that are unnecessary for a given application.

The M.I.N.I. has been used to diagnose alcohol dependence, psychosis, anxiety disorders, and depression in studies in Europe (Bergey et al., 1999; Berlin et al., 1997; Lejoyeux, Feuche, Loi, Solomon & Ades, 1999; Lejoyeux, Haberman, Solomon & Ades, 1999; Tylee, 1996). It has also been translated into 37 languages, and tested in international studies against two of the most well-validated full-length structured and semi-structured diagnostic interviews, the Composite International Diagnostic Interview (CIDI; WHO, 1990) and the Structured Clinical Interview for DSM-III-R (SCID; Spitzer, Williams, Gibbon & First, 1990). When the M.I.N.I. was administered by a clinician, as opposed to self-administered by the patient, it has shown high levels of overall agreement with these full assessments (Sheehan et al., 1998). Using the SCID as a criterion, the sensitivity (the ability to accurately identify people who have the disorder) of the clinician-administered M.I.N.I. for individual Axis I disorders ranged from .45 to .96, with sensitivity reaching .70 or greater for all but three of the modules (i.e., dysthymia, obsessive-compulsive disorder, and current drug dependence). The specificity (the ability to identify people who do not have the disorder) was .85 or higher for all modules. When the CIDI was used as the criterion, sensitivity of the M.I.N.I. was .70 or greater for all but four modules (i.e., panic disorder, agoraphobia, simple phobia, and lifetime bulimia); specificity was .70 or greater for all modules. Reported rates of interrater agreement ranged from a *kappa* of .79 to 1.00. Rates for test-retest consistency were not as high, ranging from .35 to 1.00, but the authors note that reliability was likely attenuated by the use of a different interviewer for the second administration (Sheehan et al., 1998). In the international validation studies, the sample was 62% female, included both psychiatric patients and community comparison subjects, and drew subjects from the United States, France, Italy, Spain, and the United Kingdom. The sample was primarily white and information on socioeconomic status was not presented; the authors acknowledge this as a limitation of their work (Lecrubier et al., 1997).

The M.I.N.I. also offers an expanded version, the M.I.N.I.-Plus (Sheehan et al., 2000b), containing modules for additional disorders not included in the M.I.N.I. (e.g., ADHD or Adjustment Disorders) as well as expanded modules for disorders such as mania, substance abuse, and psychotic disorders. These expanded modules allow for further clarification of time frame or DSM-IV classifications. It is possible to use expanded modules from the M.I.N.I.-Plus selectively in place of the corresponding M.I.N.I. module without compromising the validity of either instrument.

Despite these advantages of brevity and comprehensiveness, the M.I.N.I., like other comprehensive diagnostic interviews, has not been validated with a criminal justice population. A further limitation of the M.I.N.I. for court-based diversion screening is the relatively low sensitivity and specificity for the drug and alcohol abuse modules. Although the validity of these modules is adequate for general clinical assessment, given that populations screened in court-based diversion programs are likely to have high rates of substance abuse problems, the alcohol/drug modules of the M.I.N.I. could be replaced with a substance use screening instrument that has been standardized and validated within a criminal justice population. (A discussion of screening instruments for substance use disorders follows this section.) Finally, in order to reduce false positive rates, the addition of a rule-out question could be added to each screening module for which the DSM-IV provides a substance-induced category.

Screening for Substance Use Disorders (see Table 24.2)

In their comprehensive review of screening and assessment instruments for co-occurring disorders in the justice system, Peters and Bartoi (1997) detailed the limitations of currently available materials. A substantial amount of research has focused on screening and assessing substance use disorders in the criminal justice system; however there are relatively few studies addressing the validity of these instruments in samples with co-occurring mental illness. Additionally, many of the well-studied instruments address either alcohol or drug use but not both, and few assess both frequency and severity of use, each of which can be used to measure ongoing treatment progress and to evaluate program success. An appraisal of symptom severity also may help to inform recommendations about intensity of treatment (e.g., residential versus outpatient).

Instruments that Screen for Both Alcohol and Drug Use

Texas Christian University Drug Screen (TCUDS). The Texas Christian University

Table 24.2 Summary of Substance Use Screening Instruments

Screening Instrument	Form of Admin.	Admin. Time	Language Availability	Disorders Screened	Validity and Reliability
Texas Christian University Drug Screen (TCUDS), (Texas Christian University, 1997)	Lay interviewer with training; self-admin. 8th grade reading.	5–10 min.	Spanish translation used by other researchers	Items closely tied to DSM-IV criteria; screen yields score of likelihood of substance dependence; assesses frequency not quantity	Validated in forensic settings; not formally validated in co-occurring population; inter-rater reliability good for "ever used," marginal to good for drug related problems; very good sensitivity and specificity on earlier version (BBA)
Simple Screening Instrument (SSI), (CSAT, 1999)	Lay interviewer and self-admin. version	Approx. 10 min.	No translations cited in current literature	Alcohol and drug use; yields scores for likelihood of abuse and need for assessment; does not assess frequency or quantity	Validated with high sensitivity and specificity in a forensic population; good internal consistency found in at least one study; other forms of reliability not reported

303

Table 24.2 *(continued)*

Screening Instrument	Form of Admin.	Admin. Time	Language Availability	Disorders Screened	Validity and Reliability
Dartmouth Assessment of Lifestyle Instrument (DALI), (Rosenberg et al., 1998)	Lay interviewer with training	Approx. 10 min.	No translations available	Screens for alcohol, cannabis, and cocaine use only; yields cut-off score for substance use disorder; does not assess frequency or quantity	Validated in psychiatric inpatient population against patients' SCID diagnosis with high sensitivity and specificity; a new instrument and authors did not present reliability
Alcohol Use Disorders Identification Test (AUDIT), (Bohn et al., 1995)	Lay interviewer	Approx. 5 min.	Four languages, including Spanish	Alcohol use and associated symptoms; assesses both frequency and quantity of alcohol consumption	Validated among men and women alcoholics in treatment; compared well to biological and self-report data. Internal consistency good in several studies; test-retest and parallel forms reliability not reported. High sensitivity, poor specificity for lifetime use, but good for current use

Table 24.2 (*continued*)

Screening Instrument	Form of Admin.	Admin. Time	Language Availability	Disorders Screened	Validity and Reliability
Addiction Severity Index-Drug Use Section (ASI-Drug), (McLellan et al., 1992)	Lay interviewer with training	Approx. 10 min.	Spanish and eight other language	Assesses drug use and associated symptoms; yields score of need for intervention; assesses frequency and route of administration, but not quantity	Initial validation studies with male veterans in treatment for substance abuse; ASI validated in forensic settings. Inter-rater and test-retest reliability good in former settings; mixed results reported among psychiatric patients
Michigan Alcohol Screening Test (MAST), (Selzer, 1971)	Lay interviewer or self-admin.	Approx. 10 min.	No translations cited in current literature	Alcohol use only; yields cut-off scores on likelihood of current alcoholism; does not assess frequency or severity	Validated against other alcohol screens in forensic, substance using, and psychiatric populations; adequate internal consistency; sensitivity and specificity vary widely per studies

Table 24.2 (continued)

Screening Instrument	Form of Admin.	Admin. Time	Language Availability	Disorders Screened	Validity and Reliability
Drug Abuse Screening Test (DAST) (Skinner, 1983)	Lay interviewer	Approx 10 min.	French	Drug use only; yields cut-off scores on likelihood of current drug problems	Proprietary instrument. Validated in psychiatric populations with acceptable results; internal consistency was good; other forms of reliability not assessed
TWEAK (Russell & Bigler, 1979) & CAGE (Mayfield et al., 1974)	Lay interviewer	Less than 5 min.	TWEAK: No translations cited; CAGE: Spanish	Alcohol use only; yields cut-off scores on likelihood of current alcohol problems; neither instrument assesses frequency or severity of consumption	TWEAK: Validated among low-income minority women; showed good sensitivity and specificity; reliability not presented. CAGE: standardized among alcoholic, primarily white men; since used in diverse populations; and in psychiatric populations; not standardized in forensic settings; reported to have good internal consistency; excellent specificity

Drug Screen (TCUDS; Texas Christian University [TCU] Institute of Behavioral Research, 1997) is a substance abuse screening measure derived from an earlier instrument, the Brief Background Assessment (BBA; Broome, Knight, Joe & Simpson, 1996; Simpson, Knight & Hiller, 1997). The TCUDS is a brief (15 item), easily scored scale that probes for alcohol and drug use. It was one of the top recommendations of Peters and Bartoi (1997), and was found by Peters and Greenbaum (1996) to be one of the most sensitive and specific measures for identifying substance dependent versus non-dependent inmates (overall accuracy rates of 82% were based on the BBA). The earlier version (BBA) was tested within a population of probationers convicted of drug-related crimes to determine whether differences arose between self-administration and administered interviews. They found that results were similar for the two different modes of administration; *kappa* coefficients for the "ever used" drug and alcohol section ranged from .65 to .94; *kappa* coefficients for drug-related problem items ranged from .38 to .81 (Broome et al., 1996). A distinct advantage of the TCUDS is that it is closely tied to DSM-IV criteria for substance dependence. The TCUDS has an eighth-grade reading level (TCU Institute of Behavioral Research, 1998) and has been translated into Spanish by the Texas Department of Criminal Justice, although no formal translations have been evaluated (K. Knight, personal communication, October 25, 1999). A large (expected N=4,000) validation study is currently being conducted using data collected by the Texas Department of Criminal Justice, which selected the TCUDS as its primary screening instrument.

Like most other instruments, the TCUDS has not been systematically validated within a sample of individuals previously known to have co-occurring mental illness. An additional limitation of the instrument is that while it does assess frequency of substance use it does not assess severity of use, thus limiting its usefulness for monitoring ongoing treatment progress or identifying "problem drinking/drug use" that does not meet diagnostic criteria for substance dependence. This limitation could be addressed by adding a "quantity" column to the existing frequency table. Although the frequency portion of the interview is not formally scored (and thus changing it would not affect the score a client would obtain), the addition of information on severity could assist the interviewer/case manager in forming a more complete impression of the client's overall substance use pattern.

Simple Screening Instrument (SSI). The Simple Screening Instrument for Alcohol and Other Drug Abuse (SSI), developed by the Center for Substance Abuse Treatment [CSAT] (CSAT, 1999), is composed of items derived from other well-known instruments. No foreign language translations are cited in current literature for the SSI. There are currently no reliability data available for the SSI, but Peters and Greenbaum (1996) found that, of the instruments studied, it had the highest sensitivity for alcohol or drug dependence among the inmate population. A small study was done with an instrument slightly modified from the SSI, called Screening for Alcohol and Drug Abuse (SADA; Winters, 1995). Although there are differences between the two versions (mainly in the time frame— the SADA uses a 12-month time frame while the SSI uses six months), the scoring sections for the two are almost exactly the same. In this small sample of subjects in a drug evaluation program, the SADA showed high internal consistency (.91 males, .89 females) and high sensitivity (.97); specificity was moderate (.55). Other measures of reliability were not presented.

A limitation of the SSI is that it does not assess frequency and severity of use. This limitation could be partially overcome with the addition of an instrument such as the Drug/Alcohol six-month Follow-Back Calendar developed by the Dartmouth Psychiatric Research Center (1997) which, although not scored or formally validated, would assist the interviewer in forming a more complete impression of the client's overall substance use patterns and severity. Further, this instrument could be re-administered throughout treatment to monitor symptom severity over time. The reliability and validity of the time-line follow-back approach, using a calendar and other cues to prompt memory, has been documented among psychiatric outpatients (Carey, 1997), and a similar format is used in a number of proprietary and non-proprietary drug and alcohol screening measures.

Dartmouth Assessment of Lifestyle Instrument (DALI). The Dartmouth Assessment of Lifestyle Instrument (DALI; Rosenberg et al., 1998) is a promising new measure developed to assess the presence of substance use disorders among people with severe mental illness. The instrument is composed of 18 items, derived from six widely used screening instruments that had been administered to a psychiatric inpatient sample. Those items that predicted a SCID substance abuse diagnosis were selected for the DALI, and the resulting instrument was validated on an independent psychiatric inpatient sample. The 18-item DALI showed higher sensitivity (.80) and specificity (1.00) in the validation sample than any of the six instruments from which it was derived. The authors did not present information on the internal consistency, test-retest, or inter-rater reliability of the instrument.

Because the DALI has only recently been developed, no additional validation studies have been reported in the literature, although the authors report that it is currently being studied in a large outpatient psychiatric sample in New York State (S.D. Rosenberg, personal communication, September 3, 1999). An additional limitation of the DALI is that the sample on which the instrument was developed was composed mainly of white subjects from rural areas. These demographic limitations indicate the need for future validation in more diverse populations before it could be recommended for routine use within an urban, ethnically and racially diverse population. The instrument is also currently only available in English. A more substantive limitation to the instrument is that it only screens for alcohol, cannabis, and cocaine use, limiting its usefulness in communities where opioid use, for example, is prevalent. Additionally, it does not assess quantity or frequency of use.

Combinations of Instruments to Screen for Drug and Alcohol Use

Alcohol Use Disorders Identification Test (AUDIT). The AUDIT is a 10-item instrument for detecting alcohol abuse (National Institute on Alcohol Abuse and Alcoholism [NIAAA], 1999); it asks questions for both frequency and severity of use. The AUDIT has been translated into four languages, including Spanish, and been used and validated among diverse populations, including both female (Davis & Wood, 1999) and male (Luckie, White, Miller & Icenogle, 1995) veterans, Hispanics (Cherpitel, 1999), patients in treatment for drug and alcohol abuse (Lennings, Scott, Harris, Kingsbury & Andrew, 1998), male general medical patients (Bradley, McDonell, Kivlahan, Diehr & Fihn, 1998), and black, white, and Hispanic emergency room patients (Cherpitel, 1998).

The initial validation study of the AUDIT was conducted on a sample of alcoholics in rehabilitation treatment who were compared to a general medical sample. Roughly equal numbers of men and women were recruited, with a mean age of 32 years and mean education of 13.8 years; racial and ethnic breakdown of the sample was not provided (Bohn, Babor & Kramzler, 1995). In this study, the AUDIT was found to have good concurrent validity, correlating significantly with several self-report and biological measures of alcohol dependence and with information from clinical records and presenting complaints. The reliability of the AUDIT has been evaluated in several studies using different samples including substance abusers and alcoholics, primary care patients and college students. Internal consistency has been high, with *alpha* coefficients ranging from .77 to .94 among substance abusers (Allen, Litten, Fertig & Babor, 1997). Test-retest and parallel forms reliability, however, have not been reported.

A number of subsequent validity studies have already been conducted on this relatively new instrument. In an extensive review Allen et al. (1997) note the AUDIT, when measured against DSM-III-R criteria, tends to show high sensitivity (.78 to 1.00) for lifetime and current abuse or dependence, but lower specificity particularly for lifetime use (.25 to .29) though adequate for current/recent abuse or dependence (.59 to .96), generating a moderate rate of false positives. The levels of sensitivity and specificity appear comparable for men and women, thus making the measure equally useful in both groups. Likewise, no differences in sensitivity and specificity have been reported for different racial/ethnic groups; the AUDIT has performed similarly among blacks, Hispanics, and whites in the few studies that have examined this variable. An additional advantage of the AUDIT is that the World Health Organization is currently developing a corresponding screening instrument for drug abuse that is similar in form and brevity. This instrument, currently being field tested, will be called the Alcohol and Substance Involvement Screening Test (ASIST; T.F. Babor, personal communication, September 16, 1999). Until this instrument is evaluated, however, the Drug Use section of the Addiction Severity Index (McLellan et al., 1992) serves as a reasonable companion instrument.

Addiction Severity Index-Drug and Alcohol Scale (ASI-Drug). The second part of this combination screen, the Addiction Severity Index Drug and Alcohol Scale (McLellan et al., 1992), has been found to have high levels of sensitivity and specificity within criminal justice populations (Peters & Greenbaum, 1996). No other study has examined the psychometric properties of the Drug Use Subscale specifically; however, a large number of studies have been conducted using the ASI generally. The instrument is available in nine languages, but as previously noted, the ethnic and socioeconomic breakdown of the original validation sample is not presented (Cosden, 1994). The initial reliability studies on the ASI were based on a sample of male veterans on a substance abuse unit in a VA hospital. Interrater and test-retest reliabilities were .83 or greater for the most recent version of the test (McLellan et al., 1992). The validity of the ASI has been examined among diverse populations. It has been found to be reliable in a sample of women in substance abuse treatment (Cosden & Cortez-Ison, 1999) and among alcohol and/or cocaine dependent men (Cacciola, Koppenhaver, McKay & Alterman, 1999). The ASI has also been shown to provide a valid measure of drug and alcohol abuse among black men and women and Hispanic men and women with an average age of 37 years and an average education of 11 years (Brown, Alterman, Rutherford & Cacciola, 1993). Additionally, Joyner, Wright and Devine (1996) used the ASI among homeless substance users and found in this sample, which was 70% men, 80% African-American, with an average age of 30 years and an average education of 11 years, that the ASI provided reliable and valid data regarding patients' substance use. In forensic settings, the ASI was administered to male prisoners, mean age 27 with 42% belonging to an ethnic minority, and was found to be both reliable (internally consistent) and valid as compared to the individual's DIS diagnosis (Amoureus, van den Hurk, Schippers & Breteler, 1994). Vigdal and Stadler (1996) also report on its use for program and treatment planning within the Wisconsin Department of Corrections. The ASI measures frequency of drug use and route of administration, but not severity.

Among psychiatric patients, the drug and alcohol section of the ASI has been widely used, but mixed results have been reported in the literature. Dyson et al. (1998) report that among a primarily black psychiatric inpatient sample, the ASI demonstrated high reliability and good validity relative to other alcohol screens. In their study discussed in the previous section, Appleby et al. (1997) found that among inpatients in a public psychiatric facility, the drug and alcohol section of the ASI correlated significantly and meaningfully with other substance use instruments as well as with DSM-III-R diagnosis. On the other hand, poor reliability (inter-rater and test-retest) of the instrument was found among community mental health center patients (in treatment for both psychiatric and substance abuse problems) (Zanis, McLellan & Corse, 1997); patients in this sample were 74% male, 57% black, with a mean age of 37 years. Among homeless mentally ill persons averaging 37 years old, 71% of whom were men and 50% of whom were black or Hispanic, the ASI was found to underestimate the severity of substance abuse as compared to caseworker observations (Goldfinger, Schutt, Seidman & Turner, 1996). Although they found adequate reliability and validity for the drug and alcohol sections of the ASI among outpatients with severe mental illness, Carey, Cocco and Correia (1997) conclude that the ASI should be used with caution among patients who have severe mental illness.

Alcohol Use Disorders Identification Test (AUDIT) and Addiction Severity Index Drug Use Section (ASI-Drug). Another top choice of Peters and Bartoi (1997) was the combination of the Alcohol Dependence Scale (ADS; Skinner & Horn, 1984) with the drug use section of the ASI. However, the ADS is a proprietary instrument and is not available for free use. One alternative is to use the AUDIT, which, together with the ASI-Drug Use Section, would comprehensively screen for alcohol and other substance use disorders, as well as measure frequency and severity for alcohol use and frequency and route of drug administration, though not severity for drug use.

Michigan Alcohol Screening Test (MAST). The Michigan Alcohol Screening Test (MAST; Selzer, 1971) has several versions. The original is a 25-item instrument that can be self-administered or read by a lay interviewer in approximately 10 minutes. There is also a Short version (SMAST) consisting of 13 items and a Brief MAST consisting of 10 items (NIAAA, 1999). The original validation sample (Selzer, 1971) consisted exclusively of white males drawn from a range of socioeconomic strata (Hollingshead & Redlich, 1958). Five groups were included in the sample: "hospitalized alcoholics, a control group, drivers convicted of driving under the influence of alcohol, persons convicted of drunk and disorderly behavior, and drivers who had incurred 12 penalty points in two years for moving violations and accidents" (Selzer, 1971). Validity was assessed by a record review of medical facilities, social agencies, and arrest and traffic records. Sensitivity and specificity rates were not calculated; only percentages were reported. Most notably, 98% of hospitalized alcoholics scored five or more points, the recommended cut-off score; however, only 55% of drunken drivers and 59% of the drunk and disorderly obtained a score in this range. In addition, 15 false negatives were reported, but Selzer notes that later record review indicated that these respondents had not accurately answered questions related to prior arrests and hospitalizations.

The psychometric properties of the MAST have been extensively evaluated. Zung (1979) determined the internal consistency of the 25-item version of the test was adequate (alphas greater than .83) in two samples of DWI arrestees with an average age of 41 years and average education of 10 years; approximately 20% were black, 14% Latino, and less than 10% were women. Other measures of reliability of the instrument were not presented. In a large sample of female offenders with an average age of 28 years (other demographic information not provided), internal consistency was .88 (Saltstone, Halliwell, & Hayslip, 1994). Other measures of reliability were not presented for these two studies. This instrument also correlates highly with the ADS (Ross, Gavin, & Skinner, 1990), the alcohol screening instrument recommended most highly by Peters and Bartoi (1997). It has been used widely with both forensic, substance using and psychiatric populations (Blevins, Morton, & McCabe, 1996; Firestone et al., 1998; Saltstone et al., 1994; Searles, Alterman, & Purtill, 1990). Across numerous studies, the MAST has shown sensitivity rates between .36 and .98 and specificity rates from .36 to .96 (Storgaard, Nielsen & Gluud, 1994). The MAST, however, does not assess frequency or severity and no foreign language translations have been identified. In addition, the lifetime timeframe of the questions renders it inapplicable for measuring a change in status over time (Lyons, Howard, O'Mahoney & Lish, 1997).

Drug Abuse Screening Test (DAST). Although the Drug Abuse Screening Test (DAST; Center for Addiction and Mental Health, 1999; Skinner, 1982) is widely used and has been found to have sound psychometric properties in psychiatric populations (Cocco & Carey, 1998; Staley & El Guebaly, 1990), it is not a public instrument, thus it cannot be recommended based on the stated criteria. In addition, the DAST has many of the same problems as the MAST, mainly because it was based on the MAST—it does not measure frequency, severity or type of drug used; does not address alcohol abuse, and cannot be used as a change measure due to the lifetime nature of the questions. The original sample was drawn from individuals who sought help at the Clinical Institute of the Addiction Research Foundation (Skinner, 1982). Seventy-two percent of the subjects were male; no racial or ethic data was published. In this sample, internal consistency, assessed as coefficient *alpha*, was .92; no other forms of reliability were presented. In the study of incarcerated women discussed in the section on the MAST (Saltstone et al., 1994), internal consistency of the DAST was .88; no other forms of reliability were presented.

Brief Alcohol Screening Measures

The CAGE and the TWEAK. The CAGE questionnaire (Mayfield, McLeod & Hall, 1974) consists of four items that ask whether the patient feels that they should Cut down on their drinking, whether they have felt Annoyed by criticism of their drinking, Guilty about their drinking, or needed an Eye-opener (a drink in the morning). This instrument is easy to administer and score, and requires no special training. Published versions have appeared in several translations, including French (e.g., Chignon et al., 1998) and Spanish (e.g., Garcia-Campayo, Lobo, Perez-Escheverria & Campos, 1998). The authors found the test to have good internal consistency (i.e., correlations coefficients ranged from .60 to .89), excellent specificity (i.e., .89 when cut off was established for two to three positive responses) and criterion validity in the initial validation sample, which was primarily male (99%), white (77%), middle aged (63% were between 35 and 55 years), and from lower socioeconomic classes (Mayfield et al., 1974). The instrument was initially normed on alcoholic men, and is currently used mainly in primary care settings (Chan, Pristach & Welte, 1994). Although it has been used to screen for alcohol disorders among mentally ill patients, it has not been normed in forensic settings. Additionally, current research suggests that it is less accurate in classifying women than men (Peters & Bartoi, 1997).

The TWEAK Test (Russell & Bigler, 1979) consists of five questions that ask about alcohol *T*olerance, whether friends or relatives have *W*orried about the patient's drinking, whether the patient ever uses alcohol as an *E*ye-opener in the morning, about alcohol related *A*mnesia or blackouts, and whether the patient has ever felt the need to *C(K)*ut down on their drinking. The test takes less than two minutes to administer with no training required and scoring is simple. To date, this screen has not appeared in any published foreign language translation (M. Russell, personal communication, October 25, 1999). This is one of the few alcohol screening tests to be developed and normed among primarily black, inner-city women, although norms have subsequently been developed (with adjusted scoring criteria) for many other groups including general household participants and hospital clinic and emergency room patients (Chan, Pristach, Welte & Russell, 1993). Relative to other brief alcohol screens such as the CAGE, Brief MAST and AUDIT, it shows good sensitivity (.84) and specificity (.86) at a three-item cut-off (Cherpitel, 1995; Russell, 1994). The TWEAK does not assess frequency or quantity of substance use, and there are no reports in the literature on its use or evaluation in any forensic or psychiatric setting.

Screening for Personality Disorders (see Table 24.3)

Comprehensive assessment of personality disorders is difficult and time consuming. Several instruments have been developed for the assessment of personality disorders, but for a variety of reasons, most are not amenable to use in court-based diversion programs. Principally, these are comprehensive diagnostic measures not screening instruments, and thus require a significant investment of time and other resources to administer (Langbehn et al., 1999). Furthermore, many are proprietary instruments, making their cost prohibitive to some public sector agencies. There is no known screening instrument for identifying personality disorders that has demonstrated adequate levels of sensitivity and specificity in a criminal justice sample. The ideal screening instrument—particularly, one normed within criminal justice samples—is thus unavailable. Future research efforts should focus on developing a brief measure to screen for the likely presence or absence of specific personality disorder clusters in criminal justice populations.

There are additional practical and conceptual limitations to the development of such a screen, however, due to the ongoing, long-term nature of personality disorders. The DSM-IV states that the diagnosis of a personality disorder requires the clinician to assess the stability of the traits over time and across different situations and goes on to caution that "although a single interview with the person is sometimes sufficient for making the diagnosis, it is often necessary to conduct more than one interview and to space these over time" (APA, 1994, p. 630). This task is further complicated by numerous difficulties inherent in assessing personality disorders among a substance abusing population (DeJong, Van den Brink, Harteveld & Van der Wielen, 1993; Lehman, 1996). Current best practice recommendations for personality disorder assessment suggest the use of self-report inventory as a screening device and a semi-structured interview for follow-up in making a definitive diagnosis (Widiger & Sanderson, 1995). Despite these limitations, it is nevertheless plausible that there may be clinical and predictive value in trying to screen for personality disorders within a treatment court setting. While there is research on antisocial and borderline personality disorders in the forensic population, there is no available peer reviewed research on the impact of personality disorders on treatment matching and retention for the co-occurring, seriously mentally ill, substance abusing criminal justice population. However, clinical observation suggests that the presence of personality disorders has significant impact on treatment retention and efficacy for this population. In the following section, four possible options for screening for personality disorders are described. Finally, the relevance of screening for antisocial personality within a criminal justice population is briefly addressed.

Table 24.3 Summary of Personality Disorder Screening Instruments

Screening Instrument	Form of Admin.	Admin. Time	Language Availability	Disorders Screened	Validity and Reliability
Iowa Personality Disorder Screen (Langbehn, et al., 1999)	Lay interviewer	Approx. 10 min.	No translations available (SIDP-IV available in Italian)	Screens for any DSM-IV personality disorder, not for specific disorders	Validity of screen assessed relative to full SIDP-IV; screen shows good sensitivity and specificity relative to full assessment. Inter-rater reliability of full screen acceptable; other reliabilities not presented
Structured Clinical Interview for DSM Personality Disorders Screen (SCID II Screen) (First, et al., 1997a)	Clinician administered or self-administered with follow -up by clinician	At least 30 min.	Full SCID available in Spanish	All DSM-IV personality disorders	Reliability and Validity analyses of the screen alone have not been evaluated; authors do not recommend the screen be used alone without the full SCID II assessment instrument

Table 24.2 *(continued)*

Screening Instrument	Form of Admin.	Admin. Time	Language Availability	Disorders Screened	Validity and Reliability
Personality Diagnostic Questionnaire-4+ (PDQ-4+) (Hyler, 1994)	Lay administered	At least 30 min.	Translated into Spanish, Dutch, and Chinese	All DSM-IV personality disorders	Validation studies against the SCID-II varied from poor to acceptable results and with differing versions; used in forensic, substance using, and psychiatric populations; test-retest and internal consistencies not reported
M.I.N.I Antisocial Personality (Sheehan, Lecrubier, Janavs, et al., 2000a)	Lay interviewer with training; also has a self-administered version	Less than 5 min.	Translated into 36 languages	Antisocial Personality Disorder	M.I.N.I. validated against full versions of the SCID and CIDI; sensitivity and specificity poor relative to these instruments for this module; validation studies not conducted among co-occurring or forensic populations. Inter-rater reliability was good, with test-retest being somewhat lower. Question validity of this form of assessing ASPD.

Iowa Personality Disorder Screen

The Iowa Personality Disorder Screen (Langbehn et al., 1999) is an 11-item mini structured interview composed of items derived from the Structured Interview for DSM-IV Personality (SIDP-IV). This new screening instrument shows promising levels of specificity and sensitivity as compared with the full SIDP-IV assessment instrument. The full SIDP has shown moderately good inter-rater reliability (*kappa* = .66) (Green, 1987), and convergent validity (Stangl, Pfohl, Zimmerman, Bowers & Corenthal, 1985). With training, this screening instrument can be administered by a lay interviewer.

The sample used to develop the screening instrument was drawn from six research sites, five of which were in the United States and Canada and one of which was in Italy (Langbehn et al., 1999). In this last site, an Italian version of the SIDP was used (this is the only reference available to any foreign language translation of the SIDP or the Iowa Personality Disorder Screen). The authors do not provide detailed demographic information about the sample used in the development of the screener; 73% were women and they averaged more than 14 years of formal education. Pfohl (personal communication, September 9, 1999) suggests that the instrument might be useful in a court-based diversion program as a general screen for the possible presence of a personality disorder, but cautions against using it to screen for specific disorders, or even specific clusters of disorders, as it has not been validated in a comparable population. Further, he cautions that it can not be used to screen for antisocial personality as the questions in the screen do not include any specifically drawn from DSM-IV criteria. Further, the literature in this area shows limited validity for this kind of brief assessment for antisocial personality (Hare, Hart & Harpur, 1991; Hart & Hare, 1997).

Structured Clinical Interview for DSM Personality Disorders Screen (SCID II Screen)

The SCID II interview was designed to evaluate personality disorders and it is accompanied by a self-report instrument, the SCID Screen, which is used to screen an interviewee and form the basis of the clinical interview by identifying which clinical areas need follow-up (First, Gibbon, Spitzer, Williams & Benjamin, 1997a). The screen may either be self or clinician-administered; the self-administered version requires an eighth-grade reading level (First, Gibbon, Spitzer, Williams & Benjamin, 1997b). The developers of the SCID II have not recommended the use of the Screen as a stand-alone instrument and its length (more than 100 items) makes it less desirable for high volume screening in a court-based setting.

Personality Diagnostic Questionnaire-4+ (PDQ-4+)

The Personality Diagnostic Questionnaire-4+ (Hyler, 1994) is a 99-item self-report questionnaire designed to assess the 10 personality disorders of the DSM-IV. The instrument yields a total score designed to indicate the likelihood of the individual having any significant personality distur- bance, and two validity scales designed to assess underreporting or mis- representing symptoms. A score sheet facilitates organization of the responses so that specific personality disorder criteria can be assessed. The items that comprise the criteria for each personality disorder are mixed throughout the instrument in order to minimize response sets and biases. This makes scoring the PDQ-4+ somewhat complicated, but the author believes that this structure increases the test's validity. It is possi- ble to extract items to assess only certain disorders, but this practice could yield results of questionable validity, especially given the test's overall poor agreement with other assessment tools. Studies using translations of the PDQ-R (the version of the instrument based on the DSM-III-R) have been published using Spanish (Lopez et al., 1996), Dutch (Knoppert-Van der Klein & Hoogduin, 1999), and Chinese (Huang et al., 1998) versions. Hyler, Skodol, Kellman, Oldham and Rosnick (1990) compared the PDQ- R to the SCID II and reported that agreement between the two instru- ments as assessed by *kappa* was .70, but they do not report on test-retest or internal consistencies of the scales of the PDQ-R. This instrument has been used in a forensic sample (O'Maille & Fine, 1995) of male inmates, 53% of whom were black and 47% of whom were white, with a mean edu- cation of 11.2 years. In this sample, the PDQ-R yielded reliable clusters of disorders but these did not converge with the DSM-III-R clusters. While the PDQ-R has also been used with incarcerated women (Dolan & Mitchell, 1994) and among patients in substance abuse treatment (O'Boyle, 1995), these were not validation studies. The validity of the instrument has not been explicitly assessed in co-occurring populations.

A number of studies have examined the validity of the PDQ by com- paring it to comprehensive assessment instruments; however, the results from such studies are mixed. Hyler et al. (1990) found that the PDQ-R was highly sensitive, but only moderately specific for most Axis II disor- ders. They concluded that the PDQ-R was not a substitute for a structured clinical interview because it yielded too many false positives, but that it could serve as a useful screening instrument for personality disorders. Trull and Larson (1994) reached similar conclusions in their young, white, primarily female sample of psychiatric outpatients. Fossati et al. (1998) compared the PDQ-4+ to the SCID II and found low agreement between the two instruments, concluding that the PDQ-4+ was not a good substitute for a structured diagnostic interview. For application in a court-based diversion program, however, its length may limit its applicability as a screening tool.

M.I.N.I. Antisocial Personality Module

The M.I.N.I. (Sheehan et al., 2000a) includes a module that screens for antisocial personality disorder, a diagnosis with special relevance to the criminal justice population. The questions in the M.I.N.I. Antisocial Personality Module are behavioral questions, largely drawn directly from the diagnostic criteria for Antisocial Personality Disorder (ASPD) and from the diagnostic criteria for Conduct Disorder prior to age 15 (a necessary requirement for diagnosis of Antisocial Personality Disorder). Lilienfeld, Purcell, and Jones-Alexander (1997), Widiger and Corbitt (1995), and others, however, have raised questions about the conceptual and practical utility of defining a personality disorder based almost exclusively on "bad behaviors" rather than personality characteristics. A screener based on DSM criteria could produce very high rates of ASPD in a court-based diversion program, which would limit the discriminant utility of the assessment. Further, the sensitivity and specificity of this M.I.N.I. module is relatively low, largely because of the disorder's low base rate in the validation sample. Moreover, the instrument has not been validated within a criminal justice population. Although as discussed previously, this instrument has been translated into 37 languages, its validation sample had a limited ethnic and socioeconomic range.

SUMMARY AND RECOMMENDATIONS

The recommendations that follow are specifically focused on screening instruments for psychiatric disorders, including substance use disorders, that court-based programs could utilize as part of their overall screening procedures of individuals who may have mental health and substance use problems and who have involvement with the criminal justice system. This review did not include instruments solely designed for gross identification—a type of "pre-screening" merely suggesting the presence or absence of some broadly defined mental health issue—and are even briefer than the measures reviewed here. Such a brief identification instrument composed of a few questions may in fact be useful at arrest, arraignment or upon admission to a jail/correctional facility for large urban centers with a high volume of defendants and notable prevalence rates of substance use and/or mental illness (the RDS, Teplin & Swartz, 1989, has been used in this way for flagging clients who may initially present with symptoms of a severe mental illness). Further, a review of full psychiatric assessment instruments (e.g., see Broner et al., 2000), general symptom severity (e.g., for a review and critique see Maruish, 1999; Thompson, 1989) and specific symptom change measures (e.g., for trauma see Wilson and Keane (Chapter 1), 1997; van der Kolk, McFarlane and Weisaeth (Chapter 11), 1996), along with other types of specialty assessment (e.g., risk-assessment, Borum, 1999b), is beyond the scope of this chapter.

Our recommendations are guided by practical and contextual considerations that exist in most current diversion programs where clients are routinely screened and assessed. Specifically, these programs: (a) have staff with limited training; (b) require public domain instruments, available for use without cost, due to the strain that high-volume screening and assessment would have on financial resources; and (c) require brevity due to the demand for rapid screening and time needed to collect other information. Most significant, however, is the need for these programs to screen for a range of disorders given the emerging trends in court-based diversion programs to focus on treatment planning, treatment matching and monitoring, and reporting on client progress, each of which may have serious legal and medical/psychiatric consequences for the client.

There is currently no single instrument that can adequately screen for all possible mental health and substance use disorders in a court-based setting without excluding or over including people who may or may not have these problems, particularly given the contextual constraints requiring a measure that would be brief, publicly available, and that would not require much training to administer. Thus, consistent with the recommendation of Peters and Hills (1999), we suggest combining instruments to achieve the most accurate screening protocol currently available for co-occurring mental illness and substance use disorders.

MENTAL HEALTH SCREENING

It should be clear that no unqualified recommendation can be made based on currently available mental health screening instruments that fall within the parameters of this review. Most instruments have not yet been validated within the criminal justice population or in samples of people previously known to have co-occurring substance use disorders. Thus, it would be useful for programs to conduct a pilot study comparing a brief screener, such as the RDS (developed and validated within the criminal justice system, but limited in scope) to the corresponding modules of the M.I.N.I. in order to determine if the performance of the two instruments is comparable *in this specific population*. Further, if a semi-structured or structured assessment is performed as part of a follow-up assessment, the program should use this as a criterion to assess the predictive utility of the screening procedure (e.g., the issue of "false positives": too many people without disorders being identified at the screening phase). At the very least, programs that adapt these recommendations should monitor the performance of whichever instrument or set of instruments they choose so that modifications can be made, as needed, for their treatment population.

Based on the current review, however, the best recommendation for a mental health screening measure in court-based diversion programs appears to be the M.I.N.I. (without the Antisocial Personality Disorder and Substance and Alcohol Abuse modules, and with a substance use rule-out question added to reduce false positives). This instrument has the advantages of being comprehensive, easy to administer, and well-validated. If a program wanted to focus on a narrower range of disorders and did not need to discriminate between them, an acceptable alternative for cursory psychiatric screening would be the RDS.

To protect against false positive identifications of psychiatric disorders due to substance use, we recommend that an additional question be added to both instruments. We suggest including the rule-out question from the M.I.N.I.-Plus (Sheehan et al., 2000b), "Were you taking any drugs or medicines just before these symptoms began?" followed by a clarification such as, "Drugs or medicines include: alcohol, street drugs, and prescription medications taken other than as prescribed or that were not prescribed for you." We recommend the insertion of these questions in the M.I.N.I. at the end of each module for which the DSM-IV provides a substance-induced category and in the RDS following the last question in each section.

Although it could potentially shorten administration time, the substance use rule-out items should probably not be placed immediately after the skip-out exit questions, since preliminary indications from ongoing research suggest that an early rule-out may lead to an incorrect diagnosis of a substance-induced disorder, particularly with social phobia (D. Sheehan, personal communication, December 14, 1999). Until this research has been published and peer-reviewed, we recommend administering the full module to ensure that this potential problem is avoided. Differentiating between primary and secondary disorders should occur during the assessment phase, not as part of the screening, and should utilize collateral and self-report information (i.e., gathered from a thorough psychiatric, psychosocial, medical, and legal history and record review) in addition to any structured or semi-structured assessment.

Substance Use Screening

The primary purpose of a drug or alcohol screener is to flag the presence of a problem for further assessment; however, having a baseline understanding of the quantity and frequency of use contributes to the ability to distinguish substance use, abuse and dependence and allows the instrument to be used over time. Also, when screening and assessing a co-occurring population, it is important to remember the role any drug or alcohol use may play in decompensation for those with a primary mental illness. This factor could be missed if a program only screens and assesses for, and deems relevant, a full criteria diagnosis of abuse or dependence. Thus, in our review of these screening instruments, we noted information regarding the measurement of frequency and severity to aid in choosing a screener, which could then be administered periodically after baseline by the diversion and or treatment program to document change over time.

Based on the current review, we agree with Peters and Bartoi (1997) about the top three alternatives for substance abuse screening measures: the TCUDS, the SSI (adding in the Dartmouth Drug/Alcohol six-month Follow-Back Calendar), and the ADS/ASI combination (with the ADS replaced by the AUDIT for programs that require non-proprietary, publicly available instruments). Among these, the TCUDS and the SSI are more easily administered and scored, a significant consideration given the sizable case load and the lack of available time for extensive training in most criminal justice diversion or discharge planning programs. The TCUDS and the SSI both address alcohol and drug use in a single instrument, eliminating the need for two instruments. However, the TCUDS measures frequency of use, though not severity (though a quantity column can be added), but the SSI measures neither frequency nor severity, necessitating an additional instrument to measure these dimensions if a program were to seek to measure change in substance use over time with the screening instrument. Based on research currently being conducted on the TCUDS, we would expect further clarification of its reliability and validity in the near future and would be likely to choose it over the SSI, which has no large-scale studies underway. We leave open the possibility, if the AUDIT/ASI combination is selected, that the expanded AUDIT (which will have drug use questions) may, at some point in the future, eliminate the need for the ASI-Drug section supplement. Further, the AUDIT measures both frequency and severity of alcohol consumed and the ASI measures frequency and route of administration of drug use, but not severity of drug use. If another instrument or set of instruments is chosen, or for the purpose of compiling consistent information regarding frequency and severity of both alcohol and drug use, we recommend the addition of the Dartmouth Drug/Alcohol six-month Follow-Back Calendar; adding this instrument allows for the adaptation of most screeners as a change measure.

PERSONALITY DISORDERS SCREENING

As a cautionary note, we have strong reservations about the feasibility of screening for personality disorders within a substance using population in crisis. Such assessments are likely to lead to high false positive rates and could further stigmatize individuals, creating further difficulty receiving community placement due to beliefs that certain of these disorders are "difficult" or "untreatable." Finally, providing the court itself with information about the possible presence of a personality disorder could create confusion about the possible co-existence of major psychiatric disorders. With this caveat, if a court-based program decides to try to obtain this information as part of its screening we have two recommendations.

1. Funding the development or adaptation of an instrument within this population that can screen effectively for specific clusters of personality disorders.
2. If a brief screen such as the Iowa Personality Disorder Screen is used, all positive results should be interpreted with extreme caution and pending follow-up assessment with a validated structured or semi-structured interview, once the client is no longer in crisis and is psychiatrically stable.

STAFF TRAINING RECOMMENDATIONS

Screening (as well as assessment and measuring client progress over time), often performed by case managers in court-based programs, is a topic that easily folds into ongoing staff training and in essence requires additional training beyond what is strictly suggested for a specific chosen instrument. Peters and Hills (1999) describe the need for case management to be model driven and for staff to be trained in psychiatric symptom recognition, mental status, diagnostic classifications, basic understanding of psychotropic medications, their classification, benefits, and side effects, and in accessing local services. This type of training is particularly useful for cross-training drug court program staff to work with mentally ill substance using clients. By providing staff with this background, screening will be more accurate and thus have utility for determining if initial criteria for acceptance have been met, enhance the ability of case management staff to design an initial treatment plan to meet issues flagged in the screening, and make appropriate referrals for a full assessment of those accepted or for those for whom diagnostic and needs clarification is indicated to rule in eligibility. While this chapter focuses only on screening, screening as a "gateway" to services is potentially the starting point in a continuum that includes assessment and reassessment of clients' needs.

Programs often add an evaluation component to satisfy quality assurance and program monitoring procedures and secure continued and additional funding. The purpose of using reliable and valid instruments, and developing procedures for staff training, is to give a program (and those reviewing a program's data) the knowledge that the information being collected is generally consistent and meaningful. However each instrument used has its strengths and weaknesses, and the information gathered must always be placed within the context of the individual's whole presentation and history.

The level of staff training required will vary depending upon the instruments chosen and the level of staff—that is whether or not the staff has clinical training in substance abuse and mental illness, interviewing techniques and so forth—therefore, clinical staff will need little training in administering basic self-report measures, whereas lay staff will require some supervision. Described are four basic aspects of instrument training for programmatic rather than research purposes: 1) developing an understanding of the nature of the population; 2) orientation to the instrument; 3) instrument scoring and interpretation; and 4) a maintenance component to prevent interviewer drift.

1. Developing an understanding of the nature of the population. Staff should be provided with a basic orientation to mental health and substance abuse issues (including best practice integrated treatment principles (e.g., RachBeisel et al., 1999), stages of recovery (e.g., Osher & Kofoed, 1989), and so forth), along with other related risk factors such as co-morbid medical (and neurological) problems, abuse, criminal justice history, homelessness, violent behavior, past employment, education, and relationship functioning. They should understand basic clinical formulation including interactions between primary disorders and other risk factors. Further, a major theme endorsed in focus groups held in preparation for this review was staff concern about how to transfer their skills developed for working with substance using clients to their work with mentally ill clients (e.g., particularly their ability to "cheer them on" and "relate to" them); using motivational interviewing techniques for this population would not only benefit clients, but would likely facilitate the adaptation of staff skills from one client population to another.

2. Orientation to the instrument. Instruments may have a manual (such as for the SCID-II or the MINI) or a primary article, as cited in this chapter;

most screening instruments in contrast to assessment instruments, do not have a training protocol, as by their nature, they require minimum training efforts. However, a number of assessment manuals describe a gold standard for research training (e.g., First et al., 1996b, 1997b), which, while neither pragmatic for, nor necessarily relevant to most programs, could provide a variety of training method ideas for adaptation. For instance, staff could role-play the instrument in order to be comfortable with its wording and administration procedure. Then the clinician supervisor, trained on the instruments, could lead an interview with a client who has consented to be involved for training purposes, and other staff members could jointly code the interview. Scores could then be compared and discussed and recorded for future reliability. Alternatively, several audio or video tapes could be made of the full interview battery—all the instruments chosen by a program along with the program's basic intake history form—for staff to code; this latter procedure has the advantage of providing a mechanism for training new staff, as well as refreshing the training of staff over time. Finally these types of strategies complement staff training on population characteristics and related clinical and case management issues.

3. *Instrument scoring and interpretation.* Manuals and articles cited have scoring explanations; scoring programs can be built into a program's management information system to reduce staff error and time spent on this aspect. Non-clinically trained staff should initially be supervised in the interpretation of self-report instruments. When a comprehensive assessment is completed on accepted clients, information from the screening should be reviewed and if relevant incorporated; this process also aids staff in learning the benefits and limitations of the chosen instruments.

4. *Maintenance component to prevent interviewer drift.* Supervision, case conferencing, and periodic joint scoring of a taped or live interview help staff to retain the original training, address on-going or new questions, and allow the program to maintain a log of interrater performance for use when reporting program results. This type of training also serves to inform new staff and integrate them with experienced staff.

Finally, two other issues deserve brief mention, and while not directly related to staff training, they enhance the ability for staff to succeed in the goal of diverting clients to community services: services and criminal justice training. Whether a program is designed initially to focus on the mentally ill or the program is targeting a population charged with drug offenses and who may present with mental health problems, administrative staff should build dual diagnosis resources and community placement relationships in order to provide case management staff with resources and support. Otherwise, staff may resort to traditional substance abuse and mental health placements or feel defeated in their attempts to place these clients due to the length of time specialized placement can take in jurisdictions that have not yet developed well coordinated integrated service systems for this target population. Providing staff with initial strongly built contacts will create a more successful experience (for staff, clients, the courts and other collaborating stakeholders). Building such resources into the program's infrastructure also provides additional impetus to work with this challenging population that previously may not have been included in a staff's caseload.

Cross-training for the judiciary and court staff is recommended in the areas of psychiatric identification, course of recovery, flexible sanction planning, understanding of different placement options, realistic time frames for implementing treatment plans and obstacles to placement. An understanding by the judiciary and court staff of the course of mental illness and the effects of the interaction between substance use and mental illness (as well as trauma and other common co-morbid disorders) is essential in order to craft dispositions that balance public safety with individualized treatment planning. Just as the judiciary has integrated the concepts of relapse, prevention, and service and treatment needs into their understanding of drug offenders who are substance users, developing an understanding of the mentally ill client and the resources for treatment will equally benefit the goals of treatment retention and reduction in unnecessary criminal justice recidivism. Such training may also have a "trickle down" effect to diversion staff, imparting permission to work with this population in a client-centered approach.

Note

1. Considerations for screening in jail-based, as opposed to court-based, programs may be somewhat different due to the larger volume of clients. These programs might still benefit from our review of those instruments focusing on major disorders.

REFERENCES

Abram, K.M. & Teplin, L.A. (1991). Co-occurring disorders among mentally ill jail detainees: Implications for public policy. *American Psychologist, 46*(10), 1036–1045.

Allen, J.P., Litten, R.Z., Fertig, J.B. & Babor, T. (1997). A review of research on the Alcohol Use Disorders Identification Test (AUDIT). *Alcoholism: Clinical and Experimental Research, 21*(4), 613–619.

American Psychiatric Association. (1994). *Diagnostic and statistical manual of mental disorders* (4th ed.). Washington, DC: Author.

Amoureus, M.P.S.R., van den Hurk, A.A., Schippers, G.M. & Breteler, M.H.M. (1994). The Addiction Severity Index in penitentiaries. *International Journal of Offender Therapy and Comparative Criminology, 38*(4), 309–318.

Appleby, L., Dyson, V., Altman, E. & Luchins, D.J. (1997). Assessing substance use in multiproblem patients: Reliability and validity of the Addiction Severity Index in a mental hospital population. *Journal of Nervous and Mental Disease, 185*(3), 159–189.

Bergey, C., Verdoux, H., Assens, F., Abalan, F., Liraud, F., Gonzales, B., Beaussier, J.P., Gaussares, C., Etchegaray, B., Bourgeois, M. & Salamon, R. (1999). Assessment of the administrative incidence of psychotic disorders. *Encephale-Revue de Psychiatrie Clinique Biologique et Therapeutique, 25*(1), 30–36.

Berlin, I., Bisserbe, J.C., Eiber, R., Balssa, N., Sachon, C., Bosquet, F. & Grimaldi, A. (1997). Phobic symptoms, particularly the fear of blood and injury, are associated with poor glycemic control in type I diabetic adults. *Diabetes Care, 20*(2), 176–178.

Blevins, L.D., Morton, J.B. & McCabe, K.A. (1996). Using the Michigan Alcoholism Screening Test to identify problem drinkers under federal supervision. *Federal Probation, 60*(2), 38–42.

Bohn, M.S., Babor, T.F. & Kramzler, H.R. (1995). The alcohol use disorders identification test (AUDIT): Validation of a screening instrument for use in medical settings. *Journal of Studies on Alcohol, 56*(4), 423–432.

Borum, R. (1999a). *Jail diversion strategies for misdemeanor offenders with mental illness: Preliminary report.* Tampa, Florida: Department of Mental Health and Policy, Louis de la Parte Florida Mental Health Institute, University of South Florida.

Borum, R. (1999b). Advances in the assessment of dangerousness and risk. In American Psychological Association (Ed.), *Psychological expertise and criminal justice.* Washington, DC: American Psychological Association.

Borum, R., Swanson, J., Swartz, M. & Hiday, V. (1997). Substance abuse, violent behavior and police encounters among persons with severe mental disorder. *Journal of Contemporary Criminal Justice, 13,* 236–250.

Borum, R., Dean, M., Steadman, H. & Morrissey, J. (1998). *Law enforcement responses to people with mental illness: A community policing perspective.* Unpublished manuscript.

Bradley, K.A., McDonell, M.B., Kivlahan, D.R., Diehr, P. & Fihn, S.D. (1998). The AUDIT alcohol consumption questions: Reliability, validity and responsiveness to change in older male primary care patients. *Alcoholism: Clinical and Experimental Research, 22*(8), 1842–1849.

Broner, N., Borum, R. & Gawley, K. (2001). Criminal justice diversion of individuals with co-occurring mental illness and substance use disorders: An overview. In G. Landsberg, M. Rock, L. Berg & A. Smiley

(Eds.). *Serving mentally ill offenders: Challenges and opportunities for mental health professionals.* New York: Springer Publishing.

Broner, N., Borum, R., Whitmire, L. & Gawley, K. (2000, June). Screening and assessment for co-occurring mental illness & substance use in court-based diversion programs: A best practices review. (Report.) New York, NY: New York University, School of Social Work Institute Against Violence.

Broome, K.M., Knight, K., Joe, G.W. & Simpson, D.D. (1996). Evaluating the drug-abusing probationer: Clinical interview versus self-administered assessment. *Criminal Justice and Behavior (23),* 4, 593–606.

Brown, L.S., Alterman, A.I., Rutherford, M.J. & Cacciola, J.S. (1993). Addiction Severity Index scores of four racial/ethnic and gender groups of methadone maintenance patients. *Journal of Substance Abuse,* 5(3), 269–279.

Cacciola, J.S., Koppenhaver, J.M., McKay, J.R. & Alterman, A.I. (1999). Test-retest reliability of the lifetime items on the Addiction Severity Index. *Psychological Assessment, 11*(1), 86–93.

Carey, K.B. (1997). Reliability and validity of the time-line follow-back interview among psychiatric outpatients: A preliminary report. *Psychology of Addictive Behaviors, 11*(1), 26–33.

Carey, K.B., Cocco, K.M. & Correia, C.J. (1997). Reliability and validity of the Addiction Severity Index among outpatients with severe mental illness. *Psychological Assessment, 9*(4), 422–428.

Center for Addiction and Mental Health. (1999). *1999 resources.* Toronto, Canada: Author.

Center for Substance Abuse Treatment (1999). *Simple screening instruments for outreach for alcohol and other drug abuse and infectious diseases: Treatment Improvement Protocol (TIP) Series 11.* Rockville, MD: Substance Abuse and Mental Health Services Administration.

Chan, A.W.K., Pristach, E.A. & Welte, J.W. (1994). Detection by the CAGE of alcoholism or heavy drinking in primary care outpatients and the general population. *Journal of Substance Abuse, 6*(2), 123–135.

Chan, AW.K., Pristach, E.A., Welte, J.W. & Russell, M. (1993). Use of the TWEAK test in screening for alcoholism/heavy drinking in three populations. *Alcoholism Clinical and Experimental Research, 17*(6), 1188–1192.

Cherpitel, C.J. (1995). Analysis of cut points for screening instruments for alcohol problems in the emergency room. *Journal of Studies on Alcohol,* 56, 695–700.

Cherpitel, C.J. (1998). Differences in performance of screening instruments for problem drinking among blacks, whites, and Hispanics in an emergency room population. *Journal of Studies on Alcohol, 59*(4), 420–426.

Cherpitel, C.J. (1999). Gender, injury status and acculturation differences in performance of screening instruments for alcohol problems among

US Hispanic emergency room patients. *Drug and Alcohol Dependence, 53*(2), 147–157.

Chignon, J.M., Jacquesy, L., Mennad, M., Terki, A., Huttin, F., Martin, P. & Chabannes, J.P. (1998). Auto-questionnaire d'appetence alcoolique (questionnaire ECCA: échelle de comportement et de cognitions vis-à-vis de l'alcool: Traduction Francaise et validation de l'OCDS (Obsessive Compulsive Drinking Scale) / Self-assessment of alcoholic craving: Validation of the French version of the Obsessive Compulsive Drinking Scale (OCDS). *Encephale, 24*(5), 426–434.

Cocco, K.M. & Carey, K.B. (1998). Psychometric properties of the Drug Abuse Screening Test in psychiatric outpatients. *Psychological Assessment, 10*(4), 408–414.

Cosden, M.A. (1994). Addiction Severity Index. In D.J. Keyser & R.C. Sweetland (Eds.), *Test critiques, Vol X.* Austin, TX: Pro-ed.

Cosden, M. & Cortez-Ison, E. (1999). Sexual abuse, parental bonding, social support, and program retention for women in substance abuse treatment. *Journal of Substance Abuse Treatment, 16*(2), 149–155.

Dartmouth Psychiatric Research Center (1997). *Drug/Alcohol 6-Month Follow-Back Calendar.* Hanover, NH: Author.

Davis, T.M. & Wood, P.S. (1999). Substance abuse and sexual trauma in a female veteran population. *Journal of Substance Abuse Treatment, 16*(2), 123–127.

Deane, M., Steadman, H., Borum, R., Veysey, B. & Morrissey, J. (1998). Police/ mental health system interactions: Program types and needed research. *Psychiatric Services, 50*, 99–101.

DeJong, C.A., Van den Brink, W., Harteveld, F.M. & Van der Wielen, E.G. (1993). Personality disorders in alcoholics and drug addicts. *Comprehensive Psychiatry, 34*(2), 87–94.

DiCataldo, F., Greer, A. & Profit, W.E. (1995). Screening prison inmates for mental disorder: An examination of the relationship between mental disorder and prison adjustment. *Bulletin of the American Academy of Psychiatry and the Law, 23*(4), 573–585.

Dixon, L., Myers, P., Johnson, J. & Corty, E. (1996). Screening for mental illness with the Addiction Severity Index. *American Journal on Addictions, 5*(4), 301–307.

Dolan, B. & Mitchell, E. (1994). Personality disorder and psychological disturbance of female prisoners: A comparison with women referred for NHS treatment of personality disorder. *Criminal Behaviour and Mental Health, 4*(2), 130–142.

Drake, R.E., Alterman, A.I., & Rosenberg, S.R. (1993). Detection of substance use disorders in severely mentally ill patients. *Community Mental Health Journal, 29*(2), 175–192.

Drake, R.E., Bartels, S.J., Teague, G.B., Noordsy, D.L. & Clark, R.E. (1993).

Treatment of substance abuse in severely mentally ill patients. *Journal of Nervous and Mental Disease, 181*(10), 606–611.

Dyson, V., Appleby, L., Altman, E., Doot, M., Luchins, D.J. & Delehant, M. (1998). Efficiency and validity of commonly used substance abuse screening instruments in public psychiatric patients. *Journal of Addictive Diseases, 17*(2), 57–76.

El-Bassel, N., Gilbert, L., Schilling, R.F., Ivanoff, A. & Borne, D. (1996). Correlates of crack abuse among drug-using incarcerated women: Psychological trauma, social support and coping behavior. *American Journal of Drug and Alcohol Abuse, 22*(1), 41–56.

Fabrega, H., Mezzich, J. & Ullrich, R.F. (1988). Black-white differences in psychopathology in an urban psychiatric population. *Comprehensive Psychiatry, 29,* 285–297.

Fiander, M. & Bartlett, A.E.A. (1997). Missed "psychiatric" cases? The effectiveness of a court diversion scheme. *Alcohol and Alcoholism, 32*(6), 715–723.

Firestone, P., Bradford, J.M., McCoy, M., Greenberg, D.M., Curry, S. & Larose, M.R. (1998). Recidivism in convicted rapists. *Journal of the American Academy of Psychiatry and the Law, 26*(2), 185–200.

First, M.B., Gibbon, M., Spitzer, R.L. & Williams, J.B.W. (1996a). *User's guide for the Structured Clinical Interview for DSM-IV Axis I Disorders Research Version (SCID-I, Version 2.0, February 1996, FINAL Version).* New York: Biometrics Research.

First, M.B., Gibbon, M., Spitzer, R.L., & Williams, J.B.W. (1996b). *User's guide for SCID-101 instructional videotapes for SCID for DSM-IV.* New York: Biometrics Research.

First, M.B., Gibbon, M., Spitzer, R.L., Williams, J.B.W. & Benjamin, L.S. (1997a). *Structured Clinical Interview for DSM-IV Axis II Personality Disorders (SCID-II).* Washington, DC: American Psychiatric Press.

First, M.B., Gibbon, M., Spitzer, R.L., Williams, J.B.W. & Benjamin, L.S. (1997b). *User's guide for the Structured Clinical Interview for DSM-IV Axis II Personality Disorders (SCID-II).* Washington, DC: American Psychiatric Press.

First, M.B., Spitzer, R.L. Gibbon, M. & Williams, J.B.W. (1998). *Structured Clinical Interview for DSM-IV Axis I Disorders Patient Edition (SCID-I/P, Version 2.0, 8/98 Revision).* New York: Biometrics Research.

Fossati, A., Maffei, C., Bagnato, M., Donati, D., Donini, M., Fiorilli, M., Novella L. & Ansoldi, M. (1998). Criterion validity of the Personality Diagnostic Questionnaire-4+ (PDQ-4+) in a mixed psychiatric sample. *Journal of Personality Disorders, 12*(2), 172-178.

Fullilove, M.T., Fullilove, R.E., Smith, M., Winkler, K., Michael, C., Panzer, P.G. & Wallace, R. (1993). Violence, trauma, and post-traumatic stress disorder among women drug users. *Journal of Traumatic Stress, 6,* 533–543.

Garcia-Campayo, J., Lobo, A., Perez-Escheverria, M.J. & Campos, R. (1998). Three forms of somatization presenting in primary care settings in Spain. *Journal of Nervous and Mental Disease, 186*(9), 554–560.

Goldfinger, S.M., Schutt, R.K., Seidman, L.J. & Turner, W.M. (1996). Self-report and observer measures of substance abuse among homeless mentally ill persons in the cross-section and over time. *Journal of Nervous and Mental Disease, 184*(11), 667–672.

Green, C.J. (1987). The Structured Interview for DSM-III Personality disorders (SIDP): A review. *Journal of Personality Disorders, 1*(3), 288–290.

Hare, R.D., Hart, S.D. & Harpur, T.J. (1991). Psychopathy and the DSM-IV criteria for antisocial personality disorder. *Journal of Abnormal Psychology, 100*(3), 391–398.

Hart, S.D. & Hare, R.D. (1997). Psychopathy: Assessment and association with criminal conduct. In D.M. Stoff & J.Breiling (Eds.), *Handbook of antisocial behavior* (pp. 22–35). New York: John Wiley & Sons.

Hart, S.D., Roesch, R., Corrado, R.R. & Cox, D.N. (1993). The Referral Decision Scale: A validation study. *Law and Human Behavior, 17*(6), 611–623.

Haywood, T.W., Kravitz, H.M., Goldman, L.B. & Freeman, A. (2000). Characteristics of women in jail and treatment orientations. *Behavior Modification, 24*(3), 307–324.

Henderson, D.J. (1997). Drug abuse and incarcerated women: A research review. *Journal of Substance Abuse Treatment, 15*(6), 579–587.

Holden, P., Rann, J. & Van Drasek, L. (1993). *Unheard voices: A report on women in Michigan jails.* Lansing, MI: Michigan Women's Commission.

Hollingshead, A.B. & Redlich, F.C. (1958). *Social class and mental illness: A community study.* New York: John Wiley & Sons.

Huang, Y., Dong, W., Wang, Y., Cui, Y., Xu, Y. & Han, Q. (1998). A pilot evaluation on the Personality Diagnostic Questionnaire–Revision in China. *Chinese Mental Health Journal, 12*(5), 262–264.

Hyler, S.E. (1994). *PDQ-4+: Personality Diagnostic Questionnaire-4+.* New York: New York State Psychiatric Institute.

Hyler, S.E., Skodol, A.E., Kellman, D., Oldham, J.M. & Rosnick, L. (1990). Validity of the Personality Diagnostic Questionnaire-Revised: Comparison with two structured interviews. *American Journal of Psychiatry, 147*(8), 1043–1048.

Jacobson, A. & Herald, C. (1990). The relevance of childhood sexual abuse to adult psychiatric inpatient care. *Hospital & Community Psychiatry, 41*, 154–158.

Jordan, B.K., Schlenger, W.E., Fairbank, J.A. & Caddell, J.M. (1996). Prevalence of psychiatric disorders among incarcerated women. *Archives of General Psychiatry, 53*(6), 513–519.

Joyner, L.M., Wright, J.D. & Devine, J.A. (1996). Reliability and validity of the Addiction Severity Index among homeless substance misusers. *Substance Use and Misuse, 31*(6), 729–751.

Kessler, R.C, Andrews, G., Mroczek, D., Ustun, B. & Wittchen, H. (in press). The World Health Organization Composite International Diagnostic Interview Short-Form (CIDI-SF). *International Journal of Methods in Psychiatric Research.* Abstract on WHO website.

Knoppert-van der Klein, E.A. & Hoogduin, C.A. (1999). Persoonlijkheids-stoornissen volgens de Personality Diagnostic Questionnaire-Revised (PDQ-R) bij patieenten met een bipolaire stoornis. Een replicatieon-derzoek/Personality disorders by the Personality Diagnostic Questionnaire-Revised (PDQ-R) in bipolar patients. *Tijdschrift voor Psychiatrie 41*(2), 67–73.

Lamb, H.R. & Weinberger, L.E. (1998). Persons with severe mental illness in jails and prisons: A review. *Psychiatric Services, 49*(4), 483–492.

Langbehn, D.R., Pfohl, B.M., Reynolds, S., Clark, L.A., Battaglia, M., Bellodi, L., Cadoret, R., Grove, W., Pilkonis, P. & Links, P. (1999). The Iowa Personality Disorder Screen: Development and preliminary validation of a brief screening interview. *Journal of Personality Disorders, 13*(1), 75–89.

Lecrubier, Y., Sheehan, D.V., Weiller, E., Amorim, P., Bonora, I., Sheehan, K.H., Janavs, J. & Dunbar, G.C. (1997). The Mini International Neuropsychiatric Interview (MINI). A short diagnostic structured interview: Reliability and validity according to the CIDI. *European Psychiatry, 12*, 224–231.

Lehman, A.F. (1996). Heterogeneity of person and place: Assessing co-occurring addictive and mental disorders. *American Journal of Ortho-psychiatry, 66*(1), 32–41.

Lejoyeux, M., Feuche, N., Loi, S., Solomon, J. & Ades, J. (1999). Study of impulse-control disorders among alcohol-dependent patients. *Journal of Clinical Psychiatry, 60*(5), 302–305.

Lejoyeux, M., Haberman, N., Solomon, J., & Ades, J. (1999). Comparison of buying behavior in depressed patients presenting with or without compulsive buying. *Comprehensive Psychiatry, 40*(1), 51–56.

Lennings, C.J., Scott, L., Harris, J., Kingsbury, A. & Andrew, M. (1998). Dual diagnosis (comorbidity) among clients of a drug and alcohol outpatient service. *Alcoholism Treatment Quarterly, 16*(3), 79–87.

Lilienfeld, S.O., Purcell, C. & Jones-Alexander, J. (1997). Assessment of antisocial behavior in adults. In D.M. Stoff, J. Breiling, & J.D. Maser (Eds.), *Handbook of antisocial behavior* (pp. 60–74). New York: John Wiley & Sons.

Lopez, J., Paez, F., Apiquian, R., Sanchez de Carmona, M., Fresan, A., Robles, R. & Nicolini, H. (1996). Estudio sobre la traduccion y la val-idacion del Cuestionario Revisado del Diagnostico de la Personalidad (PDQ-R) / Study on the translation and validation of the Personality

Diagnostic Questionnaire-Revised (PDQ-R). *Salud Mental, 19*(3, Suppl.), 39–42.

Luckie, L.F., White, R.E., Miller, W.R. & Icenogle, M.V. (1995). Prevalence estimates of alcohol problems in a Veterans Administration outpatient population. *Journal of Clinical Psychology, 51*(3), 422–425.

Lyons, J.S., Howard, K.I., O'Mahoney, M.T. & Lish, J.D. (1997). *The measurement and management of clinical outcomes in mental health.* New York: John Wiley & Sons.

Malgady, R.G., Rogler, L.H. & Tryon, W.W. (1992). Issues of validity in the Diagnostic Interview Schedule. *Journal of Psychiatric Research, 26*(1), 59–67.

Maruish, M.E. (1999). *The use of psychological testing for treatment planning and outcomes assessment.* Mahwah, NJ: Lawrence Erlbaum Associates.

Mayfield, D., McLeod, G. & Hall, P. (1974). The CAGE questionnaire: Validation of a new alcoholism instrument. *American Journal of Psychiatry, 131*, 1121–1123.

McFarland, B. Faulkner, L., Bloom, J. & Hallaux, R. (1989). Chronic mental illness and the criminal justice system. *Hospital and Community Psychiatry, 41*, 718–723.

McLellan, A.T., Kushner, H., Metzger, D., Peters, R.H., Smith, I., Grissom, G., Pettinati, H. & Argeriou, M. (1992). The Fifth Edition of the Addiction Severity Index. *Journal of Substance Abuse Treatment, 9*, 199–213.

Monahan, J. (1995). Clinical and actuarial predictions of violence. In D. Faigman (Ed.), *Modern science evidence: The law and science of expert witness testimony, Vol. 1.* St. Paul: West Publishing.

Mueser, K.T., Drake, R.E. & Miles, K.M. (1997). The course and treatment of substance use disorder in persons with severe mental illness. In L.S. Onken, J.D. Blaine, S. Genser, & A.M. Horton (Eds.), *Treatment of drug-dependent individuals with comorbid mental disorders* (pp. 86–109). Rockville, MD: National Institute on Drug Abuse.

National Institute on Alcohol Abuse and Alcoholism (NIAAA) (1999). www.niaaa.nih.gov.

O'Boyle, M. (1995). DSM-III-R and Eysenck personality measures among patients in a substance abuse programme. *Personality and Individual Differences, 18*(4), 561–565.

O'Maille, P.S. & Fine, M.A. (1995). Personality disorder scales for the MMPI-2: An assessment of psychometric properties in a correctional population. *Journal of Personality Disorders, 9*(3), 235–246.

Osher, F.C. & Kofoed, L.L. (1989). Treatment of patients with psychiatric and psychoactive substance abuse disorders. *Hospital and Community Psychiatry, 40*(10), 1025–1030.

Paradis, C.M., Horn, L., Yang, C.M. & O'Rourke, T. (1999). Ethnic differences in assessment and treatment of affective disorders in a jail population. *Journal of Offender Rehabilitation, 28*(3–4), 23–32.

Peters, R.H. & Bartoi, M.G. (1997). *Screening and assessment of co-occurring disorders in the justice system*. Delmar, NY: The National GAINS Center.

Peters, R.H. & Greenbaum, P.E. (1996). *Texas Department of Criminal Justice/Center for Substance Abuse Treatment Prison Substance Abuse Screening Project*. Millford, MA: Civigenics, Inc.

Peters, R.H. & Hills, H.A. (1997). *Intervention strategies for offenders with co-occurring disorders: What works?* Delmar, NY: The National GAINS Center.

Peters, R.H. & Hills, H.A. (1999). Community treatment and supervision strategies for offenders with co-occurring disorders: What works? In E. Latessa (Ed.), *Strategic solutions: The international community corrections association examines substance abuse*, (pp. 81–137). Lanham, MD: American Correctional Association.

RachBeisel, J., Scott, J. & Dixon, L. (1999). Co-occurring severe mental illness and substance use disorders: A review of recent research. *Psychiatric Services, 50*(11), 1427–1434.

Rayburn, T.M. & Stonecypher, J.F. (1996). Diagnostic differences related to age and race of involuntarily committed psychiatric patients. *Psychological Reports, 73*, 881–882.

Richie, B.E. & Johnsen, C. (1996). Abuse histories among newly incarcerated women in a New York City jail. *Journal of the Medical Women's Association, 51*(3), 111–114.

Robins, L., Cottler, L., Bucholz, K. & Compton, W. (1998). *Diagnostic Interview Schedule for DSM-IV (DIS-IV)*. September 11, 1998 version. St. Louis, MO: Washington University.

Robins, L., Helzer, J., Croughan, J. & Ratcliff, K. (1981). National Institute of Mental Health Diagnostic Interview Schedule: Its history, characteristics, and validity. *Archives of General Psychiatry, 38*, 381–389.

Robins, L., Marcus, L., Reich, W., Cunningham, R. & Gallagher, T. (1998). *Diagnostic Interview Schedule Version IV (DIS-IV): Question-by-question specifications*. September 11, 1998 revision. St. Louis, MO: Washington University.

Rock, M. & Landsberg, G. (1998). County mental health directors' perspective on forensic mental health developments in New York State. *Administration and Policy in Mental Health, 25*(2), 327–332.

Rogers, R., Sewell, K.W., Ustad, K., Reinhardt, V. & Edwards, W. (1995). The Referral Decision Scale with mentally disordered inmates. *Law and Human Behavior, 19*(5), 481–492.

Rosenberg, S.D., Drake, R.E., Wolford, G.L., Mueser, K.T., Oxman, T.E., Vidaver, R.M., Carrieri, K.L. & Luckoor, R. (1998). Dartmouth Assessment of Lifestyle Instrument (DALI): A substance use disorder screen for people with severe mental illness. *American Journal of Psychiatry, 155*, 232–238.

Ross, H.E., Gavin, D.R. & Skinner, H.A. (1990). Diagnostic validity of the MAST and the Alcohol Dependence Scale in the assessment of DSM-III alcohol disorders. *Journal of Studies on Alcohol, (51)*6, 506–513.

Russell, M. (1994). New assessment tools for risk drinking during pregnancy: T-ACE, TWEAK, and others. *Alcohol Health and Research World, 18*(1), 55–61.

Russell, M. & Bigler, L. (1979). Screening for alcohol-related problems in an outpatient obstetric-gynecologic clinic. *American Journal of Obstetrics and Gynecology, 134,* 4–12.

Saltstone, R., Halliwell, S. & Hayslip, M. (1994). A multivariate evaluation of the Michigan Alcoholism Screening Test and the Drug Abuse Screening Test in a female offender population. *Addictive Behaviors, (19)*5, 455–462.

Searles, J.S., Alterman, A.I. & Purtill, J.J. (1990). The detection of alcoholism in hospitalized schizophrenics: A comparison of the MAST and the MAC. *Alcoholism: Clinical and Experimental Research, 14*(4), 557–560.

Segal, D.L., Hersen, M. & Van Hasselt, V.B. (1994). Reliability of the Structured Clinical Interview for DSM-III-R: An evaluative review. *Comprehensive Psychiatry, 35*(4), 316–327.

Selzer, M.L. (1971). The Michigan Alcoholism Screening Test: The quest for a new diagnostic instrument. *American Journal of Psychiatry, 127*(12), 1653–1658.

Sheehan, D.V., Lecrubier, Y., Janavs, J., Knapp, E., Weiller, E., Hergueta, T., Bonora, L.I., Amorim, P., Lepine, J.P., Sheehan, M.F., Baker, R.R. & Sheehan, K.H. (2000a). *Mini International Neuropsychiatric Interview (M.I.N.I Version 5.0.0.).* (Copyright 1992, 1994, 1998, 2000 by Sheehan, D.V. & Lecrubier, Y.) Tampa, FL and Paris: University of South Florida Institute for Research in Psychiatry and INSERM-Hôpital de la Salpêtrière.

Sheehan, D.V., Lecrubier, Y., Janavs, J., Knapp, E., Weiller, E., Hergueta, T., Bonora, L.I., Amorim, P., Lepine, J.P., Sheehan, M.F., Baker, R.R. & Sheehan, K.H. (2000b). *Mini International Neuropsychiatric Interview (M.I.N.I. PLUS Version 5.0.0).* (Copyright 1994, 1998, 2000 by Sheehan, D.V. & Lecrubier, Y.) Tampa, FL and Paris: University of South Florida Institute for Research in Psychiatry and INSERM-Hôpital de la Salpêtrière.

Sheehan, D.V., Lecrubier, Y., Sheehan, K.H., Amorim, P., Janavs, J., Weiller, E., Hergueta, T., Baker, R. & Dunbar, G.C. (1998). The Mini-International Neuropsychiatric Interview (M.I.N.I.): The development and validation of a structured diagnostic psychiatric interview for DSM-IV and ICD-10. *Journal of Clinical Psychiatry, 59(suppl. 20),* 22–57.

Simpson, D.D., Knight, K. & Hiller, M.L. (1997). *TCU/DCJTC Forms Manual: Intake and during-treatment assessments.* Fort Worth, TX: Texas Christian University, Institute of Behavioral Research.

Skinner, H.A. (1982). Drug abuse screening test. *Addictive Behavior, 7,* 263–371.

Skinner, H.A. & Horn, J.L. (1984). *Alcohol Dependence Scale: User's Guide.* Toronto: Addiction Research Foundation.

Spitzer, R.L. (1983). Psychiatric diagnosis: Are clinicians still necessary? *Comprehensive Psychiatry, 24*(5), 399–411.

Spitzer, R.L., Williams, J.B.W., Gibbon, M. & First, M.B. (1990). *Structured Clinical Interview for DSM-III-R.* Washington, DC: American Psychiatric Press.

Staley, D. & El Guebaly, N. (1990). Psychometric properties of the Drug Abuse Screening Test in a psychiatric patient population. *Addictive Behaviors, 15*(3), 257–264.

Stangl, D., Pfohl, B., Zimmerman, M., Bowers, W. & Corenthal, C. (1985). A structured interview for the DSM-III personality disorders. *Archives of General Psychiatry, 42,* 591–596.

Steadman, H.J., Morris, S.M. & Dennis, D.L. (1995). The diversion of mentally ill persons from jails to community-based services: A profile of programs. *American Journal of Public Health, 85*(12), 1630–1635.

Steadman H.J., Mulvey, E.P., Monahan, J., Robbins, P.C., Appelbaum, P.S., Grisso, T., Roth, L.H. & Silver, E. (1998). Violence by people discharged from acute psychiatric inpatient facilities and by others in the same neighborhoods. *Archives of General Psychiatry, 55,* 339–401.

Storgaard, H., Nielsen, S.D. & Gluud, C. (1994). The validity of the Michigan Alcoholism Screening Test (MAST). *Alcohol & Alcoholism, 29*(5), 493–502.

Substance Abuse Mental Health Services Administration (SAMHSA) (2000). *Cultural Competence Standards.* Rockville, MD: U.S. Department of Health and Human Services, SAMHSA.

Swartz, M., Swanson, J., Hiday, V., Borum, R. & Wagner, R. (1998). Violence and severe mental illness: The effects of substance abuse and nonadherence to medication. *American Journal of Psychiatry, 155,* 226–231.

Swartz, M., Swanson, J., Wagner, R., Burns, B., Hiday, V. & Borum, R. (1999). Can voluntary outpatient commitment reduce hospital recidivism? Findings from a randomized controlled trial in severely mentally ill individuals. *American Journal of Psychiatry, 156*(12).

Teplin, L.A. (1994). Psychiatric and substance abuse disorders among male urban jail detainees. *American Journal of Public Health, 84,* 292–293.

Teplin, L.A., Abram, K.M. & McClelland, G.M. (1996). Prevalence of psychiatric disorders among incarcerated women. *Archives of General Psychiatry, 53,* 505–512.

Teplin, L.A. & Swartz, J. (1989). Screening for severe mental disorder in jails. *Law and Human Behavior, 13*(1), 1–18.

Texas Christian University Institute of Behavioral Research. (1997). *TCU Drug Screen.* Fort Worth, TX: Author.

Texas Christian University Institute of Behavioral Research. (1998). *Research roundup: IBR's quarterly newsletter.* Fort Worth, TX: Author.

Thompson, C. (1989). *The instruments of psychiatric research.* New York: John Wiley & Sons.

Torrey, E.F., Steiber, J., Ezekiel, J., Wolfe, S.M., Sharfstein, J. & Flynn, L.M. (1993). Criminalizing the mentally ill: The abuse of jails as mental hospitals. *Innovations & Research, 2,* 11–14. Washington, DC: Public Citizen's Health Research Group.

Trull, T.J. & Larson, S.L. (1994). External validity of two personality disorder inventories. *Journal of Personality Disorders, 8*(2), 96–103.

Tylee, A. (1996). Depression research in European society (DEPRES) study. *International Journal of Methods in Psychiatric Research, 6*(S), S33–S37.

Van der Kolk, B., McFarlane, A. & Weisaeth, L. (1996). *Traumatic stress: The effects of overwhelming experience on mind, body, and society.* New York: Guilford.

Veysey, B.M., Steadman, H.J., Morrissey, J.P., Johnsen, M. & Beckstead, J.W. (1998). Using the Referral Decision Scale to screen mentally ill jail detainees: Validity and implementation issues. *Law and Human Behavior, 22*(2), 205–215.

Vigdal, G.L. & Stadler, D.W. (1996). Assessment, client treatment matching, and managing the substance abusing offender. In K.E. Early (Ed.), *Drug treatment behind bars: Prison-based strategies for change* (pp. 17–43). Westport, CT: Praeger/Greenwood.

Wexler, H.K. & Graham, W.F. (August, 1993). *Prison-based therapeutic community for substance abusers: Six month evaluation findings.* American Psychological Association, Toronto, Canada.

Widiger, T.A. & Corbitt, E.M. (1995) Antisocial personality disorder. In W.J. Livesley (Ed.), *The DSM-IV personality disorders: Diagnosis and treatment of mental disorders* (pp. 103–126). New York: Guilford Press.

Widiger, T. & Sanderson, C. (1995). Assessing personality disorders. In J. Butcher (Ed.), *Clinical personality assessment: Practical approaches* (pp. 380–394). New York: Oxford University Press.

Wilson, J. & Keane, T. (1997). *Assessing psychological trauma and PTSD.* New York: Guilford Press.

Winters, K.C. (1995). *Clinician's guide to self-evaluation workbook for alcohol and drug abuse: Screening for alcohol and drug abuse (SADA).* Center City, MN: Hazelden Press.

World Health Organization. (1990). *Composite Diagnostic Interview (CIDI), version 1.0.* Geneva, Switzerland: Author.

Zanis, D.A., McLellan, A.T. & Corse, S. (1997). Is the Addiction Severity Index a reliable and valid assessment instrument among clients with severe and persistent mental illness and substance use disorders? *Community Mental Health Journal, 33*(3), 213–227.

Zung, B.J. (1979). Psychometric properties of the MAST and two briefer versions. *Journal of Studies on Alcohol, 40*(9), 845–859.

Conclusion

Gerald Landsberg

The key issue of the "criminalization of mental illness," as well as the problem of "victimization of family and non-family members by the mentally ill," are increasingly recognized in the United States as significant social problems. They figure prominently in the discourse of mental health care and criminal justice professionals, family members, and mental health advocates, as well as victims assistance and aging professionals, among others. In this book we have examined the challenges and opportunities for social workers and other mental health care professionals in building systemic responses to these problems. We have reviewed promising practices with respect to jail/prison services, community-based diversion, the special needs of emotionally disturbed women, and the complex problems facing victims of mentally ill offenders. And finally, we have presented pertinent perspectives from the legal system as well as a comprehensive review of screening instruments for co-occurring mental illness and sustance use in criminal justice programs.

It is now our task to identify immediate and future action that could improve the quality of life for the mentally ill, victims and society at large.

In his testimony before Congress on September 21, 2000, Dr. Bernand S. Arons, Director of the SAMSHA Center for Mental Health Services, conceptualized the problem in bold strokes:

> The mental health and criminal justice systems have a big, common problem: persons with mental illness are increasingly involved in the criminal justice system, resulting in greater burden on criminal justice and less effective treatment for persons with mental illness. . . . We need to emphasize that as a society we have created this situation. Inadequate treatment and services leaves people unprotected from the force of their illness, and we wait and watch until they do something, often a non-violent misdemeanor, to put them in trouble with the law. Jails and prisons are not set up to help ameliorate the force of these illness, and a vicious cycle is often set in place creating high rates of recidivism for these people.

Regarding solutions for the development of needed services, Dr. Arons envisions a two-pronged goal for mental health and criminal justice vis-a-vis persons with mental illness. This is defined as follows:

> In order to minimize involvement of persons with mental illness in the criminal justice system while protecting the public, the degree of criminal justice involvement should be directly proportional to the extent to which an individual poses a danger to society. Therefore, two compatible goals can be stated:
>
> - For persons with mental illness who are non-dangerous, they should be diverted to effective treatment at the earliest practical stage of the criminal justice process.
> - For persons with mental illness who are dangerous, provide humane care and treatment during incarceration and explicit linkage to community-based treatment on release.

Several strategies can be deduced from this goal statement:

1. Criteria defining dangerous or non-dangerous persons need to be formulated and adopted by consensus of both the mental health and criminal justice system and applied fairly.
2. Persons involved in the criminal justice system should be screened for mental illness.
3. Efficient diversion mechanisms should be available.
4. Availability of effective community-based and humane jail/prison-based treatment should be assured.
5. Provision for necessary supervision should be arranged through the criminal justice system.

The need for collaborative initiatives forms the basis of successful programs. The publication, "The Courage to Change: A Guide for Communities to Create Services for People with Co-Occurring Disorders in the Justice System," reports that:

> When these successful communities were examined, it was found that many of their innovations reflected an investment in the concept of system integration. The essence of this concept is that people in all three systems recognize the need for a holistic approach to treating each person and that they are willing to share information, money, and clients across the three systems. These promising innovations were not without major barriers, however.

Before system integration can occur, personnel in the mental health, substance abuse, and criminal justice systems must be convinced of three things: (1) people with co-occurring disorders present a significant and ongoing management dilemma within their systems; (2) they can be more effective in treating this population if they combine their efforts with personnel in other systems and devise complementary services; (3) they should undertake integration efforts not only with the goal of making their own systems more effective, but also in the best interest of people with co-occurring disorders, and the communities in which they will be living. (GAINS, 1999)

The same philosophic mind set needs to be adopted for jail or prison services. Both require a strong emphasis on integrated treatment for co-occurring disorders. Jails, which are usually operated by counties or localities, need linkages between their facilities—usually under the management of the sheriffs or chiefs of police departments—and locally- or county-based mental health providers. Prisons, which are stated-operated, often have self-contained services but need both mental health and substance abuse staff providing on-site treatment. For incarcerated individuals, the ultimate key to success is the availability of excellent discharge planning that hopefully will link them to a well-developed and integrated community-based system for co-occurring disorders.

We also need to address emerging issues in this field beyond those concerning offenders. We need to ask how we may best intervene and serve the victims of mentally ill offenders, especially when there is violence involved. Addressing this problem not only requires an effective community-based system of care for the defendant but also a system that is *responsive to victims*. Repeatedly, in his work on the problem of victimization, the author found that victims, especially family members, had reached out to the mental health system, only to be rebuffed. Frequently, they made attempts for help as they were increasingly incapable of aiding their family members who began to deteriorate and become violent. Therefore, it is imperative that the creation of new community systems actively engage family members. Some progressive agencies have developed family support groups either solely operated by the agency or in collaboration with several chapters of the Alliance for the Mentally Ill. We also greatly stress the importance of community education regarding problems facing victims. Educational activities for family members, advocates, agency providers and staffs are essential. Further, as discussed in earlier sections of this book, broad-based collaborations are important tools for developing an effective community response.

Two of the key problems in addressing the issue of criminalization of mental illness have been the difficulty in bringing it to the fore as a major national issue, and the paucity of funding resources for new program development. However, there is cause for significant optimism on both fronts. A series of conferences and meetings on this problem have been sponsored on a federal level, and this has resulted in the passage of new legislation. This legislation includes the Mental Health Early Intervention, Treatment and Prevention Act of 2000 (part of the Children's Health Act of 2000) and America's Law Enforcement and Mental Health Project; it provides for funding for diversion programs, integrated treatment and mental health courts. Thus, needed expansion of services may be forthcoming.

For social workers and other mental health professionals, the future is now. These new developments and initiatives offer opportunities for creative clinical and program initiatives. Outreach—a skill whose importance is well recognized by mental health professionals, criminal justice and substance abuse providers, families and advocates, agency and victims assistance providers—needs to be increasingly honed. It is a crucial first step toward change. Hopefully, the information in this book will be an important source as new opportunities unfold.

INDEX

Abuse, implications of, 162–163, 175–178. *See also specific types of abuse*
Abuser, *see* Batterer
  dependency theory, 198
  pathology, 198–199
Access to care, 66–67, 134
Accountability, 119, 130, 263
Acting out, 235
Active Neglect, of elderly, 196
Active treatment, dual disorders, 97
Addiction, responsibility for, 178
Addiction Severity Index
  Drug and Alcohol Scale (ASI-Drug), 306–307, 312, 322
  Psychiatric Subscale (ASI-Psychiatric Subscale), 296–297, 302
Adequate mental health program, requirements of, 34
Ad Hoc Mental Health Task Force, 261–262, 264
Administration, screening instruments, 294
Administrative segregation, 234–235
Admission criteria, 29, 51, 93, 138
Admitting physician, role of, 29
Adolescents, support for, *see* Friends of Island Academy (FOIA), youth support program
Adult children:
  abusive, 203. *See also* Elder abuse
  impaired, 198, 204, 219
Adult Protective Services, 201
Advocacy:
  after arrest, 237–238
  importance of, 67, 236
  Kendra's Law and, 283
  prior to arrest, 236–237
  social workers and, 238
Advocate, role of, 16–17
Affective disorders, 84, 92
Aftercare services, 145, 221

Aggression, 162
Agoraphobia, 85
Alcohol abuse, 7, 242. *See also* Substance abuse disorders
Alcoholics Anonymous, 140
Alcohol Use Disorders Identification Test (AUDIT), 305–307, 309, 311, 322
Alliance for the Mentally Ill, 340
Alternative sentencing programs, 209, 272
American Association of Suicidology, 59
American Bar Association, 87
America's Law Enforcement and Mental Health Project, 341
Amnesty International USA, 59
Anderson, Mary Elizabeth, 16–17
Antisocial Personality Disorder, 85, 201, 317
Anxiety disorders, 85–86, 176, 298–299
Arizona Council on Offenders with Mental Impairments (ACOMI), 111, 115, 119
Arizona Health Care Cost Containment System (AHCCCS), 109
Arizona jail diversion program, managed care environment:
  Department of Health Services (ADHS), Division of Behavioral Health Services (DBHS), 108–115
  three-tiered model, 115–117
Arons, Dr. Bernard S., 338–339
Arraignment, 227
Arrests:
  advocacy strategies, 236–237
  incidence of, 64
Assertive community treatment (ACT), 139
Assisted Outpatient Treatment (AOT), New York State, 147, 274, 276–280, 284
At-risk elderly, elder abuse preventive

services, 200–201
Attention deficit hyperactivity disorder, 85
Attitudinal change, 63
Attorney:
    client's best interests, 241–242
    court appointment of, 29, 240–243
    in private practice, 241
    social worker, relationship with,
        239–241, 253–255
Attorney-client privilege, 253–254, 256
Attorney General, role of, 33
Auditory hallucinations, 176

Baker Act, 267
Baker-Miller, Jean, 180
Barriers, generally:
    to care, 65–66
    to change, 68
    to training, 55–56
Batterer, service remedies for, 204
Bipolar disorders, 2, 85, 177, 216, 291
Birmingham Police Department, com-
    munity service officer (CSO) unit:
    answering calls, guidelines for, 74
    case study, 75–76
    casework functions of CSO, 73–74
    education and community service, 72
    historical perspective, 70–72
    mission statement, 70
    1999 CSO statistics, 77–78
    operations, 73
    professional knowledge, 72
    total calls, statistics, 79
Borderline Personality Disorder, 201
Boundary spanners, 95–96
Brokerage model of intervention, 136
Brooklyn Treatment Court (BTC),
    91–92, 293
Broward Mental Health Court:
    features of, 131, 264
    functions of, generally, 11, 14, 17,
        128–129
    goals of, 130
    in-court prosecutor prospective,
        265–266
    Mental Health Court team, 131–132
    participants in, 266
Bureau of Justice Statistics, 2
Byren Grant, 32

CAGE questionnaire, 309, 313

Call response, CSO guidelines, 74
Capitation, 118–119
Caregivers, elder abuse and, 197, 204
Case advocacy, Project Link, 136–138
Case management strategies, 9, 14, 62,
    67, 112, 124, 146, 149, 182
Center for Substance Abuse Treatment
    (CSAT), 293
Childhood abuse, impact of, 176–177
Children of female prisoners:
    childcare for, 161
    impact of substance abuse on, 178
    reunification with, 161
    visitation, 162
Children's Health Act (2000), 341
Civil commitment, 5, 226, 248
Class action lawsuits, 32
Co-morbidity, 7. *See also* Co-occurring
    mental illness and substance abuse
    in criminal justice programs
Composite International Diagnostic
    Interview-Short Form (CIDI-SF),
    296, 301
Co-occurring mental illness and
    substance abuse in criminal
    justice programs:
    boundary spanners, 95
    breadth of disorders, 85–86
    case management services, 96–97
    diversion, 86–92
    early identification, 96
    implementing diversion, 94–97
    implications of, generally, 63
    incidence of, 84–85
    integrated services/treatment, 92–95
    key agency representatives, meetings
        of, 95
    leadership, 95–96
    overview, 17, 83–85, 97–98
    prevalence of, 84, 290
    scope of problem, 290–291
    screening instruments for, 291–326
Code of silence, 8
Cohen, Lee, 17
Collaboration:
    as goal, 338–340
    law enforcement response, 48
    meeting process, 95
    multi-systems, co-occurring mental
        illness and, 87
    as success factor, 164

trends in, 97–98
Commitment orders, 283
Community-based care/treatment, 9, 62
Community-based diversion programs:
  Birmingham Police Department
    Community Service Officer Unit,
    70–79
  Broward Mental Health Court,
    128–132
  community programs, 81–154
  criminal justice diversion, individuals
    with co-occurring mental illness
    and substance abuse disorders,
    83–98
  Friends of Island Academy,
    120–127
  jail diversion in managed care
    environment, Arizona experience,
    107–119
  law enforcement response to social
    problems, 47–49
  Memphis CIT model, 59–68
  New York City, criminal justice
    mental health services, 144–154
  police/mental health linked
    programs, 45–79
  police/mental health training
    program, development and imple-
    mentation of, 51–58
  Project Link, 133–142
Community Corrections Act, 32
Community Mental Health Center Act
  (1963), 9, 133
Community mental health services,
  218–219
Community Partnership of Southern
  Arizona (CPSA), 115–117
Community programs:
  Broward's mental health court,
    128–132
  criminal justice mental health serv-
    ices, New York City's system,
    144–154
  Friends of Island Community,
    providing youth with positive
    opportunities after jail, 120–127
  individuals with co-occurring
    mental illness and substance abuse
    disorders, criminal justice diver-
    sion, 83–98
  managed care environment in

Arizona, jail diversion, 107–119
Project Link, preventing incarcera-
  tion of adults with severe mental
  illness, 133–142
Community Service Officer (CSO)
  Unit:
  Birmingham police department,
    12–13, 70–79
  Memphis CIT model, 61
Competency exam, 231–232, 248
Comprehensive Employment Training
  Act (CETA), Title II program, 71
Comprehensive Psychiatric Emergency
  Programs (CPEP), 153
Comprehensive Service Providers
  (CSPs), role of, 117
Conduct Disorder, 317
Confidentiality, 96
Continuity of care/services, 6, 87, 95,
  145–146
Convention Against Torture, 5
Coordination of services, 31, 95, 131
Corrections environment, impact of,
  3–5
County jails, jail diversion programs
  and, 111
Court appearances, 30
Court backlogs, 87
Court release officers, roles of, 31
Covington, Stephanie, 179
Crack cocaine, 229, 242
Criminal charges, 238
Criminal defense attorney:
  observations of, 249–256
  role of, 246–249
Criminalization of mental illness:
  future directions of, 81, 338, 341
  historical perspective, 3
  termination of, 243–244
Criminal justice interventions, elder
  abuse, 202–203
Criminal Justice Mental Health Standard, 87
Crisis centers, suicide prevention, 36, 38
Crisis intervention counseling, 73
Crisis intervention team (CIT), *see*
  Memphis CIT model
Crisis management delivery system, 71,
  76–77

Dartmouth Assessment of Lifestyle
  Instrument (DALI), 304–305, 311,

322

Day treatment programs, 135

Dean, Joette, 11

Debriefing, importance of, 38, 73

Decision-making process, 181

Defense attorney, role of, 16, 226. *See also* Attorney; Criminal defense attorney

Defense strategies, 17

Deinstitutionalization, 9, 51, 84, 23

Department of Social Services (DSS), role of, 140

Depression, *see* Major depression
  in abused women, 176–177
  in adolescents, 124
  in caregivers, 204

Depressive disorders, 85

Detoxification, 28

Developmental disabilities, 63, 216

Diagnostic and Statistical Manual of Mental Disorders, 2

Diagnostic and Statistical Manual (DSM-IV), 216, 314, 316

Directly Observed Therapy (DOT) Program, 281–282

Discharge planning, 146, 149–150, 209, 291

Discipline and Publish (Foucault), 8

Domestic violence:
  batterer, assistance for, 204
  elder abuse and, 206–207
  implications of, 15, 48, 125, 177–178, 183

Drug use, screening for, *see* Substance use disorders, screening instruments

Drug Abuse Screening Test (DAST), 308, 313

DTAP model, 90–91

Dual diagnosis, 7, 10, 84

Early identification, importance of, 96

Eating disorders, 177, 299

Education initiatives, Friends of Academy, 123

Ehrenkranz School of Social Work, Institute Against Violence, 215, 221

Elder abuse:
  at-risk elderly, preventive services for, 200–201
  case example, 193–195
  criminal justice system, 206–209

defined, 195–197
  discharge planning and, 209
  diversion, 210
  incidence of, 15, 193
  intervention strategies, 200–203
  mandatory reporting, 208
  prevention strategies, 200
  social service interventions, 203–206
  theories of, 197–199
  treatment, 210

Emergency Psychological Technicians, 55

Emergency Service Unit (ESU), New York City Police Department, 52–57

Emotional abuse, impact of, 178

Emotionally disturbed children, 109–110

Employment:
  preparation and placement, Friends of Island Academy, 123
  status, implications of, 31, 93

Emotionally disturbed women:
  gender-based network of services, 159–164
  Maryland's programs for incarcerated women with mental illness and substance abuse disorders, 165–171
  VOICES program, 172–185

Empowerment model:
  challenges of, 181
  characteristics of, 180–181
  program design, phase-oriented approach, 181–183

Engagement, in dual disorder treatment, 97

Epidemiological Catchment Area (ECA), 86

Episodic care, 6

Ethnic differences, 5, 15, 86

Experiential-based learning, 63

Family:
  role in treatment, 31, 64
  as victims, 217–219

Fee-for-service providers, 109

Feedback, importance of, 63, 74

Felony offenses, 137

Female offenders, statistics, 2

Female prisoners:
  children of, 161
  common life themes, 161
  motivations for change, 161–162, 176

profile of, 161, 174–175
reasons for incarceration, 160
Financial abuse of elderly, 196
Finkelstein, Howard, 130
Florida Mental Health Act, 267
Focus groups, 218–219
Follow-up contact, importance of, 74
Forensic planning council, functions
    of, 37
Frail elderly, 197
Friends of Island Academy (FOIA),
    youth support program:
background, 120–121
counseling services department, 124
education initiatives, 123
employment preparation and place-
    ment, 123
GIIFT Pack, 125–126
leadership, 125–126
Mentoring Program, 122
Milestones Plan, 121–122, 126
mission, 127
objectives and goals, 13, 121
preventive intervention, adolescent
    link, 124
Rosewood Program for female ado-
    lescents, 125
Youth Development Model, 127
Fundamental mental health services, 34
Funding sources, types of, 32–34, 93, 109

Gatekeepers, 67
Gender differences, 5, 15, 86
Gender-sensitive programs, female
    prisoners:
Hampden County Correctional
    Center, 179–185
profile of offenders, 174–175
target population, 173–174
General Education Development
    (GED) exam, 123, 125
Generalized anxiety disorder, 85–86
GIIFT Pack (Guys and Girls Insight on
    Imprisonment for Teens), 125–126
Gilligan, Carol, 180–181
Gilligan, James, 10
Goal-setting, importance of, 37,
    121–122
Goldstein, Andrew, 272–273, 275
Grant funding, 32–33, 109, 137, 139,
    166, 168

Group counseling, 125
Guardianships, 202–203
Guilt, 178
Guilty but mentally ill (GBMI), 219

Hallucinations, 176–177, 232
Hampden County Correctional
    Center, gender-specific interven-
    tion program
empowerment model, 180–181
evaluation, 185
participant selection, 184
program design, 181–184
relational model, 180–181
social work, implications for, 184–185
staffing, 184
theoretical construct, 179
Health Care Financing Administration
    (HCFA), 109
Health maintenance organizations
    (HMOs), 4, 109. *See also* Jail diver-
    sion in managed care environ-
    ment, Arizona experience
Hinkley, John, 271–272
HIV, 84
Home health care, 202
Homelessness, implications of, 14, 84–85,
    137, 145, 149
Hospital incentives, 282
Hospitalization:
admissions, 29
length of stay, 14, 17
utilization rates, 134
Hostage Negotiation Team (HNT), 53
Hotlines, 148

Ideology, implications of, 8
Imagining Robert (Neugeboren), 8
Impulsivity, 7
Incarceration:
as community mental health system,
    230–244
historical perspective, 8–10
Information sharing, 95
Initial Assessment Screening Form,
    27–28
Injuries, police officers', 64–65
Inpatient psychiatric care, 226
Insanity defense, 17, 220, 225, 231–232
Institutionalization, 234
Integrated services/treatment, 62,

93–95, 140–141, 151
Intensive Case Management (ICM), 47, 209–210
Inter-agency Narcotics Enforcement Team (Lane County, OR), 32
Interpersonal needs, in female prisoners, 161–162
Interpersonal relationships, problems with, 93
Involuntary admission, 51
Iowa Personality Disorder Screen, 315, 318

Jail diversion programs, effectiveness of, 13. *See specific programs*
Jail/prison population statistics:
    ethnic differences, 5, 15, 86
    gender differences, 5, 15, 86
    growth in, 2
    mentally ill, prevalence rates, 2, 134
Jail/prison services for incarcerated populations:
    Lane County Adult Corrections Mental Health Services (Lane Co., Oregon), 25–33
    Oswego Mental Health Forensic Mental Health Program (Oswego, NY), 35–41
Job Readiness training, 123
John Jay College of Criminal Justice, 54
Judge, role of, 16, 30–31, 225–228, 246–247

Karopkin, Judge, 5, 11, 16
Kendra's Law:
    applications of, 5, 16–17, 201
    Directly Observed Therapy (DOT) Program, 281–282
    enactment of, 275–276
    implementation of, 274–285
    initial results, 276–281
    recommendations for implementation, 282–283

Lamberti, Steven, 13
Lane County Adult Corrections Mental Health Services (Lane Co., Oregon):
    behavioral problems, 31
    community context, 25–26

Community Corrections Center, 31
    funding sources, 32–34
    jail physical plant, 26–27
    lessons for professionals, 34–35
    purpose of program, 11, 25
    residential substance abuse treatment program, 31
    services provided, 27–32
Lane County Psychiatric Hospital, 32
Law enforcement, *see* Police/mental health linked programs
    elder abuse interventions, 200–201, 209
    Memphis CIT model, 61
    response to social problems, 47–49
    training programs, 113
    working relationship with mental health provider system, 57–58
Law Enforcement Administration Act (L.E.A.A.), 32
Leadership:
    significance of, 67, 95–96
    skills development, 125–126
Learned helplessness, 178
Learning disabilities, 216
Lee's Summit, 62
Legal Aid Society, The, 16
Legal system, mental health professionals and:
    judge's perspective, 225–228
    social workers as advocates, 229–244
Lerner-Wren, Judge Ginger, 11, 262–263
LifeNet, 148
Life Skills program, 123
LINK services, New York City's system of criminal justice mental health services:
    development of, 146–147
    overview, 14, 125, 144
Literacy programs, 123, 125
Low-level offenses, 30

Madness and Civilization (Foucault), 8
Major depression, 2, 85, 216, 291
Managed care environment, Arizona experience:
    behavioral health care trends, 108–109
    collaboration of state and local agen-

cies, 110–111
crisis services, 111, 113
outreach, 111–112
Regional Behavioral Health System
(RBHAs), 109–114
service delivery issues, 109
Management information systems, 87
Mandatory drug sentences, 10
Mania, 2
Maryland Community Criminal Justice
Treatment Program (MCCJTP), 166
Medicaid, 107–108, 148
Medications, prescriptions for, 84, 150
Medicine in Psychiatry Service (MIPS),
139, 141
Memory impairment, 176
Memphis CIT (Crisis Intervention
Team) model:
background, 60–61
barriers to implementation, 65–66
evaluation, 64–65
mental health professionals, implica-
tions for, 66–68
operational components, 61–62
partnership, 63–64
purpose of, 12, 59–60
replication of, 60
selection and training, 62–63
targets of, 59–60
Memphis TACT (Tactics Apprehension
and Containment Team), 65
Mental Disability law, 128
Mental health assessment, 29
Mental Health Association of New
York, 148–149
Mental health block grant funds, 109
Mental Health Court:
development of, 261–262
effectiveness of, 262–264, 269
future directions for, 264–265
in-court prosecutor, perspective of,
265–266
participation considerations, 267–269
screening process, 266
Mental Health Early Intervention,
Treatment and Prevention Act of
2000, 341
Mental health interventions, elder
abuse, 202
Mental health professionals, role of, 39
Mental illness/chemical addiction

(MICA):
elder abuse and, 207
residential services, 137, 139–140
treatment plan, 242
Mentally ill, generally:
institutionalization, 234
legal rights of, 54, 112, 130
offenders, prevalence of, 2, 136
segregation of, 236–237
victimization of, 234
Mentoring Program, 122
Michigan Alcohol Screening Test
(MAST), 307–309, 311
Milestones Chart, 125
Milestones Plan, 121–122, 126
M.I.N.I. Antisocial Personality Module,
317, 319
Mini-International Neuropsychiatric
Interview (M.I.N.I.), 298–300, 302,
320–321
Misdemeanors, 2–3
Misdiagnosis, 162
Mobile crisis response teams, 117
Mobile treatment team services, Project
Link, 133, 139
Model Penal Code, 231–232
Mood disorders, 54, 208

Narcissistic Personality Disorder, 201
Narcotics Anonymous, 140
Nathaniel Project, 14, 89, 149
National Alliance for the Mentally Ill
(NAMI), 59–60, 129, 203, 263
National Association of People of Color
Against Suicide, 59
National GAINS Center, 199
National Institute of Corrections, 175
National Institute of Justice (NIJ), 89,
293
National Institute of Mental Health, 9
National Institute on Alcohol Abuse
and Alcoholism (NIAAA), 293
National Institute on Drug Abuse
(NIDA), 293
Neglect:
childhood, impact of, 177
of elderly, 195–196
Neugeboren, Jay, 8
New York City, criminal justice mental
health services:
collaborated services, 151

community case management, 150
New York City, criminal justice mental
    health services *(continued)*
    development of, 146–147
    discharge planning, 147, 149–150
    diversion, 147–149
    hospitalization recommendations,
        151, 153
    housing recommendations, 151
    illustration of, 152
    integrated services, 151
    jail mental health services, 149
    LINK transition services, 14, 150
    overview, 144–145
    police crisis response, 153
    scope of problem, 145
New York City Center for Court
    Innovation (CCI), 91–92, 293
New York City Department for the
    Aging (DFTA), 199–200, 205–206
New York City Department of Mental
    Health, 51–58, 85, 124, 145,
    149–150, 282
New York City Police Department,
    51–57
New York State Office of Mental
    Health, 57
Non-violent offenders, 2, 10, 12
Not Guilty by Reason of Insanity
    (NGRI), 220, 231–232
Nuisance crimes, 83–84
Nurse practitioners, functions of, 92

Office for the Victims of Crime (OVC),
    215–216
Older American Act, 200
OMH certification, 38
Oswego Corrections Facility, 11
Oswego Mental Health Forensic Mental
    Health Program (Oswego, NY):
    community resources, linkages to, 39
    forensic planning council, initiation
        of, 37
    geographic area, 36
    goal-setting, 37
    nature of services, 37–40
    operationalizing, 38–39
    physical plant, 40
    policies and procedures, develop-
        ment of, 37
    purpose of program, 35–36

results, 40–41
staffing changes, 39–40
staff training, 38
Suicide Prevention/Crisis
    Intervention Program, 35
target population, 36
Outpatient mental health services, 30,
    137
Outreach programs, 113, 114 118, 341

Panic disorder, 85
Paranoid Personality Disorder, 201
Parenting skills, 162, 183
Parole, 117–118
Partnerships:
    law enforcement response, 48, 88
    Memphis CIT model, 63–64
Passive Neglect, of elderly, 196
Patient compliance, 30, 130
Patient "dumping," 62
Patient rights, 66, 112
Patterson, George, 12
Peer counseling, 125
Personality Diagnostic Questionnaire4+
    (PDQ4+), 316–317, 319
Personality disorders, implications of,
    216. *See also* Personality disorders
    screening instruments
Personality disorders screening instru-
    ments:
    Iowa Personality Disorder Screen,
        315, 318
    M.I.N.I. Antisocial Personality
        Module, 317, 319
    overview, 314
    Personality Diagnostic
        Questionnaire4+ (PDQ4+),
        316–317, 319
    Structured Clinical Interview for
        DSM Personality Disorders Screen
        (SCID II Screen), 315, 319
    Structured Interview for DSM-IV
        Personality (SIDP-IV), 315, 318
Persuasion, in dual disorder treatment,
    97
Petitions of commitment, 74
Phobic disorders, 83, 176, 178
Phoenix Project:
    background, 166–167
    diversion, 167
    evaluation, 167–168

Physical abuse:
  of elderly, defined, 196. *See* Elder
    abuse
  implications of, 75, 125, 178
  incidence of, 175
Physical health, problems with, 93
Physicians, licensure requirements, 4
Ping-pong therapy, 93
Police crisis response, 153
Police Executive Research Forum, 53
Police/mental health linked
    programs:
  Birmingham police department
    community service officer unit,
    70–79
  development of police/mental
    health training program in large
    urban environment, 51–58
  law enforcement response to social
    problems, 47–49
  Memphis CIT model, 59–68
Police/mental health training program,
    development process:
  background to, 51–52
  barriers to training, 55–56
  curriculum, 54–55
  follow-up activities, 56–57
  initial developmental steps, 52–54, 57
Police officers, *see* Law enforcement;
    Police/mental health linked
    programs
Post-booking, 14, 88–92, 116–117
Post-traumatic stress syndrome, 85–86,
    178
Poverty, impact of, 3, 85–86
Power of attorney, 203
Primary substance abuse disorder, 216
Pre-booking, 14, 87–88
Privatized health services, 4, 65
Probation, 117–118
Progress reports, 118
Project Link:
  admission criteria, 138
  background of, 133–134
  case advocacy services, 138
  Collaborative Management Team,
    137, 141
  cultural training, 137
  description of, 133
  development of, 13–14, 136–137
  enrollment, 141

  mental illness/chemical addiction
    (MICA) residential services, 137,
    139–140
  mobile treatment team services, 139
  program effectiveness, 141–142
  Rochester State Hospital experience,
    134–136
  service integration, 140–141
  services and operations, overview,
    138–141
Prosecutor, role of, 16, 258–269
Provider networks, in managed care,
    109–110
Psychiatric examination, 226
Psychiatric treatment, during incarcera-
    tion, 233, 237, 272
Psychiatric security review board, 112
Psychiatric syndromes, screening
    instruments:
  Addiction Severity Index, Psychiatric
    Subscale (ASI-Psychiatric Subscale),
    296–297, 302
  Composite International Diagnostic
    Interview-Short Form (CIDI-SF),
    296, 301
  Mini-International Neuropsychiatric
    Interview (M.I.N.I.), 298–300, 302,
    320–321
  Referral Decision Scale (RDS),
    297–298, 302, 320–321
  Structured Clinical Interview for
    DSM-IV Screen (SCID Screen),
    295–296, 301
Psycho-education, 31
Psychological abuse, of elderly,
    196–197
Psychosis, 6, 28, 216
Psychotropic medications, 28
Public defenders, role of, 240–243, 247,
    250–251
Public safety, 5, 9–10, 16
Punitive segregation, 234–235

Quality of life, 129, 131
Quality-of-life crimes, 233

Rape, prevalence of, 4
Recidivism, 25, 87, 127
Recovery process/steps, 98, 130
Referral Decision Scale (RDS),

297–298, 302, 320–321
Referrals, 39, 61, 73–74, 110, 118, 124, 131, 138, 151
Regional Behavioral Health System (RBHAs):
  collaboration of state and local agencies, 110–111
  crisis services, 111, 113
  overview, 13, 109–110
  parole, responsibilities with, 117–118
  probation, responsibilities with, 117–118
  three-tiered jail diversion model requirements, 114–115, 118
Rehabilitation programs, 52
Reintegration, into society, 9, 14
Relapse:
  prevention, 97
  rates of, 93
Relational model, 180–181
Relationship-building, importance of, 162
Relationships, significance of, 180–181
Residential Substance Abuse Treatment Grant, 33
Resource building, 162
Restraints, use of, 34
Rikers Island, adolescent programs, *see* Friends of Island Academy (FOIA), youth support program
Robbery, of elderly, 197
Robert Wood Johnson Foundation, Local Initiative Funding Partner's Program, 137
Rochester State Hospital, 134–136
Rock, Marjorie, 12
Role modeling programs, 122, 126, 178
Role-play, 55, 123
Rosewood Program, female adolescents, 125
Ross, Chief Circuit Judge Dale, 130, 261

Salasin, Susan, 15
Satz, Michael J., 261
Schizo-affective disorders, 216
Schizophrenia, 2, 84–85, 92, 199, 216, 229, 291
Screening instruments, co-occurring mental illness and substance use:
  characteristics of, 291–293
  instrument selection principles,

294–295
  mental health screening, 320–322
  methodology, 293–294
  personality disorders, 314–320, 323
  psychiatric syndromes, 295–302
  scoring and interpretation, 325
  staff training, 323–326
  substance use disorders, 302, 305–315, 324–325
Screening process, 162
Segregation, 234–235
Self-awareness, importance of, 180
Self-harm, 177
Self-neglect, 179
Service delivery, coordination of, 112, 130
Severely and persistently mentally ill (SPMI), 210, 274–275, 282–283
Sexual abuse:
  impact of, 125, 178
  incidence of, 175
Shame, 178
Sherman, Richard, 11
Simple Screening Instrument (SSI), 303–304, 310, 322
Skills development, 162
Skolnick, Andrew A., 4
Sliding fee scale, 110
Social exchange theory, 198–199
Social service intervention strategies:
  elder abuse, 202
  overview, 16
Social work, law enforcement collaboration, 48
Social workers:
  as advocate, 236–238
  defense attorney, relationship with, 238–243, 253–255
  role of, 15–16
Solitary confinement, 8
Somatization, 177
Specialization, resistance to, 66
Specialized courts, 14
Specialized response, co-occurring mental illness, 88
Speiser, Circuit Judge Mark A., 129
Staffing considerations, 35
Staff training, 38, 93
State mental hospitals, reform of, 9
State prisons, population statistics, 233
Steadman, Henry J., 1

Stigma, impact of, 7, 235–236
Stress management, 55
Strong Ties Community Support
    Program, 136, 139
Structured Clinical Interview:
  DSM Personality Disorders Screen
      (SCID II Screen), 315, 318
  for DSM-IV Personality (SIDP-IV),
      315, 318
  for DSM-IV Screen (SCID Screen),
      295–296, 301
Substance abuse, generally:
  in adolescents, 124
  elder abuse and, 210
  in female prisoners, 177–178
  mental illness and, screening for,
      291–326
Substance Abuse and Mental Health
    Services Administration
    (SAMHSA), 10, 33, 59, 64–65, 166,
    168–169, 293, 338
Substance abuse disorder, 6–7, 15
Substance use disorders, screening
    instruments:
  Addiction Severity Index-Drug and
      Alcohol Scale (ASI-Drug),
      306–307, 312
  Alcohol Use Disorders Identification
      Test (AUDIT), 305–307, 309, 311,
      322
  CAGE questionnaire, 309, 313
  Dartmouth Assessment of Lifestyle
      Instrument (DALI), 304–305, 311
  Drug Abuse Screening Test (DAST),
      308, 313
  Michigan Alcohol Screening Test
      (MAST), 307–309, 312
  Simple Screening Instrument (SSI),
      303–304, 310, 322
  Texas Christian University Drug
      Screen (TCUDS), 300, 303, 310,
      322
  TWEAK Test, 309, 313
Substandard treatment, 4
Suicidal behavior, 176, 178
Suicidality, 7
Suicide:
  in adolescents, 124
  risk assessment, 28–29, 39
  segregation of mentally ill and, 235
Summary probation, 117

Supportive social services, 62
SWAT program, 65
System integration, 339

Tactics Apprehension and
    Containment Team (TACT), 65
TAMAR Project:
  background, 168–169
  characteristics of, 15
  evaluation, 171
  services, 169–171
  VOICES program compared with,
      163–164
Texas Appleseed Foundation, 3
Texas Christian University Drug Screen
    (TCUDS), 300, 303, 310, 322
Thinking disorders, 54
Third-party supervision, 116–117
Three-tiered jail diversion model,
    115–117
Torrey, E. Fuller, 4, 7
Torture, 7
Tough-on-crime legislation, 2
Training:
  case management, co-occurring men-
      tal illness, 97
  Memphis CIT model, 62–63
  Oswego Mental Health Forensic
      Mental Health Program, 38
  police/mental health training pro-
      gram, 52–57
  screening instruments administra-
      tion, 323–326
  substance abuse counselors, 210
Transinstitutionalization, 84, 145, 230
Transition therapist, role of, 31
Trauma, female prisoners and, 176–177
Treatment Alternatives for the Dually
    Diagnosed (TADD), 91
Treatment Alternatives to Street Crime
    (TASC), 89–91
Treatment strategies, *see specific pro-
    grams*
TWEAK Test, 309, 313

U.N. Committee against Torture, 5
United States Marshals, 33
Urban Justice Center/Mental Health
    Project, 16

Urgent Care Centers, 115
Urinalysis screenings, 30

Vacco, Attorney General Dennis, 126
Validity, in screening instruments, 294.
  See also specific screening
  instruments
ValueOptions (VO), 115, 117
Value systems, significance of, 181
Victimization:
  characteristics of, 15–16
  education programs, 220–221
  of elderly, 193–195, 197
  of female prisoners, 161–162
  of incarcerated mentally ill, 234
Victims of Elder Abuse, interventions:
  aging service programs, 205–206, 208
  criminal justice system, 206–209
  social services, 203–206
Victims of Mentally Ill Offenders,
    services for:
  elder abuse, 193–211
  family members, 218–219
  generally, 15, 193
  needs, identification and address of,
    215–221
  non-family victims, 217–220
Videotapes, training, 67
Violence, generally:
  dealing with, 84
  in female prisoners, 176
  to inmates, 4–5
  intergenerational cycle, 198
  link with mental illness, 5–8
Violence Prevention programs, 126
Violent Crime Control and Law
    Enforcement Act (1994), 33
Violent crimes, 3
Visitation, with children, 162
Visual presentations, in training
    programs, 67
Vocational skills, 162
VOICES (Validation, Opportunity,

Inspiration, Communication,
    Trauma, Addictions, Mental
    Health, and Recovery) program:
  characteristics of, 15, 162–163,
    172–173
  community integration phase,
    183–184
  evaluation planning, 163–164
  exploration/discovery phase, 182–183
  information, education, and more
    phase, 182–183
  planning steps, 162–163
  TAMAR program compared with,
    163–164
  target population, 173–174
  treatment/healing phase, 183–184
Voluntary disposition, 87–88
Vulnerability, 15, 87

Wachtler, Judge Sol, 9–10, 270–273
Webdale, Kendra, 275
Weisman, Robert, 13
Well-being, importance of, 17, 112
White House Conference on Mental
    Health, 59
Women, *see* Female prisoners
  Hampden County Correctional
    Center program, 179–185
  mentally ill offenders, prevalance of,
    5, 15
  network of services for, 159–162
  Phoenix Project, 166–168
  substance abuse in, 86
  TAMAR program, *see* TAMAR
    program
  VOICES program, *see* VOICES
Work release programs, 31
Workshops:
  CIT training format, 63–64
  Friends of Island Academy program,
    123, 125

CPSIA information can be obtained at www.ICGtesting.com
Printed in the USA
BVOW041644140612

292703BV00003B/1/A

9 780826 115041

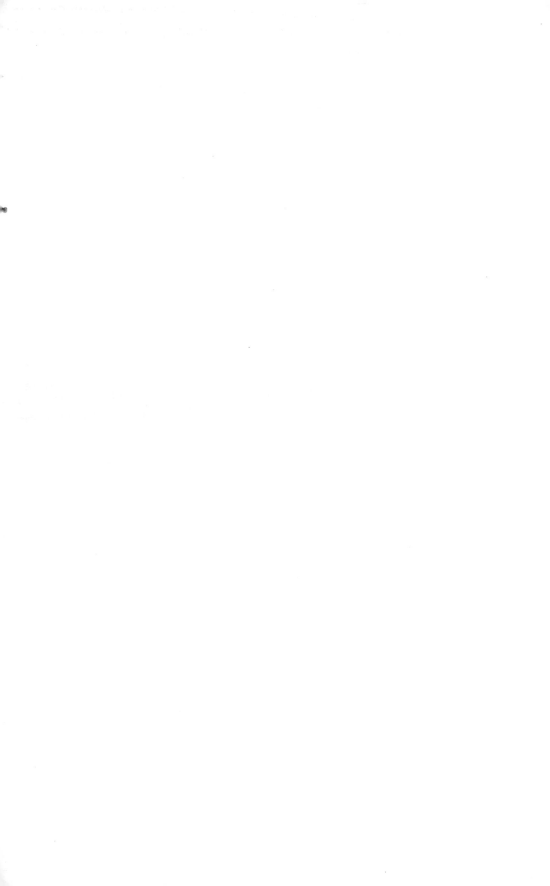